# The Hormones

# The Hormones
## Endocrine Physiology

Clark T. Sawin, M.D.

Assistant Professor of Medicine, Tufts University School of Medicine; Chief, Endocrine Section, Medical Service, Veterans Administration Hospital, Boston

Foreword by E. B. ASTWOOD, M.D., Professor of Medicine, Tufts University School of Medicine; Chief, Endocrinology Service, New England Medical Center Hospitals, Boston

ILLUSTRATIONS BY BARRY T. O'NEIL

Little, Brown and Company
Boston

To A. G. Olsen, E. B. Astwood, and my wife who aroused, encouraged, and sustained my interest in endocrinology

# Foreword

PROBABLY the best reason for doing something is that it needs to be done. After some six years of consideration Dr. Sawin decided that the need was great enough and has now written a concise book on endocrinology. The need for a short, authoritative text was borne upon him by his experience in teaching the subject to first-year medical students. When first confronted with this task he could find no text that seemed to suit. So by dint of hard labor and voluminous reading he drew up a series of outlines of the various topics to be covered in his course.

These mimeographed outlines distributed to the class were an immediate success with the students, and doubtless this favorable reception spurred him on to the continuing task of revising and updating them every year since. Finally, Dr. Sawin was led to see that these synopses would be of value to a readership much wider than just the first-year class of Tufts University School of Medicine, and he undertook the hardest revision of all, to make them suitable for publication in a book of broadly useful scope. The product is a volume that should be welcomed by students in the medical and biological sciences as well as by clinicians and established scientists in other fields. It is an up-to-date account of the subject, and such an account is not easily found in reviews or textbooks.

The subject is approached in a logical sequence by a consideration of what a hormone is, how hormones are studied, how measured, and how they may possibly act. Discussions of these matters embrace the most modern points of view. Consideration is then given to the neurohumoral control of the anterior pituitary and to the regulation of the hypothalamoneurohypophyseal complex. The major endocrine glands are dealt with in order: the adrenal cortex and medulla, the thyroid and parathyroid glands, the gonads and reproductive physiology, and the endocrine pancreas and diabetes mellitus. Finally, there is a discussion of growth and development, with a consideration of their relation to growth hormone and its effects, and of the hormonal regulation of energy metabolism and obesity. The whole field of endocrinology as we know it today is thus encompassed, and no major areas are left untouched.

The writing of a small textbook of endocrinology is no ordinary task. Endocrinology is a broad subject spreading over many disciplines and encompassing various fields of biology, morphology, chemistry, pharmacodynamics, and medicine; a treatise on endocrine physiology would be thin and superficial were these wide ramifications of the subject neglected. Dr. Sawin has had to draw upon an extensive mass of literature to round out his account, and has done a masterful job of condensation in keeping the text within this small compass.

The book reflects the author's views on teaching, a subject long of interest to him. *The Hormones* is written in a straightforward manner in good, clear English. It is eminently understandable, and what seems at present to be established fact is distinguished and set apart from what is problematical, uncertain, or unknown. To some readers the manner of presentation of parts of the subject may be regarded as dogmatic, but where should one draw the line between dogmatism and cautious uncertainty, between plain statement and circumlocution?

Although the aim throughout is to explain the subject as simply and as clearly as possible, facts have not been neglected; the book is crammed with facts, but they do not unbecomingly obtrude. The book is a quick and ready reference. What one finds is a concise and up-to-date answer to the question one seeks out, or he finds that an answer is not yet possible with the data currently at hand. The carefully prepared index makes it a useful reference work when a brief, authoritative statement is what is wanted.

E. B. Astwood

# Preface

THIS book is aimed primarily at medical students who are introducing themselves to endocrinology for the first time. I suspect, though, from my experience with older students, physiologists, and physicians, that the book may be of some interest to a wider readership both as an introduction and as a reasonably up-to-date review. The main emphasis is on human endocrine physiology, and the values noted throughout the book are from measurements made in man. However, while the hormonal actions and relationships are taken from human investigation whenever possible, such work has often not been done or is in fact impossible to do. Much of the information comes from work on other animals and can be only tentatively applied to human beings. Having to use nonhuman data may be a limitation from a human viewpoint, but it also means that the material can be used by those with a more general interest in mammalian endocrinology. I have assumed a certain acquaintance with anatomy, histology, and biochemical terms and pathways.

A textbook is not a fountain of all knowledge. Any text, in an effort to synthesize and simplify, tends to be somewhat dogmatic and to resemble a small encyclopedia, sometimes challenging only the reader's memory. This book of necessity has a bit of both tendencies. Facts, and fair numbers of them at that, must be readily at hand if one is to judge the validity of general concepts; dogma has its uses in clarifying a concept provided one is amenable to change when new facts demand it. But a mass of facts and dogmatic conclusions alone do not make for good teaching; I have tried to emphasize another tendency as well, a tendency toward uncertainty.

Although many of the concepts of endocrine physiology are reasonably well understood, many are not at all clear. Much of the factual matter has been included here precisely because of this; one cannot show loose ends and expose areas of controversy without giving enough experimental findings to show the present state of knowledge and to point out areas of ignorance and disagreement. Such uncertainty may make the reader vaguely uneasy and somewhat dissatisfied, but he cannot avoid it in real life and might as well get used to it. Aimed properly, this uncertainty may point to new challenging and interesting problems to be solved, and it will help in cultivating an open-minded approach to new data and ideas.

A textbook, then, is a tool. The reader should use this book to develop his understanding of concepts, marking and underlining, making his own outlines, and concentrating on the brief summary paragraphs scattered throughout various chapters. Of the mass of facts and figures used in each chapter to flesh out the bare concepts, the reader should know only that these facts exist and where to find them when needed. In a course this text should ideally be used in such a way that the student is always asking questions and pointing toward the unknown; instructors must respond in kind by admitting ignorance when that is in fact appropriate. The student would do well to attempt to synthesize the information in his own way; I have tried to demonstrate this approach in Chapter 12 on the hormonal control of energy metabolism.

One of the most serious problems facing me in writing these chapters was what to leave out, not (as an occasional student may wonder) what to put in. I have tried to select only what seemed important and to hold to the admonition of St. Paul: πάντα δοκιμάζετε το καλὸν κατέχετε (Examine everything, keep what is good). The facts presented are taken from current work up to late 1968 and early 1969, but each issue of such journals as *Endocrinology* and the *Journal of Clinical Endocrinology and Metabolism* raises new questions. There seems to be, moreover, no easy way of reconciling the major differences that sometimes appear in various published reports. Many of these differences will disappear with time and repetition, but for the moment a reasonable guess is often all that is possible, and much of what I have written is interpretation and opinion. When there seems to be severe conflict, I have tried to present both sides of the question without unduly confusing the reader. Critical letters from readers who strongly object to some of my opinions might help to broaden my horizons. I would also offer some cheer to the occasional researcher who wonders what happens to all those reprints he sends out; here at least they did not simply wind up in a bottomless reprint file but were actually used, and, I think, to good purpose.

In general the reader should note that the discussion of each hormone follows, but with great variations, the skeletal outline shown on page 4. Appendix I is a bibliographic listing of fairly general and inclusive works, including basic physiology, clinical endocrinology (although these two often overlap), methods in endocrine research, and a bit of history. Appendix II is a glossary of abbreviations, acronyms, units, and weights, small items that students (and others) always ask about.

No detailed clinical discussion of the treatment of endocrine diseases is given; at this stage, even for medical students, it may be enough to learn normal physiology. However, it seems clear to me that medical students—and often candidates for degrees in physiology—learn endocrine physiology best when it is related in some way to endocrine disease. So most of the common endocrine diseases are mentioned briefly, and when the pathophysiology of one of these disorders flows easily from the discussion of normal physiology, the disease is discussed in more detail (e.g., diabetes mellitus).

Each chapter ends with selected recent references which seem to me either to be conceptually important, to point out areas of controversy, or simply to be useful. They are intended, along with Appendix I, to direct the student in delving further into a problem—something often avoided because of academic pressures; they might still be used later on when things are more relaxed. Also, I have successfully used references of this type as sources for student discussion groups, in which students orally present constructive critical reviews of a published work after which their colleagues criticize their reviews. When this is done with a reasonably informed moderator (he need *not* be an expert), the students enjoy it and, perhaps more important, improve their analytic thinking, an aim that often seems neglected.

I hope the reader will perceive the broad outlines of endocrine physiology, become aware of the many advances of recent years, and realize that many questions remain unanswered. The last point seems to me most important. The main product of a good education is a questioning mind; without this it is hard to recognize ignorance in oneself or in others. Recognizing that one cannot know everything makes for a certain modesty, insures against dogmatism, and allows the development of a certain amount of confidence in the face of uncertainty. Recognizing that someone else may be wrong is necessary to keep everyone honest, though the matter must be handled tactfully if for no other reason than because the other person may be right after all. Awareness of the unknown and the uncertain provides, then, a constant source of ideas for new studies and investigations.

. . . to myself I seem to have been only like a boy playing on the seashore, and diverting myself in now and then finding a smoother pebble or a prettier shell than ordinary, whilst the great ocean of truth lay all undiscovered before me.—SIR ISAAC NEWTON, from Brewster's *Memoirs of Newton*

C. T. S.

# Acknowledgments

Drs. James C. Melby, George A. Bray, Kenneth E. W. Melvin, H. Maurice Goodman, and Marvin L. Mitchell read one or another chapter in varying states of readiness; my thanks to them for their critical help. Mrs. Esther Arra types faster without error than anyone I know.

# Contents

# The Hormones

# 1. Approach to Endocrinology

The humours that do abound
. . . either be sanguine, or
cholericke, or flegmaticke, or
melancholious.
—PHILIP BARROW,
*The Method of Physick*

WHEN individual cells decided to stop going their own separate ways and to join together both anatomically and functionally, the multicellular organisms that were formed had to develop some means for their cells to tell one another what was going on and what to do. Unless this was done, there would be no coordination of the activities of the various parts of the organism and its existence would be constantly threatened. In animals, the coordination is provided by the nervous and endocrine systems, working in concert. The endocrine system also plays a role in the behavior of the group, or "supraorganism." For example, when population density rises in many natural populations, the reproductive ability or fertility of the members of the group decreases, thus limiting the growth of the population. While it is true that animals as diverse as the rat and the elephant follow this rule, man, with his present "population explosion," may be an exception to it.

Historically, the idea that the fluids of the body are important to proper bodily function is ancient. The "four humors" (blood, phlegm, bile, and "black bile") were the basis for a whole system of medicine lasting in one form or another for centuries. Without adequate experimental facts, however, its predictive value was small and thus it fell into disrepute. In the mid-nineteenth century Claude Bernard demonstrated that the liver releases glucose to the blood, which in turn carries it to the tissues of the body. He first used the term *internal secretion.* Once again the idea that the blood carries important substances from one part of the body to another became widespread, based this time on the firmer foundation of fact.

In the late nineteenth and early twentieth centuries specific glandular structures without secretory ducts were nevertheless recognized as having a secretory function. The idea had been in the air for a century, and Berthold had shown experimentally (1849) that something made in the testis caused a cock's comb to grow. Berthold's work was not widely known, however, and it was another 40 to 50 years before structures such as the thyroid, parathyroid, and pituitary were accepted as secreting into the blood materials which have specific effects on distant tissues. These glands of internal secretion became known as *endocrine glands* and the substances secreted were called *hormones.* The term *hormone* was first used by E. H. Starling in June, 1905, while

1

describing secretin and gastrin; it was suggested initially by W. B. Hardy and is derived from the Greek ὁϱμάω ("I excite").

## PROPERTIES OF A HORMONE

A hormone as presently conceived is:

*secreted by living cells* in
*trace amounts* from
*within the organism* and is
*transported usually by the blood* to a
*specific site of action* where it is
*not used as a source of energy* but acts to
*regulate and not initiate reactions* in order to
*bring about an appropriate response by the organism.*

Thus, vitamins, major energy sources, enzymes, and the like are not hormones.

The definition may turn out to be unduly restrictive, however, since some humoral substances may be formed from precursors in the blood stream or at the site of action and so are not themselves secreted. Others may act locally by diffusion without ever getting into the blood stream at all. Nevertheless, it is a useful working definition.

Since there is no direct cellular connection between the cells of secretion and the effector site, the endocrine system differs from the other great regulatory system, the nervous system. Nevertheless, the ties with the nervous system are extensive and are now recognized as being of great importance, so important that neuroendocrinology is a separate field of study.

A major point, one that is easy to lose sight of in the forest of facts to follow, is that most hormones are present in the circulation at all times, albeit in greater or lesser amounts. While it is necessary to discuss them one at a time, this is an arbitrary and artificial separation from the body's point of view. One must try to see what the combined effects of the hormone "soup" are and imagine the final response of the body to the mixture of the moment.

## DISCOVERY AND STUDY OF HORMONES

The discovery of most hormones, in the basic sense of finding out that they exist, stems from two main sources. The *clinical observation* of diseased patients still provides stimulation and knowledge for the understanding of endocrine physiology, particularly since not all endocrine relationships are known nor are all aspects of endocrine disease explained by the known effects of the recognized hormones. The other source, the *laboratory animal*, is often the only means of obtaining information because of obvious limitations in experiments on human beings. Yet care must be used in transferring information learned from animals to man because there are often vital differences between species.

A comparison among present-day animals suggests that hormones have evolved over the course of time in several possible ways.

1. There may be a change in the use to which a hormone is put; for example, prolactin is concerned with lactation in mammals but may act as a growth hormone in amphibians and reptiles and seems involved in salt and water balance in some teleost fishes.
2. The molecular structure of a hormone may change, and the change may or may not affect its action; there is a tendency for mutated forms to be effective in all species but for the original form to be inactive in "higher" species. This phenomenon has been termed *species specificity*. Perhaps it is most strikingly seen in the case of growth hormone. Growth hormone from humans or primates works well enough in humans, but no other growth hormone is effective. However, other mammals will respond to human growth hormone. Yet the many differences in the insulin molecule that occur in different species seem not to affect its activity in other species.
3. Finally, it is possible that the receptors at the site of action of the hormone have evolved and become more specific; although never described, this development could account for some of the species specificity noted above.

How does one study a hormone? The main approach is to remove a suspected endocrine gland, observe a defect in the animal, and try to correct the defect by administering a presumed hormonal preparation. One may give an extract of the gland or an analogous synthetic hormone either by mouth or by injection.

A slightly different approach is to examine the effects of extracts of suspected endocrine tissue. This may lead to the discovery of effects due to unsuspected hormones, in which case the question of the physiologic importance of the observed actions must be answered. An effect produced by large doses of an extract may have no meaning to the body because such large amounts of hormone are not found in vivo.

In either instance proof of physiologic importance most often depends on the demonstration of the hormone in the blood and on showing appropriate changes in the concentration of the hormone in response to appropriate stimuli.

Having established the probable existence of a hormone and, at least grossly, its main effects, one can now investigate the detailed biochemistry and physiology of the hormone. Ideally, one would like to know:

1. What is the hormone *chemically*? Is this isolated substance the same as that actually *secreted* to the blood stream? Ultimately, *synthesis* is required to prove structure.
2. What is the *source* of the hormone? That is, what cell or cell fraction makes it?
3. How is it *synthesized* and *stored* in the gland?
4. What is the *secreted form* of the hormone and *how much is secreted*?
5. How is it *carried* in the blood?
6. How does it *act* on its target tissue?
7. How is it *metabolized* either at site of action or elsewhere?
8. What *controls* the *secretion* of the hormone and its *action* on a target organ?

This, of course, is the ideal. No hormone is well characterized on all points, and for the protein hormones only a few of these questions can be answered. In the discussion of each hormone, the reader will note that the above sequence of eight queries is generally followed insofar as possible.

## MECHANISM OF HORMONE ACTION

The problem of the mechanism of hormone action is difficult. The precise mode of action on the cell, assuming there is only one, is not known for any hormone. Many hormonal effects, on the other hand, are well known, and there is a tendency for the earliest of these to be called the mechanism of action. This is a proper approach but does not necessarily define mechanism. As in any field, endocrinology has its fashions, and the following possible modes of action for hormones have been proposed at one time or another. The hormone, very often after *binding* to a specific tissue or tissue component, might then:

1. *Affect membrane transport* of various substances.
2. *Affect the activity of the gene* in running the cell by changing DNA-directed mRNA synthesis, perhaps by decreasing intrastrand bonds of DNA or by regulating which area of DNA is to be active. (DNA = deoxyribonucleic acid; mRNA = messenger ribonucleic acid.)*
3. *Affect protein synthesis* at some point beyond mRNA synthesis, probably at the ribosome-polysome level.

*See Appendix II for list of abbreviations.

4. *Change the amount or activity of enzyme(s)* or other specific proteins.
5. *Change the amount or availability of a cofactor.* Adrenocorticotropic hormone (ACTH) and thyroid-stimulating hormone (TSH) are thought by some to do this.
6. *Act itself as a coenzyme.*
7. *Exert an allosteric effect* on a membrane, nucleic acid, polysome, or enzyme. Here the hormone binds to one part of a molecule or membrane, causing a molecular rearrangement whereby actions are changed at a distant part of the molecule or membrane.
8. *Affect the entire cytoskeleton* or some of the structural elements of the cell in a subtle way, thus causing some or all of the above.
9. *Stimulate or inhibit the formation of a hormonal mediator,* for example, cyclic 3′,5′-adenosine monophosphate (cyclic AMP or cAMP) or perhaps a prostaglandin, which then brings about the observed effect.

Despite all these thoughts, which are by no means mutually exclusive, few clear-cut answers have emerged and most of the area is still open to investigation. Factors usually not tested may be important; for instance, a hormone may have more than one mechanism for affecting the same or different tissues, or the specificity of response by different tissues may play more of a role than we think.

Furthermore, the evidence supporting some of the mechanisms noted is not as firm in retrospect as it was thought to be initially. The evidence for 1 and 2 above derives mainly from the fact that the synthesis of mRNA is blocked by actinomycin D, and the synthesis of protein by puromycin or cycloheximide (Fig. 1). Thus, if these poisons (or antimetabolites) block a hormonal action, it is presumed that the hormone acted via mRNA synthesis, protein synthesis, or both. The problem is that the antimetabolites may have other unknown effects;

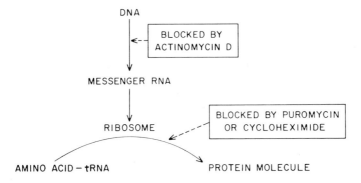

Fig. 1. Antimetabolites and the synthesis of mRNA and protein.

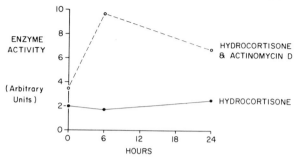

FIG. 2.   Effect of actinomycin D on the response of leukocyte alkaline phosphatase to hydrocortisone. (From E. E. McCoy, and M. Ebadi. *Biochem. Biophys. Res. Commun.* 26:265, 1967.)

if so, theses such as 1 or 2 would then be open to question. An example: The white-cell enzyme, alkaline phosphatase, is slightly stimulated by hydrocortisone. Actinomycin D was added to see whether the effect would be blocked. If it was, one would say that hydrocortisone acts in this instance by stimulating mRNA synthesis; if the effect was not inhibited, one would say that mRNA synthesis is not necessary. In fact, the enzyme activity was markedly stimulated, making interpretation most difficult (Fig. 2). Similar results occurred with the lipoprotein lipase of adipose tissue, suggesting that this is not an isolated finding.

## Cyclic AMP

The concept and discovery of intracellular hormonal mediators (see 9 above) is perhaps the most exciting development in basic endocrinology in recent years. First described in 1957 by Rall, Sutherland, and Berthet, *cyclic AMP* (Fig. 3) has been intensively studied to the point where it is now implicated in the action of adrenocorticotropin

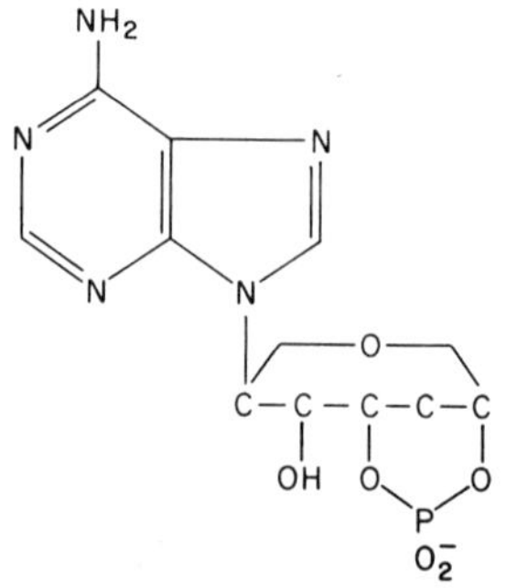

FIG. 3.   Cyclic 3′,5′-adenosine monophosphate.

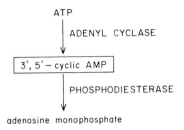

FIG. 4.   Synthesis and breakdown of cyclic AMP.

(ACTH), luteinizing hormone (LH), thyrotropin (TSH), melano-cyte-stimulating hormone (MSH), antidiuretic hormone (ADH), thyroid hormone, glucocorticoids, parathyroid hormone (PTH), insulin, glucagon, catecholamines, estradiol, and serotonin. No one would be surprised if this list were outdated by the time it is read. The length of the list suggests that *cAMP may be a universal mediator of hormonal stimulation.*

Cyclic AMP is formed from adenosine triphosphate (ATP). The reaction is catalyzed by the enzyme adenyl cyclase. cAMP is broken down in turn fairly rapidly by a phosphodiesterase to 5′-AMP (Fig. 4).

For the most part, hormones that act by stimulating the formation of cAMP do so by stimulating the activity of adenyl cyclase. Since adenyl cyclase is usually found in the cell membrane, mechanisms 4, 8, and 9 above (and perhaps others) are involved. A hormone may also stimulate cAMP formation by inhibiting the phosphodiesterase.

Even here, however, there is more than meets the eye, for the hormones that increase cAMP do so only in the tissues where they act and not in other tissues. There must be a high degree of specificity for the hormone in the receptor sites of the responding tissue at some

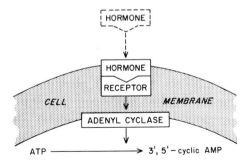

FIG. 5.   Postulated mechanism for hormonal stimulation of cyclic AMP synthesis.

point before the stimulation of adenyl cyclase (Fig. 5). Almost nothing is known about these receptor sites.

*Prostaglandins*

Another candidate for an intracellular hormonal mediator is the group of substances called *prostaglandins*. Not much is yet known about them, so it is probably premature to assign them this role with any certainty. While cAMP acts as a stimulator of actions, in many instances the *prostaglandins seem to act as inhibitors*. The prostaglandins may also be true hormones, circulating in the blood and acting in a way unrelated to intracellular hormonal mediation. They are most potent substances and a few micrograms cause a maximal response.

Although observed in 1913, when prostatic extracts were seen to lower blood pressure, and in 1930, when seminal fluid was found to cause contraction of uterine muscle, the prostaglandins were not named until 1934, when von Euler showed that extracts of the prostate gland and seminal vesicles also contracted uterine muscle. Since 1957 a great deal of work by Bergstrom and his colleagues has shown that they are found in many other tissues, but the name has stuck.

The prostaglandins are derived from the essential fatty acids and have a basic 20-carbon fatty acid structure containing a 5-membered ring (Fig. 6). Those found in tissues are mostly prostaglandins E (PGE) and F (PGF). PGE has a ketone group at $C_9$ and a hydroxyl group at $C_{11}$; PGF is the same except for a hydroxyl group at $C_9$ instead of a ketone group. They are further named according to the number of double bonds in the aliphatic chains; $PGE_2$, for example, has two double bonds. All are metabolized quickly to other, less active prostaglandins. The "secretion rate" of $PGF_1$ has been estimated at roughly 100 to 200 nanograms (ng) per day.

Overall, knowledge of the prostaglandins is too new for us even to be sure that they play a role in normal physiology, but since they are found in many tissues and can have many different effects they are probably important and in some instances may be hormonal mediators. To date, prostaglandins have been involved in:

1. Reproduction. Depending on the dose, they can inhibit or stimulate uterine contraction. They may play a role in the transport

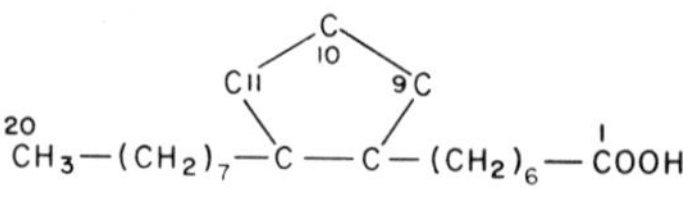

FIG. 6.   Basic carbon structure of prostaglandins. Some of the carbon atoms in the fatty acid chain are numbered for convenience (numbers 1, 9, 10, 11, and 20).

of sperm to the site of fertilization, the fallopian tube, since some infertile men have less PGE in their seminal fluid than normal men. They may also be important in stimulating uterine contraction during delivery of the fetus.

2. Gastrointestinal function. Gut motility, for example, can be stimulated with PGE or PGF, and PGE can block the secretion of acid and enzymes by the stomach.

3. Synthesis of adrenal cortical hormones. The prostaglandins can stimulate the synthesis of adrenal corticoids.

4. Regulation of blood pressure. PGE can lower the blood pressure and block the hypertensive response to norepinephrine. Recently it has been shown that a hypotensive substance found in extracts of renal medulla, called medullin, is in fact a $PGE_2$. The kidney may secrete the $PGE_2$, which then lowers blood pressure by peripheral vasodilation.

5. Salt and water resorption by the kidney. PGE causes a decrease in sodium and water resorption resulting in an increase in free water clearance and in urinary volume and sodium excretion. It is not clear whether this is all intrarenal, with renal $PGE_2$ exerting its effects locally, or whether circulating prostaglandin plays a role. We do know that PGE inhibits the action of ADH on the isolated toad bladder (see Chap. 4, under The Neurohypophysis). More to the point, PGE has recently been shown to block the action of ADH on water resorption by isolated mammalian renal tubules by interfering with the production of cAMP. Whether this inhibitory effect or the action on vasodilation or both account for the effect of PGE on sodium and water resorption is not resolved.

6. Energy supply. They inhibit the lipolysis (free fatty acid release) stimulated by norepinephrine in human adipose tissue as well as in the rat and the dog. There is still some uncertainty regarding this effect in vivo, since PGE given to humans without norepinephrine causes a slight *rise* in plasma free fatty acids (indicating some increase in lipolysis). Strongly suggesting a role in vivo is the fact that rats deprived of essential fatty acids, the precursors of the prostaglandins, show an increased lipolysis, implying that the prostaglandins act as a normal inhibitor of lipolysis.

The last two effects of prostaglandins listed, those on the kidney and on lipolysis, are to date the best examples of the inhibitory action of these substances. In both cases PGE probably inhibits the formation of cAMP, perhaps by interfering with the function of adenyl cyclase. cAMP is thus a mediator of hormonal stimulation while the prostaglandins may be a mediator of hormonal inhibition, acting to block cAMP synthesis (Fig. 7). Nevertheless, proof that the prosta-

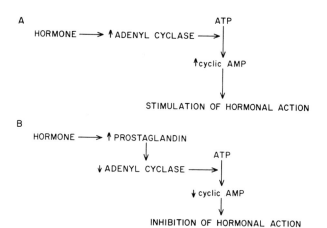

Fig. 7.   A. Cyclic AMP as a mediator of hormonal stimulation (reasonably well proved). B. Prostaglandin as a mediator of hormonal inhibition (highly speculative).

glandins play a physiologic role as intracellular inhibitors depends on the measurement of prostaglandins in the affected tissues, and this has not yet been done.

### Concept of Permissive Action

Most hormonal actions are directly related to the amount of hormone present, at least within a certain range. That is, there is a good dose-response relationship. More hormone gives a bigger response. However, it often appears that a hormone has to be present for some body process to work, yet the hormone itself does not stimulate that process and adding more of the hormone does not make it work better. Hormones that act in this way are said to have a permissive action. Best described for hydrocortisone, permissive actions have also been described for growth hormone and thyroid hormone and may exist for other hormones as well. For example, hydrocortisone's presence is needed for the optimal action of other hormones such as thyroxine, growth hormone, norepinephrine, and insulin.

The label *permissive action* is useful but it does not really explain the action and in fact simply hides our ignorance. It may, however, point the way to some common cellular effect, as yet unknown.

## Control of Secretion and Action of Hormones

The *control* of the secretion and action of a hormone is one of the most important aspects of endocrinology. It is implicit in the idea of a hormone as a regulator, one of the characteristics of a hormone. If a hormone is to regulate, its secretion must be under some kind of control; sometimes its action is controlled as well. A useful concept in *regulating secretion* is the idea of *negative feedback*, whereby the effect of a hormone tends to shut off further secretion of that hormone. At its simplest, the result of a hormonal stimulation directly affects the secreting gland and stops secretion. For example, a drop in serum calcium causes an increased secretion of parathyroid hormone, which in turn raises the serum calcium. When the serum calcium rises to a normal level, it directly inhibits the secretion of parathyroid hormone by the parathyroid gland. In its more complex form, a negative feedback system operates indirectly and involves several steps; for example, hydrocortisone shuts off ACTH secretion, but does so by acting on the hypothalamus and not on the pituitary. Other variants on the theme include regulation of hormonal secretion by several hormonal effects instead of by one, inhibition or stimulation by effects other than those of the hormone or by environmental factors outside hormonal control, and regulation of two or more hormones by one or more hormonal effects. Sometimes a negative feedback mechanism becomes so complex that it is difficult to perceive the mechanism; see, for example, the regulation of gondadotropin secretion by gonadal hormones in the female.

Sometimes one can demonstrate *control of hormonal action*. A given amount of hormone may have varying effects depending on what else is going on; for example, insulin increases the uptake of glucose by muscle, but not as much uptake occurs if extra hydrocortisone is present at the same time. Or a hormone may have to be converted to something else before it can act; testosterone apparently must be changed to dihydrotestosterone by the receptor tissue before that tissue can respond to the testosterone, and anything affecting that change will obviously affect the hormonal action.

## Assay of Hormones

The assay of hormones is rapidly yielding to new techniques that are more sensitive and more specific than before. At one time some form of bioassay was the only approach. Bioassays, or assays dependent on the response of a living tissue or an entire animal, are necessary to show that the substance being measured has biologic activity, but they are subject to wide variation. Relatively insensitive, they are of limited use in assaying the small amounts of hormone found in body fluids. Furthermore, in many cases they lack a high degree of specificity, so that the response may be due to substances other than the hormone. As more hormones became chemically recognizable, reliable chemical assays were developed for thyroxine and hydrocortisone, and more recently for testosterone, estradiol, aldosterone, and the catecholamines.

Note that no protein or peptide hormone is on this list. These hormones have been much harder to characterize chemically. Moreover, with the available chemical reactions, it has been impossible to tell the tiny amount of a particular peptide hormone from all the other peptides and proteins floating around in the blood or excreted into the urine. For a long while, therefore, the bioassay remained the only approach for peptide hormones.

In order to attack the problem of assaying peptide hormones, many bioassays have been refined to the point where they are useful in detecting hormones in blood, particularly in a large volume of blood. But the problem of specificity remains. They are also of use in analyzing urine, since an entire day's output of hormone can be processed at once. For example, for the gonadotropins, the urinary bioassay remains the only practical assay for most practicing physicians despite its relative crudity, its tediousness, and its inability to distinguish follicle-stimulating hormone (FSH) from LH unless special modifications are used.

A few years ago a new approach in the assay of peptide and protein hormones resulted in a major advance. Instead of attempting to use a chemical or biologic property as the end point, the new approach, the radioimmunoassay, is based on the immunologic properties of these hormones.

It is characteristic of peptides and proteins, whether hormonal or not, to stimulate antibody formation when injected into an appropriate animal. The antibody is another protein that binds specifically to its antigen (the peptide or protein injected) and to no other. If one could isolate a peptide hormone in reasonably pure form, an antibody specific for that hormone could be developed. This has now been done for many of the peptide hormones and is the basis of the various highly sensitive radioimmunoassays. It should be clear, however, that what is being measured is immunologic and not biologic activity. The possibility exists that a given immunoassay may detect substances that are not biologically active. To date, radioimmunoassays have been devised for insulin, glucagon, FSH, LH, prolactin, GH, TSH, ACTH, α-MSH, β-MSH, vasopressin, PTH, thyrocalcitonin, gastrin, secretin, angiotensin, and bradykinin. Most have been applied to the assay of these hormones in blood.

### The Radioimmunoassay

As we have said, a pure hormone is required for a radioimmunoassay. Then one must have an animal capable of making high concentrations of antibody to the hormone. With these requirements met, it is time to set up the assay.

Some of the pure hormone is labeled with radioactive iodine and a small but known amount placed in a test tube. A small, measured amount of the antibody goes into the same tube, and the plasma sample to be assayed is also added. After a while, an equilibrium will be reached at which some of the labeled hormone and some of the un- labeled hormone in the plasma sample will be bound to the antibody. Since only a small amount of antibody is present, its binding capacity for the hormone is limited and constant. Therefore, if there are bind- ing sites in the test tube for four molecules of hormone (whether labeled or unlabeled) and if four molecules of labeled hormone are added, all the labeled hormone will be bound to the antibody. If, in addition, there are four molecules of unlabeled hormone in the test tube, the antibody will be able to bind only half of the total of eight molecules. Since the molecules are uniformly distributed and both forms of hormone compete for a constant amount of antibody, only two molecules of labeled, radioactive hormone will be bound to anti- body along with two of unlabeled hormone (Fig. 8). Therefore, in general, *the more unlabeled hormone present in the plasma sample, the less labeled hormone will be bound to the antibody* and vice versa.

The hormone bound to antibody is then separated from the un- bound, or free, hormone and, after the radioactivity in each fraction has been counted, the ratio of bound to free hormone (the B/F ratio)

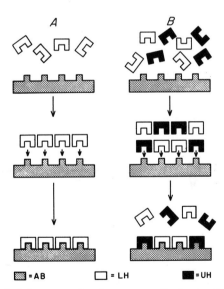

FIG. 8.    A. Labeled hormone binding to antibody in the absence of un- labeled hormone. B. Labeled hormone binding to antibody in the presence of an equal number of molecules of unlabeled hormone. LH = radioactively labeled hormone; UH = unlabeled hormone; AB = binding sites on anti- bodies.

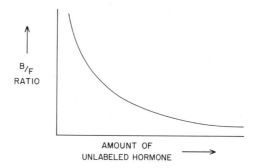

Fɪɢ. 9.　Relation of bound to free hormone (B/F) ratio to amount of unlabeled hormone in unknown plasma sample or in standard curve.

is calculated. A low ratio indicates that a low amount of labeled hormone was bound to the antibody and, as seen above, a high amount of hormone in the original unknown plasma. A high B/F ratio indicates the opposite (Fig. 9). Comparison of the B/F ratio with a standard curve gives the exact result, usually in millimicrograms per milliliter (mμg/ml), or nanograms per milliliter.

The principle of the radioimmunoassay has recently and elegantly been applied to the assay of nonprotein hormones, including progesterone, testosterone, hydrocortisone, corticosterone, thyroxine, and triiodothyronine. Basically, the technique is the same except that a natural binding protein, a synthetic resin, or finely ground charcoal instead of an antibody acts as the binding agent. These techniques have greatly increased the sensitivity of the assays for these hormones and opened areas for investigation that were difficult to approach before. An excellent example of how important advances in science often are critically dependent on new techniques.

## Bɪʙʟɪᴏɢʀᴀᴘʜʏ

Bergström, S.　Prostaglandins: Members of a new hormonal system. *Science* 157:382, 1967.

Berson, S. A., and Yalow, R.　Radioimmunoassays of peptide hormones in plasma. *New Eng. J. Med.* 277:640, 1967.

Davidson, E. H.　Hormones and genes. *Sci. Amer.* 212:36, 1965.

Grantham, J. J., and Orloff, J.　Effect of prostaglandin $E_1$ on the permeability response of the isolated collecting tubule to vasopressin, adenosine 3',5'-monophosphate, and theophylline. *J. Clin. Invest.* 47:1154, 1968.

Haynes, R. C., Jr., Sutherland, E. W., and Rall, T. W.　The role of cyclic adenylic acid in hormone action. *Recent Progr. Hormone Res.* 16:121, 1960.

Hechter, O., and Lester, G.   Cell permeability and hormone action. *Recent Progr. Hormone Res.* 16:139, 1960.

Karlson, P.   New concepts on the mode of action of hormones. *Perspect. Biol. Med.* 6:203, 1963.

McCoy, E. E., and Ebadi, M.   The paradoxical effect of hydrocortisone and actinomycin on the activity of rabbit leucocyte alkaline phosphatase. *Biochem. Biophys. Res. Commun.* 26:265, 1967.

Rall, T. W., Sutherland, E. W., and Berthet, J.   The relationship of epinephrine and glucagon to liver phosphorylase: IV. Effect of epinephrine and glucagon on the reactivation of phosphorylase in liver homogenates. *J. Biol. Chem.* 224:463, 1957. (The classic article on the subject.)

Samuels, L. D.   Actinomycin and its effects. *New Eng. J. Med.* 271:1252, 1964.

Sutherland, E. W., Robison, G. A., and Butcher, R. W.   Some aspects of the biological role of adenosine 3',5'-monophosphate (cyclic AMP). *Circulation* 37:279, 1968.

Turtle, J. R., and Kipnis, D. M.   An adrenergic receptor mechanism for the control of cyclic 3', 5' adenosine monophosphate synthesis in tissues. *Biochem. Biophys. Res. Commun.* 28:797, 1967.

# 2. Recognized Endocrine Glands and Other Glands and Humors

THE *recognized endocrine glands* are the anterior pituitary, posterior pituitary, thyroid, parathyroid, adrenal cortex, adrenal medulla, ovary, testis, placenta, and pancreas. Nevertheless, this is not the limit of endocrinology. For example, the thymus, the heart, and the uterus are reported to have endocrine functions, which at present are not at all clear. Several other substances and structures are involved in a hormone-like action although in some cases there may be no recognized gland or cell type as the source.

## PLASMA KININS

Rocha e Silva and his co-workers noticed in 1949 that a mixture of snake venom and plasma caused a slow contraction of the isolated guinea pig intestine. They coined the name *bradykinin* to describe the responsible substance. A similar material had been described before that by Werle in 1937 and named *kallidin*. These kinins also caused dilation of peripheral small blood vessels and, as one might expect, hypotension; they are probably related to hypotensive substances found in the urine as long ago as 1909.

Three kinins have been found in blood and are probably formed there. One is bradykinin, a nonapeptide:

$$NH_2–ARG–PRO–PRO–GLY–PHE–SER–PRO–PHE–ARG$$

Another is kallidin, which has 10 amino acids; the structure is the same as bradykinin plus an N-terminal lysine. The third kinin, as yet unnamed, has 11 amino acids and is identical to kallidin plus an N-terminal methionine.

All three kinins are probably formed from common precursors, the *kininogens*. Several kininogens are known, one with a molecular weight of more than 100,000 and two others of about 50,000 mol. wt. The hydrolytic enzyme *kallikrein* acts on the kininogen to cause the release of kinins. Some of the enzyme or its activator may come from granulocytic leukocytes in the blood. Normally, blood levels of brady-kinin are about 0.2 to 0.9 mμg/ml.

Several actions of the kinins have been described:

1. Stimulation of most smooth muscle contraction—for example, small intestinal, venous, or bronchial. They are effective at very low concentrations, e.g., 0.1 mμg/ml.
2. Dilation of arteries (an exception to the general rule of smooth muscle), especially in the periphery. This may result in a lower blood pressure. Physiologically, this action may be essential for survival of the newborn by opening the pulmonary arterial vessels and allowing all of the blood to circulate through the lungs (blood levels of bradykinin in the newborn are clearly elevated: 13 mμg/ml).
3. Increase in the stroke volume of the heart, perhaps secondary to action 2 above.
4. Increase in capillary permeability.
5. Increase in migration rate of leukocytes.
6. Pain, when the kinin is placed on the base of a blister.

Their physiologic role is completely unsettled, but they may play a part in regulating blood flow (see 2 and 3 above) although this seems unlikely for skeletal muscle. They may be important in the inflammatory response (see 4, 5, and 6 above). Whether or not the gut is significantly affected in vivo is even less clear. Increased activity of the sympathetic nervous system may, in some unknown way, lower the plasma level of bradykinin, but again, the significance is not clear.

## SEROTONIN

Serotonin is a derivative of tryptamine (Fig. 10). About 97% of the serotonin in plasma is bound to platelets. There is about 200 mμg/ml bound to platelets and only 6 mμg/ml in the rest of the plasma.

Although it is found in the pineal, no specific gland is known to secrete serotonin. However, some tumors, called malignant carcinoid tumors, do secrete both serotonin and bradykinin. One may find levels of bradykinin as high as 0.4 to 1.2 μg/ml. The combination results in

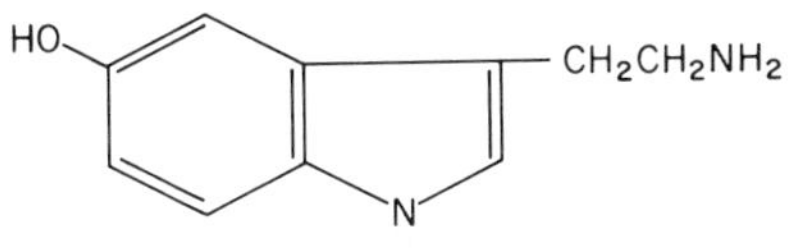

FIG. 10.    Serotonin or 5-hydroxytryptamine.

peripheral vasodilation, bronchoconstriction, and hypotension and is called the carcinoid syndrome.

Serotonin may have a role in peristalsis since it increases bowel smooth muscle motility; it may be a neurohumor since it is found in the pineal gland and central nervous system; and it may play a part in the regulation of blood flow since it causes peripheral vasodilation in many areas and increases capillary permeability.

## PINEAL GLAND

The pineal has been assigned many roles over the centuries. It was, for instance, called the seat of the "rational soul" by Descartes. Today, we know it contains *melatonin* (5-methoxy, N-acetyltryptamine), which can be synthesized only in the pineal; melatonin (Fig. 11) is similar in structure to its precursor, serotonin. In the frog, melatonin lightens the skin by concentrating the granules in the melanophores and counteracts the effect of MSH; hence its name. In mammals, the skin does not have melanophores but melatonin is still important. In the female rat, for example, it decreases ovarian weight and frequency of estrus. These effects are related to the effect of light on estrus and are mediated by changes in gonadotropin secretion. Decreased exposure to visible light, mediated by the cervical sympathetic ganglia, causes an increase in the pineal synthesis of melatonin. The extra melatonin, in turn, brings about a decrease in the secretion of gonadotropin by the pituitary (perhaps by blocking the secretion of hypothalamic releasing factors) and ultimately results in less frequent estrus. A similar mechanism in male rats results in small testes. In man, however, melatonin's role is not clear since light seems to have little effect on ovulation and, if anything, appears to decrease rather than increase ovarian activity.

The pineal gland may also have something to do with the adrenal cortex. Although older work had suggested that the pineal might stimulate the secretion of aldosterone, it more probably (if anything) acts to inhibit the basal secretion of aldosterone and perhaps of glucocorticoids as well.

Finally, melatonin may inhibit the secretion of thyroid hormones. Whether any of the effects of melatonin or the pineal have physiologic

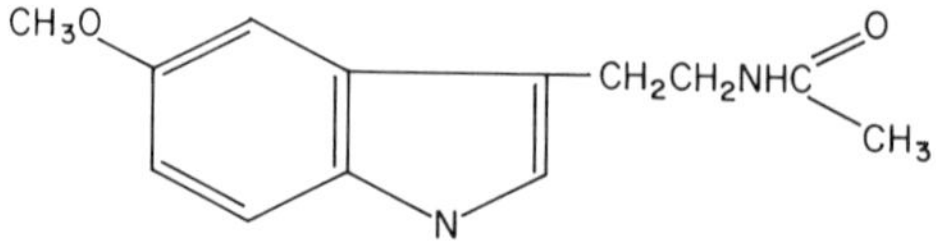

FIG. 11.   Melatonin.

meaning is not at all certain; more time must pass and more experiments be done before any judgment can be made.

## THE KIDNEY

Although not commonly thought of as an endocrine gland, the kidney is probably the site of formation of several hormones:

1. Medullin. This is a $PGE_2$ and is discussed in Chap. 1.
2. Erythropoietin. Red cell production in the bone marrow is increased by erythropoietin.
3. Renin. The juxtaglomerular apparatus near the glomerulus is composed of the *juxtaglomerular body* (specialized cells of the afferent and probably efferent glomerular arterioles) and the *macula densa* (a group of specialized cells of and near the distal tubule located close to the juxtaglomerular body). The whole probably plays a role in the autoregulation of renal blood flow, the mechanism whereby the kidney maintains a constant blood flow in the face of fairly wide variations in blood pressure. More pertinent is the fact that the apparatus makes renin, a protein (42,000 mol. wt.) discovered independently by Page and by Braun-Menendez in 1940. The stimulus for its secretion probably comes in part from the macula densa, which seems to act as a sensing device for the amount of sodium in the distal tubule. Renin has a major part in aldosterone secretion (see Chap. 5), and may be important in maintaining or raising the blood pressure.

## GASTROINTESTINAL HORMONES

Although covered in discussions of the gastrointestinal tract, these are mentioned here as a reminder that they are indeed hormones and that they are historically important to endocrinology since gastrin and secretin were the first substances to be called hormones.

Secretin was discovered in 1902 by Bayliss and Starling. We now know it to be a single-chain peptide containing 27 amino acids. Gastrin was described by Edkins in 1905, but for many years he was not believed and only in 1938 was gastrin's existence definitely established by Komarov. Today, gastrin is well known and has been purified and synthesized. It is a 17-amino acid peptide (gastrin I) of 2114 mol. wt.:

$$GLU\text{--}GLY\text{--}PRO\text{--}TRP\text{--}MET\text{--}(GLU)_5\text{--}ALA\text{--}$$
$$TYR\text{--}GLY\text{--}TRP\text{--}MET\text{--}ASP\text{--}PHE\text{--}CONH_2$$

The terminal amide group is important for activity, which includes not only stimulation of gastric acid production but also stimulation of enzyme secretion by the pancreas. However, most of the rest of the peptide is *not* important for good activity; the last five amino acids seem to be all that is needed for potent stimulation. Normal plasma levels of both secretin and gastrin I are 400 μμg/ml or less.

## The Thymus

The thymus is thought to contain a lymphocyte-stimulating factor, which may thus increase antibody production. This substance may be humoral, and the thymus may soon resume its place as a more or less orthodox endocrine gland, a place widely accepted many years ago but recently in disfavor.

## Bibliography

Cohen, R. A., Wurtman, R. J., Axelrod, J., and Snyder, S. H.   Some clinical, biochemical, and physiological actions of the pineal gland. *Ann. Intern. Med.* 61:1144, 1964.

Melmon, K. L., and Cline, M. J.   Kinins. *Amer. J. Med.* 43:153, 1967.

Pierce, J. V.   Structural features of plasma kinins and kininogens. *Fed. Proc.* 27:52, 1968.

Sjoerdsma, A.   Serotonin. *New Eng. J. Med.* 261:181, 231, 1959.

# 3. The Hypothalamus and the Anterior Pituitary Gland

ONCE called the "master gland," the anterior pituitary gland is now known to be subject to influences from a still higher level, the central nervous system, via the hypophyseal portal blood flow. Nevertheless, its removal leads to multiple widespread effects, all of decreased function. After hypophysectomy one sees a decline in function of the ovary, testis, lactating breast, thyroid, and adrenal cortex, along with decreased growth in the young. There is perhaps less mobilization of fatty acids, as well as a tendency toward a lower blood glucose and paler skin.

When extracts of the pituitary gland were made, one of the above effects was used as an end point in controlling and guiding the isolation of specific pituitary hormones. Thus, a purified fraction which restored normal growth was called growth hormone. The name, then, derives from the effect, not from the chemistry of the substance. It is clear that other effects not implied by the given name might well be the result of such a hormone. Only in the last few years, for example, was it realized that growth hormone mobilizes fatty acids.

## RELATION OF HYPOTHALAMUS AND PITUITARY

The hypothalamus and the anterior pituitary function together as an integrated unit. Although the human hypothalamus weighs only 4 g, it is a very complex area with many functions. It controls, for example, appetite, temperature, thirst, the posterior pituitary, and the anterior pituitary. Its control over the anterior pituitary is related to the peculiar blood supply of the latter (Figs. 12 and 13). In man there is no pituitary artery, and all the blood to the anterior pituitary comes through portal vessels from the hypothalamus. The long portal vessels supply 90% of the blood and go from the median eminence to fairly discrete areas of the lateral and inferior pituitary. The short portal vessels, discovered in 1954, are largely within the pituitary gland and run from the lower part of the pituitary stalk, an extension of the

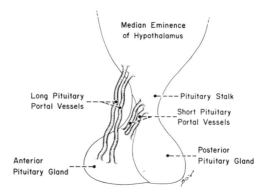

FIG. 12.   Relationship of hypothalamus and anterior pituitary gland.

hypothalamus, to the upper part of the anterior pituitary; they supply about 10% of the blood and keep a small portion of the gland alive when the stalk is sectioned. Each portal vessel seems to supply a fairly circumscribed area of the anterior pituitary.

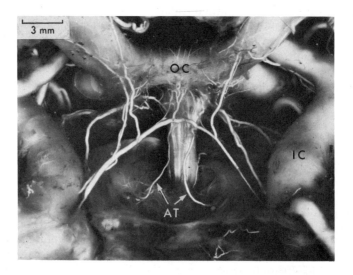

FIG. 13.   Human pituitary stalk, anterior view, with pituitary portal vessels. AT = trabecular arteries which supply little or no blood to the anterior pituitary gland. The stalk, in the center of the picture, passes just behind the optic chiasm (OC) downward to the pituitary gland. Thin white vessels on the stalk are the long pituitary portal vessels. IC = internal carotid artery. (From G. P. Xuereb, M. M. L. Prichard, and P. M. Daniel, *Quart. J. Exp. Physiol.* 39:199, 1954.)

The *hypothalamus* is now known to contain releasing or inhibiting factors for all the hormones of the anterior pituitary. Most of these factors probably arise in the lower part of the hypothalamus, the median eminence. However, higher centers in the hypothalamus or in other areas of the brain often influence the median eminence. Thus, by changing the rate of secretion of these releasing or inhibiting factors the brain and hypothalamus can increase or decrease the secretion of hormones by the anterior pituitary.

At the moment, most of these hypothalamic factors are thought to be small peptides, but this may not be the case. The human hypothalamus contains LH-releasing factor (LH-RF or LRF), FSH-releasing factor (FSH-RF), thyrotropin-releasing factor (TRF), corticotropin-releasing factor (CRF), growth hormone–releasing factor (GH-RF or GRF), and MSH-inhibiting factor (MSH-IF). In other species one can find prolactin-inhibiting factor (PIF) and MSH-releasing factor (MSH-RF) as well as all the others; these two may be present in the human hypothalamus but have not been carefully sought. Whether these factors have any systemic effect outside the pituitary is not known. This is a definite possibility since other hypothalamic substances have systemic effects, such as the neurohypophyseal hormones and a substance, sialogen, which acts directly on the salivary glands to increase the flow of saliva. The releasing factors may act by depolarizing the membrane of the anterior pituitary cell and their effects may be mediated by cAMP.

## CONTROL OF PITUITARY HORMONE SECRETION

While this topic will be discussed later with each specific hormone, we take note now of three general categories of controlling mechanisms, all of which are variants of negative feedback control. (1) The first is the classic negative feedback mechanism whereby a pituitary hormone stimulates the secretion of another hormone—for example, thyroxine—which in turn shuts off the secretion of the pituitary hormone by acting directly on the pituitary gland. (2) In the second category the same thing occurs, but indirectly. A pituitary hormone stimulates the secretion of another hormone, which then inhibits the secretion of the pituitary hormone, not by acting on the pituitary gland but by inhibiting the output of the hypothalamic releasing factor. (3) Finally, the pituitary hormone may shut off its own secretion ("short circuit feedback control") by acting directly on either the hypothalamus or the pituitary gland.

Not much is known about what goes on in the hypothalamus when changes in the secretion of the releasing factors take place. Certainly there are adrenergic and cholinergic neurons as well as neurons of a

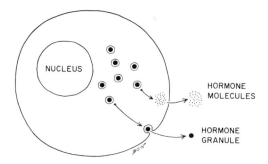

Fig. 14.   Granular and nongranular release of hormones from the anterior pituitary gland.

completely different type, perhaps with serotonin, histamine, or other polyamines as the neurotransmitter. The norepinephrine content of the hypothalamus is, for example, greater when the animal is in the dark. While one might speculate that this finding is related to the diurnal variation of CRF release (see Chap. 5), CRF release is probably controlled by cholinergic neurons. Perhaps a bit clearer is the rise in the synthesis of hypothalamic catecholamines after the gonads are removed, implying that catecholamines ultimately stimulate secretion of gonadotropins. On the other hand, it is entirely possible that hypothalamic substances such as melatonin (see above) inhibit the secretion of releasing factors and ultimately inhibit the secretion of pituitary hormones.

The *anterior pituitary* in man includes the intermediate lobe found in other species. It weighs about 500 mg (more during pregnancy) and contains seven recognized hormones. Several other possible hormones are usually spoken of as "activities" since they may be identical to one of the known hormones or even artifacts of the isolation procedure. Most are proteins of fairly large molecular weight, e.g., > 4000. In general, the hormones are stored in granules inside the pituitary cell; when the hormones are secreted, the granules themselves may be released, or perhaps the hormone comes off the granule before it is secreted (Fig. 14). The role of proteinases in the anterior pituitary is not known; they may act in controlling the release of active pituitary hormones.

## Cell Types in the Pituitary

Based on the usual acidophilic and basophilic stains, the most common usage describes three cell types: acidophil, basophil, and chromophobe.

Labeling a cell as acidophil or basophil, however, is only in part based on the routine hematoxylin and eosin stains. In the effort to describe a separate cell type for each pituitary hormone, histologists have devised a bewildering array of special staining procedures. Some of these are hard to classify as acidic or basic, and so are the cells stained. Even if a cell is labeled, for example, an acidophil, there is no necessary relation of staining intensity to cell function because the amount of stain taken up depends on the number of granules in the cell; the presence of few granules means poor staining but may be associated with either diminished or excessive secretion of hormone.

In sum, the various empirical staining procedures have no functional value unless it can be shown that certain cells are the only ones to stain in a particular way and that these same cells are the only ones secreting a certain hormone. The effort to find one cell type for each hormone by using different stains, electron microscopy, etc., has, in general, been successful, and, in a few species at least, the well-known hormones can be associated with a separate cell type. For man the best associations of hormones with cell types at present are:

Growth hormone: acidophil, alpha cell (α cell)
Prolactin: acidophil, epsilon-eta cell (ε-η cell)
Gonadotropins (FSH and LH): basophil, delta cell (δ cell)
Thyrotropin: basophil, theta cell (θ cell)
MSH: basophil, zeta cell (ζ cell)
ACTH: chromophobe, probably; gamma cell (γ cell)

This listing is the best available for man; it should not be confused with listings for other species, in which pituitary cells may stain the same but have a completely different function. As we have implied, cells without granules stain poorly, are therefore called chromophobes, and may be secreting a little or a lot of hormone. Many of these cells on closer examination actually seem to have small, lightly staining granules, and one such type is probably the human ACTH cell noted above.

In the attempt to show enough cell types in man so that there might be one for each hormone, some workers in the field may have overshot the mark, since nine different cell types have now been described. Nevertheless, FSH and LH cannot be definitely assigned different cell types, and there is some uncertainty regarding TSH and MSH. Finally, although growth hormone and prolactin are assigned, the inability to separate these two hormones completely from each other in man makes one wonder about the assignment.

There is probably no regenerative capacity of anterior pituitary cells; a few remaining cells will not multiply to replace others that have been lost.

## Hormones of the Anterior Pituitary

This section is mostly a compilation of facts about the hormones; detailed discussion of their function appears later in the appropriate chapter.

*Follicle-stimulating hormone* (FSH) is mainly concerned with stimulating development of the ovarian follicle (*not* the ovum) in the female, while in the male it is needed for development of testicular tubules and the maintenance and differentiation of spermatozoa. It is a glycoprotein with a molecular weight of about 30,000 and is probably made by the delta-basophil cell. Plasma levels in men average 0.2 mU/ml and in women 0.15 mU/ml rising after the menopause to 2.00 mU/ml (radioimmunoassay, NIH-FSH-$S_1$ standard). FSH is cleared by the kidney four times as fast as LH.

*Luteinizing hormone* (LH) has lately been recognized as a distinct entity. In 1924 it was first suggested that there might be two gonadotropins, one stimulating the follicle to grow and the other changing it to a corpus luteum. The first crude separation of FSH and LH was made in 1934, but only in recent years has there been any agreement that human FSH and LH are separate hormones. This has now been shown both in pituitary extracts and in plasma.

In the female, LH does more than cause luteinization or formation of the corpus luteum ("yellow body"). It also stimulates estrogen secretion and causes ovulation. Some LH is apparently necessary for the full effect of FSH on follicular development. In the male, LH is also called interstitial-cell-stimulating hormone (ICSH). LH stimulates the development of the Leydig cells of the testis and causes them to secrete testosterone. FSH may enhance this function.

LH is a glycoprotein of about 30,000 to 45,000 mol. wt. and may actually be a dimer of a smaller molecule. It may be made by the same cell as FSH. About 30 µg are secreted each day in men and in women, except at ovulation when women secrete more. It may be carried in the blood with a globulin; less than 5% appears unchanged in the urine. Plasma levels in men and nonovulating women are comparable: 2 to 4 mµg/ml (15 to 30 mU/ml). Values are higher in women just before ovulation and during the menopause: 10 to 20 mµg/ml (radioimmunoassay, NIH-LH-$S_1$ standard). The half-life is about 60 minutes.

Clinically, both FSH and LH can be used to stimulate gonadal function in patients who have normal gonads but poor pituitary function.

*Prolactin* or *luteotropin* has a dual action; in the female it stimulates and maintains *lactation* and maintains the *corpus luteum*, allowing it to secrete progesterone. The second action was more or less independently described; hence the second name: *luteotropin or LTH*. Later, in the rat at least, these two activities were shown to be due to the same substance. In other species the luteotropin, though they undoubtedly have one, may not be the same as prolactin; e.g., LH or estrogen may be the luteotropin in the rabbit.

In man the problem is still more complex. First of all, the same extract of human pituitary usually has both prolactin and growth hormone activities. To date, these two activities have not been consistently separated, although evidence is accumulating that the substances may indeed be different. Furthermore, some evidence suggests that no luteotropin is needed in man although prolactin is required for lactation. Another activity of prolactin, seen particularly in birds given prolactin and perhaps in rats, is the arousing of parental behavior. In the male it has no known function except a possible direct stimulation of prostatic growth or a possible synergistic action with testosterone, and it may decrease sexual activity.

Prolactin is a single-chain peptide of 23,000 mol. wt. (sheep) produced by an acidophil cell which is probably different from that producing growth hormone. There may be several closely related molecules of comparable activity. Plasma levels have been measured in sheep by radioimmunoassay and are about 100 mμg/ml; the level drops during pregnancy and increases during lactation.

*Thyroid-stimulating hormone* (TSH or *thyrotropin*) stimulates the thyroid in several ways to increase the production of thyroid hormone and stimulates the growth of the thyroid in both cell size and number. It may also have some nonthyroid effects, e.g., increased thyroxine uptake by muscle. TSH is a glycoprotein of 26,000 to 30,000 mol. wt. and is made by a basophil cell. The purest bovine preparation to date has about 30 units/mg. Human TSH preparations have about 20 units/mg when compared to bovine TSH. However, the relative potency of human versus bovine TSH varies with the bioassay used. It is better to compare human TSH preparations against a human rather than a bovine standard; the human standard has recently been set up. Referred to this standard, the better human preparations have about 1.5 units/mg.

As tested by one of these human preparations, the human pituitary contains about 300 μg of TSH and secretes each day about 110 μg. The circulating plasma contains about 1 to 2 mμg/ml, perhaps bound to a γ-globulin. The half-life of TSH in the plasma is 35 to 54 minutes, relatively long for a peptide-protein hormone. It is metabolized mainly by the liver and the kidney.

There are also TSH-like substances. Many hyperthyroid patients have an abnormal TSH called the long-acting thyroid stimulator (LATS); this substance is not of pituitary origin though it acts like TSH and probably is the cause of the hyperthyroidism. In addition, the human placenta and some human cancers seem to make a TSH-like substance, of uncertain physiologic importance.

*Adrenocorticotropic hormone* (ACTH or corticotropin) was first clearly demonstrated in 1927. It stimulates the adrenal cortex to make and secrete hydrocortisone and also maintains adrenal size. Some think the two activities represent two different hormones, but there is little convincing evidence for this idea. It is a single-chain peptide of 39 amino acids in all species examined, with a molecular weight of about 4500. It may be made by a pituitary basophil, though this is in doubt. It does not seem to be associated with granules in the pituitary cell except perhaps as a storage form.

Full activity requires only the first 20 amino acids, as was determined after chemically synthesizing compounds of varying amino acid length similar to ACTH. The full 39 amino acid hormone has also been synthesized. What do the other 19 amino acids do? Perhaps they prolong activity by delaying breakdown of the hormone. There is little species difference as far as action in mammals is concerned, and all the species differences in amino acid composition are in the part of the molecule not required for full activity, i.e., beyond amino acid 20. Some species specificity (order specificity?) exists, however, since mammalian ACTH will not stimulate the alligator's adrenals.

The human pituitary contains about 0.2 to 0.4 mg of ACTH, some of which may be in a bound form. Less than 1 unit ($< 10$ μg) is normally secreted each day. The plasma level is in the range of 0.2 to 0.5 mU/100 ml of plasma in the daytime morning hours and is lower in the evening. It represents an average level of 3 mμg/100 ml. The plasma half-life is 5 to 10 minutes, the biologic half-life, about one hour. ACTH is bound and inactivated by the adrenal and the kidney; the kidney actually takes up more ACTH per gram than does the adrenal although it has no known effect on the kidney. In some patients it may be detected in the urine.

ACTH has a number of extraadrenal or nonadrenal actions. It can:

1. Increase or decrease blood glucose depending on circumstances.
2. Support or stimulate erythropoiesis though this may be due to some other ill-defined pituitary factor.
3. Delay inactivation of hydrocortisone by the liver.
4. In excess, cause pigmentation of the skin; this may be important clinically in Addison's disease.
5. Mobilize free fatty acids from adipose tissue in vitro.
6. Slightly increase ovarian estrogen secretion.

Whether or not any of these play a role in the intact animal is uncertain, since the doses used to demonstrate the effects are usually much larger than are found in vivo. A reasonable case may be made, however, for 3 and 5, the delay of hydrocortisone inactivation and the mobilization of free fatty acids. Action 4 is actually an MSH-like action and no doubt occurs because of the similarity in molecular structure between ACTH and MSH (see MSH, below).

*Growth hormone* (GH) is also known as somatotropin or STH. It causes general tissue growth without maturation or development and has other effects to be discussed later. It is a peptide, probably a single chain looped on itself with the ends linked via a disulfide bridge. Molecular weight in humans is 21,500. The human pituitary contains a large amount: 4 to 15 mg. Each species seems to have a different GH, and the responsiveness to a given GH preparation varies from species to species. The rat will respond to growth hormones from many other species, all of differing amino acid composition, whereas man responds only to GH derived from a primate. Thus, GH demonstrates a high degree of species specificity.

GH is made in an acidophil cell but can also often be associated with a larger chromophobe cell. The acidophil stain is not taken up by the hormone itself. Its release from the pituitary is mostly under control of the hypothalamus, and GH-releasing activity can be shown in extracts of the hypothalamus. Somewhere between 0.4 and 1.0 mg per day is released. The plasma has 0 to 3 m$\mu$g/ml in the resting state, and some think it may circulate bound to an $\alpha_2$-macroglobulin. The plasma half-life is about 30 minutes in man, and turnover is about 3% per minute. GH is destroyed by blood as well as by other tissues of the body.

*Melanocyte-stimulating hormone* (MSH) is sometimes called intermedin because it seems to come from the intermediate lobe of the pituitary in those species with a distinct intermediate lobe. It darkens the pigment cells in fish and amphibians, which respond to it in minutes via increased cAMP. Its function in mammals is not clear, though it may play a role in regulating skin pigmentation. Large doses given to humans will cause darkening of the skin, and some patients with abnormally dark skin have as their only abnormality an elevated blood level of MSH. MSH may also affect the function of the central nervous system, where it causes an increased excitability.

Allen and Smith first recognized, in 1916, that MSH exists. Since then we have learned that there are two forms of MSH: $\alpha$-MSH and $\beta$-MSH. $\alpha$-MSH has 13 amino acids and is identical in sequence to the first 13 amino acids of ACTH, plus a 1-acetyl and a 13-NH$_2$. $\alpha$-MSH is the same in all species examined. $\beta$-MSH in most species has 18 amino acids, with some variation in the sequence. Man's $\beta$-MSH has 22 amino acids. All have in common a string of amino acids corresponding to Nos. 4 to 10 of ACTH, and these seem essential for activity. The molecular structures are interesting because ACTH has some intrinsic MSH-like activity and can cause pigmentation in man. MSH, however, has no ACTH-like activity.

In humans $\beta$-MSH accounts for most of the total MSH activity in plasma, and, by radioimmunoassay, there is normally less than 0.09 m$\mu$g/ml. The half-life is one to two hours.

Little is known about the control of MSH secretion. Its secretion is affected by the hypothalamus, which may either stimulate or inhibit. An MSH-inhibiting factor (MSH-IF) has been found in the hypothalamus and is probably important since the overall effect of the hypothalamus seems to be tonic inhibition of MSH secretion.

In addition to these seven generally recognized hormones, there are other substances which can be obtained from pituitary extracts but have uncertain physiologic functions:

1. A hypoglycemic peptide.
2. At least four distinct fat-mobilizing hormones different from growth hormone. Two of these have been called β-lipotropin and γ-lipotropin; both are polypeptides, the former of 9000 to 9800 mol. wt. and the latter of about 5800 mol. wt. Both have some MSH activity. There is a similar lipolytic material in hypothalamic extracts.
3. Exophthalmos-producing substance (EPS), which is closely associated with TSH but can be separated from it and seems to have a molecular weight of about 40,000. It is thought by some to cause exophthalmos in hyperthyroidism but has no known function in the normal person. One main problem in assessing its significance is that it is assayed in fish; what it may mean to a mammal is unknown.

## BIBLIOGRAPHY

Abe, K., Nicholson, W. E., Liddle, G. W., Island, D. P., and Orth, D. N. Radioimmunoassay of β-MSH in human plasma and tissues. *J. Clin. Invest.* 46:1609, 1967.

Adams, J. H., Daniel, P. M., and Prichard, M. L. Observations on the portal circulation of the pituitary gland. *Neuroendocrinology* 1:193, 1965/66.

Bajusz, E. Hormonal mechanisms and their interaction with the central nervous system. *Confin. Neurol.* 27:441, 1966.

Guillemin, R. The adenohypophysis and its hypothalamic control. *Ann. Rev. Physiol.* 29:313, 1967.

Harris, G. W. *Neural Control of the Pituitary Gland.* London: Edward Arnold, 1955. (A classic book.)

Harris, G. W., and Donovan, B. T. (Eds.). *The Pituitary Gland* (3 vols.). Berkeley: University of California Press, 1966. (Encyclopedic.)

Lippmann, W., Leonardi, R., Ball, J., and Coppola, J. A. Relationship between hypothalamic catecholamines and gonadotrophin secretion in rats. *J. Pharmacol. Exp. Ther.* 156:258, 1967.

Rinne, U. K., and Arstila, A. U. Ultrastructure of the neurovascular link between the hypothalamus and anterior pituitary gland in the median eminence of the rat. *Neuroendocrinology* 1:214, 1965/66.

Schally, A. V., Müller, E. E., Arimura, A., Bowers, C. Y., Saito, T., Redding, T. W., Sawano, S., and Pizzolato, P. Releasing factors in human hypothalamic and neurohypophyseal extracts. *J. Clin. Endocr.* 27:755, 1967.

# 4. The Hypothalamus and the Posterior Pituitary Gland: The Neurohypophysis

> What is man, when you come to think upon him, but a minutely set, ingenious machine for turning, with infinite artfulness, the red wine of Shiraz into urine?
>
> —BARONESS KAREN BLIXEN
> ("ISAK DINESEN"),
> *Seven Gothic Tales*

REMOVAL of the posterior pituitary causes a transient *diabetes insipidus* (the "tasteless" diabetes as opposed to diabetes mellitus, the "sweet" diabetes). No obvious defect occurs other than the excessive flow of dilute urine. One might talk then of a posterior pituitary hormone that prevents the excretion of a dilute urine, an antidiuretic hormone (ADH). However, with a careful hypophysectomy, diabetes insipidus lasts only a short time; on the other hand, if the hypothalamus is damaged the diabetes insipidus is permanent. Obviously, the posterior pituitary cannot be considered independently of the hypothalamus any more than can the anterior pituitary; the posterior pituitary and its hypothalamic connections are together called the neurohypophysis.

## NEUROHYPOPHYSEAL HORMONES AND THEIR SECRETION

Studies done on extracts of the posterior pituitary showed the presence of many activities besides antidiuresis. Finally, all the observed activities were explained by isolating *two* hormones; both are small peptides. Since, as usual, their chemistry was not known until later, they were named according to their actions in assay systems: oxytocin, assayed by contractility of uterine muscle (first observed by Dale in 1906), meaning literally to "stimulate birth," and vasopressin, assayed by rise in blood pressure (first observed by Oliver and Schafer in 1895). Both are somewhat misnamed. Oxytocin plays only a secondary role in the delivery of the child. Its main action is probably on the lactating breast, where it stimulates the release of milk. Vasopressin has little to do with maintaining blood pressure (an effect seen only at dose levels rarely reached physiologically) but is of prime importance in stimulating water retention by the kidney. It is preferably called antidiuretic hormone (ADH) when its physiology is discussed and vasopressin only when one is speaking of its chemistry. All mammals have both hormones. Fish and birds have similar but slightly different compounds which may have different functions.

Chemically, these hormones can be called octapeptides or nonapeptides depending on whether one thinks of cystine as one amino acid residue or two. They are numbered as if they were nonapeptides (Fig. 15). They were the first peptide hormones to be completely synthesized. Their structures are fairly similar, and there is in fact a small amount of overlap in their activities. 8-ARG vasopressin (1228 mol. wt.) has about 400 to 600 units/mg of pressor activity. It is the one found in most mammals. 8-LYS vasopressin is found in only the pig, hippopotamus, and related species.

Oxytocin and vasopressin are usually called posterior pituitary hormones since they can be extracted in the greatest quantity from the posterior pituitary gland. Yet it is likely, as we have suggested earlier, that the principal site of origin is the hypothalamus, with the posterior pituitary acting largely as a storage site. In the hypothalamus two sets of nuclei are thought to make the hormones or their precursors: the supraoptic and paraventricular nuclei. From here, the hormones, perhaps bound in tiny granules, travel down numerous axons to the posterior pituitary, where they are then stored or released to the blood stream (Fig. 16). There is strong evidence that ADH originates in the supraoptic nuclei and oxytocin in the paraventricular, but no definite proof.

While most of the synthesis may take place in the hypothalamus, recent work has shown that chronic dehydration (in the rat) can cause enlargement of the posterior pituitary, the implication being that synthesis as well as storage occurs there. Even here, as in the hypothalamus, ADH and oxytocin are probably synthesized in separate neurons.

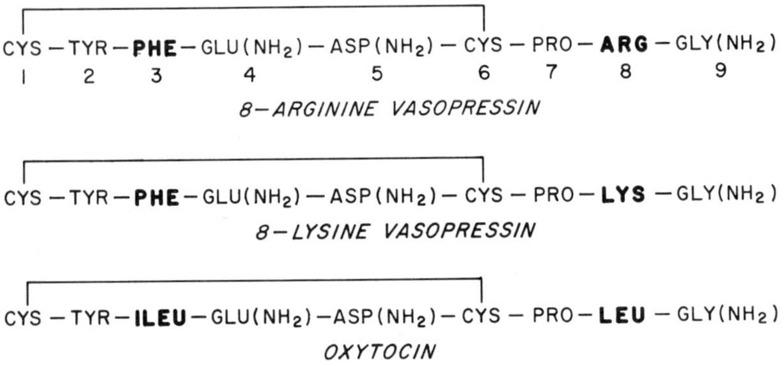

$$\text{CYS} - \text{TYR} - \textbf{PHE} - \text{GLU}(\text{NH}_2) - \text{ASP}(\text{NH}_2) - \text{CYS} - \text{PRO} - \textbf{ARG} - \text{GLY}(\text{NH}_2)$$
$$1 \quad 2 \quad 3 \quad 4 \quad 5 \quad 6 \quad 7 \quad 8 \quad 9$$

*8—ARGININE VASOPRESSIN*

$$\text{CYS} - \text{TYR} - \textbf{PHE} - \text{GLU}(\text{NH}_2) - \text{ASP}(\text{NH}_2) - \text{CYS} - \text{PRO} - \textbf{LYS} - \text{GLY}(\text{NH}_2)$$

*8—LYSINE VASOPRESSIN*

$$\text{CYS} - \text{TYR} - \textbf{ILEU} - \text{GLU}(\text{NH}_2) - \text{ASP}(\text{NH}_2) - \text{CYS} - \text{PRO} - \textbf{LEU} - \text{GLY}(\text{NH}_2)$$

*OXYTOCIN*

FIG. 15. Structures of mammalian neurohypophyseal hormones. Differences in peptide chains are noted in bold lettering.

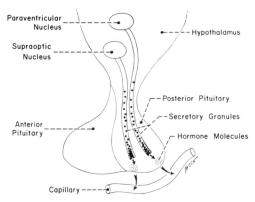

Fig. 16.   Synthesis and secretion of neurohypophyseal hormones.

The evidence for this mechanism of hormonal synthesis and release is indirect because no one has yet followed a hormone-laden granule down an axon to the posterior pituitary and shown there the release of the hormone into the blood. However, it is a good case because:

1. The hypothalamus contains both hormones in small amounts.
2. Electric stimulation of the hypothalamus can cause release of both hormones.
3. Lesions in the hypothalamus alone can cause diabetes insipidus.
4. Granules are observed along these axons which disappear under conditions in which ADH release would be expected. These granules are not the hormones—they are too big—but they presumably contain them or an immediate precursor.
5. Careful removal of the posterior pituitary leaving the hypothalamus intact (as noted) does not result in permanent diabetes insipidus. The granules go down the axons as far as possible, and the hormones are probably released from there.

The posterior pituitary contains much more of these hormones than the hypothalamus. It also has a protein, previously called the Van Dyke protein, which binds the hormones. This protein, now called *neurophysin,* has been studied recently; its molecular weight is about 20,000 to 25,000, and one molecule can bind several molecules of the hormones. The protein-hormone complex is found mostly in small granules which have either traveled down axons to the posterior pituitary or been formed there de novo. While both ADH and oxytocin are probably released from the granules and binding protein before reaching the blood stream, most workers feel that both hormones are not bound to the same protein molecule nor are they found together in the same granule. For example, centrifugation studies show that the heavier granules contain ADH and the lighter ones oxytocin. Furthermore, in humans there is good evidence that ADH and oxytocin are not secreted together into the blood stream but are released independently in response to appropriate stimuli; occlusion of the carotid artery will increase the secretion of ADH but not oxytocin, while suckling will do the opposite.

## Antidiuretic Hormone (ADH)

The primary action of ADH is to increase free water resorption from the distal renal tubules and collecting ducts. As one might expect, the camel, a desert animal, is more sensitive to this hormone than man.

ADH has a more general action on overall water balance. By itself it tends to increase intracellular water in muscle with a loss of sodium and potassium and to cause a low serum sodium. When it is combined with aldosterone, these effects are modified; the intracellular water does not go up and cellular sodium and potassium do not drop as much nor is the serum sodium so low. Thus the effects of ADH on the body as a whole not only reflect a renal action but involve actions elsewhere which are modulated by aldosterone. Neither ADH nor aldosterone acts solely on the kidney.

The posterior pituitary contains about 15 units or 25 μg of ADH. About 10% to 20% of this can be rapidly released in a few minutes; the rest is secreted more slowly, presumably because of the protein binding.

The plasma level of ADH is difficult to measure because the bioassay which must be used is not universally reliable. The radioimmunoassay that is available is not sensitive enough. Furthermore, the plasma level varies with the state of hydration. A reasonable estimate in a man who is in a state of "normal" hydration is 2 μU/ml in plasma or about 1 μU/ml in whole blood. The plasma level is the equivalent of about 3 μμg/ml (3 picograms/ml) or $3 \times 10^{-12}$ M. At about this level there is a mild antidiuretic effect; the level corresponds to a secretion rate of roughly 10 mU/hour. *Dehydration* or exercise increases the plasma level to 6 to 8 μU/ml (a secretion rate of roughly 20 to 40 mU/hour). At this plasma level the antidiuretic effect is at its height, and further increases in ADH have no extra effect on the kidney. Severe hemorrhage may cause an even more striking rise in the plasma level to 900 μU/ml; at this level there may actually be a vasopressor effect. Water-loading does just the opposite, decreasing the plasma ADH so that it is undetectable.

Little ADH circulates bound to any plasma protein, and in man the plasma half-life is about three minutes. ADH is cleared and inactivated fairly rapidly by the liver and kidney, only about 10% of secreted ADH being found in the urine in an active form.

*Action on the Kidney*

The kidney responds quickly to ADH. Within 2 to 4 minutes there is a detectable drop in free water clearance with no change in solute load or glomerular filtration rate. Antidiuresis is maximal when about 100 μU/minute is given intravenously.

How does ADH act? No theory is as yet comprehensive enough to integrate all the available observations, but the details are fairly clear. The most complete information comes from work done with a structure analogous to the kidney, the toad bladder, which happens to be about one cell thick. Some superb recent work has also been done on isolated mammalian collecting tubules. Although it does not raise the blood pressure, ADH can cause vasoconstriction of renal arterioles. This alone could increase water resorption, perhaps secondary to an increase in sodium resorption or to a decrease in medullary blood flow. However, there is little question that ADH acts directly on the renal tubular cells; any effect on blood vessels is probably of secondary importance.

It turns out that water is not the only thing being transported in response to ADH. Sodium transport and probably urea transport are increased, and these in turn play a role in water transport. Much of the following is therefore aimed at explaining the action of ADH on sodium and urea as well as on water.

At the renal tubule, although the actions of ADH are brought about by changes on the luminal side of the renal tubule cell, the ADH must be present at the "serosal" or nonluminal surface to be effective. Clearly, then, whatever ADH does, it must act somehow on the intracellular machinery of the cell since it is without effect when placed directly on the luminal surface.

ADH is probably bound to the renal cell by disulfide bonds (—S— S—). Several things then happen. After binding, ADH causes an increase in cyclic 3′,5′-AMP which in turn stimulates water and sodium resorption through unknown mechanisms. On the other hand, some evidence suggests that ADH and cAMP increase water resorption but through different mechanisms. Furthermore, other substances, such as parathyroid hormone and perhaps epinephrine (although published data are conflicting), increase renal cAMP without increasing water resorption. However, although several substances elevate cAMP, the cAMP in each instance may well be in functionally separate parts of the tissue or the cell. For example, ADH increases the activity of adenyl cyclase, and presumably the synthesis of cAMP, in the distal part of the renal tubular system, while parathyroid hormone does the same with a more proximal area. Each area's cAMP is thus more or less specific for a particular hormonal action. For the moment, with these qualifications, cAMP may be regarded as the mediator of the effect of ADH on water and sodium resorption.

Following the effect on cAMP come effects on sodium, urea, and, of course, water. There is an increased sodium resorption at a distal site with a resulting increase in sodium concentration in the renal medulla. The osmotic gradient set up probably enhances the resorption of water. The ADH effect on sodium resorption is apparently not an enhancement of the existing active transport mechanism by which sodium is pumped out of the renal tubular cell and into the interstitium of the renal medulla. It acts rather to increase the permeability of the luminal surface of the tubular cell to sodium. The active transport process simply continues to pump the sodium through the other side of the cell since its full capacity is rarely reached.

There is also an increased permeability to urea. Whether this has an effect on water transport is not clear, but an increased medullary urea concentration would increase the osmotic gradient. Urea may also delay the inactivation of ADH by the kidney and prolong the action of any ADH present.

Along with these effects, and most important for our discussion, is a separate and specific effect on water resorption. The permeability of the luminal surface of the tubular cell to water is increased, even, apparently, when no water flows through the tubular cells. For ADH to cause an actual increase in the amount of water resorbed from the tubular lumen, a change in the permeability to water is not enough. There must also be water to resorb or, in more technical language, there must be a concentration gradient down which water can flow since it seems not to be actively transported.

The work with isolated mammalian tubules mentioned before supports much of the above information, which was, in fact, derived from work done with the urinary bladder of the toad. When ADH was placed on the nonluminal surface of the tubule and the lumen contained a hypotonic solution, vacuoles appeared in the cells, the cell size increased, and the intercellular spaces became much larger; all this occurred within 5 to 10 minutes (Fig. 17). Electron microscopy of the luminal surface did not show any "holes." Thus water resorbed by ADH comes into the cell through the luminal membrane and probably leaves the cell both by going through the opposite nonluminal membrane and by going into the spaces between the luminal cells.

Precisely what happens at the luminal membrane of the cell is not known, but the membrane contains a lysolecithin-lecithin interconversion system. Since lysolecithin can act to change membrane permeability, the action of ADH might conceivably be mediated by a change

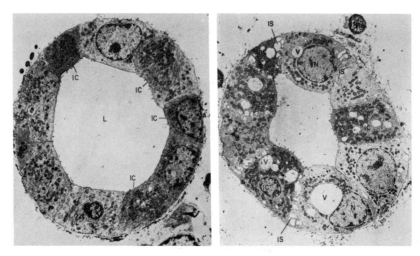

Fig. 17.   Action of ADH on mammalian renal collecting duct (rabbit). *Left,* without ADH; *right,* with ADH.

Note that with ADH the cells swell, the lumen becomes smaller because of bulging of the cells, the lateral cell membranes have separated forming large intercellular spaces, and within the cells themselves there are large vacuoles, presumably filled with water. L = tubular lumen; IC = intercalated cell; N = nucleus; IS = intercellular spaces; V = large vacuoles. (From C. E. Ganote, J. J. Grantham, H. L. Moses, M. B. Burg, and J. Orloff, *J. Cell Biol.* 36:355, 1968.)

in this system. In addition, the adrenal cortex (perhaps aldosterone) is necessary for ADH to act optimally, but again the mechanism is not clear.

Because more water flows across the cell (toad bladder experiment) under optimal stimulation by ADH than apparently can diffuse across the luminal surface of the cell, workers have suggested the existence of "pores" or "channels" in the cell membrane and inside the cell. The difference between the actual amount of water transported and the amount expected to diffuse is called "bulk flow"; because it travels in specific tiny channels, considerations of diffusion do not apply. Many of the observed facts can be explained if one postulates a double-layered luminal cell membrane. ADH would act on the outer layer to increase permeability to sodium, urea, and water and on the inner layer to increase "pore" size and therefore bulk flow of water (Fig. 18). We have then a reasonable explanation of the end effects of ADH, at least in physical terms.

One problem is that the "pores" have never been observed, even by electron microscopy, as noted above. It may be that the size of the pores is less than can be measured by present methods and that ADH

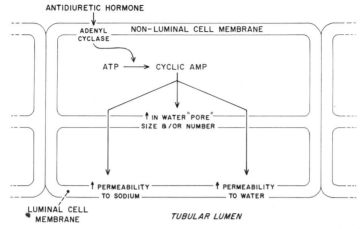

ANTIDIURETIC HORMONE

ADENYL CYCLASE    NON-LUMINAL CELL MEMBRANE

ATP ⟶ CYCLIC AMP

↑ IN WATER "PORE"
SIZE & /OR NUMBER

↑ PERMEABILITY TO SODIUM    ↑ PERMEABILITY TO WATER

LUMINAL CELL MEMBRANE    *TUBULAR LUMEN*

FIG. 18.  Outline of the postulated actions of ADH on the renal tubular cell.

does not increase their size but their number. If so, one can still explain the observed transport of water assuming that the "pores" are less than 10 Angstrom units (Å) in diameter.

In sum, ADH, mediated by cAMP, causes an increased permeability to water, sodium, and possibly urea. The effect on water, in the presence of a proper gradient, is enhanced by an increase in "pore" size or number, and therefore one sees a greater bulk flow of water; that on sodium and urea tends to increase the osmotic gradient (nonluminal/luminal) and thus enhance the resorption of water.

It should be noted that the action of a given amount of ADH can be modulated by other factors; with an increased solute load, less water will be resorbed, while with a decreased glomerular filtration rate (GFR) more water will be resorbed. How much water is resorbed varies directly with the amount of ADH and inversely with the amount of solute in the tubule. Finally, both norepinephrine and the prostaglandins can inhibit the action of ADH on the kidney. Nothing is known about how norepinephrine does this, but the prostaglandins may act by blocking the formation of cAMP (see Chap. 1, under Cyclic AMP and Prostaglandins).

## Control of ADH Secretion

As we have said, the hypothalamus is clearly important because lesions of the hypothalamus can cause a total lack of ADH secretion. Probably the main stimulus to ADH secretion is a *rise in plasma osmolality*. An increase of only 1 to 2 mOsm/kg (<1% of plasma osmolality) raises ADH output, providing the osmotic threshold of about 285 to 290 mOsm/kg is exceeded. Changes in osmolality affect the plasma

ADH within the range of about 0.3 to 6.0 μU/ml. The increase in osmolality must be perceived by the appropriate neurons in the supraoptic nucleus; however, not just any increase in plasma osmolality will do. Hypertonic saline solution is excellent; hypertonic glucose has no effect. Whether the same neurons sensing the rise in osmolality also secrete ADH is not known; they may be different. The thirst center is quite near and probably overlaps the supraoptic nucleus. While they may be affected by the same osmotic stimulus, the thirst receptor and the osmoreceptor for ADH secretion are in slightly different locations.

A *fall in plasma volume* also acts as an effective stimulus to ADH secretion through decreasing distention of vascular receptors located in the atria of the heart and the carotid sinuses, the impulses being transmitted to the brain via the vagus nerve. In addition, a drop in plasma volume probably increases the sensitivity of the hypothalamus to a given osmotic stimulus. The relative importance of changes in plasma volume compared to changes in osmotic stimuli is not yet well established for man; under most circumstances the osmotic stimulus is probably controlling.

In both instances the response is ultimately an increase in water resorption, lowering plasma osmolality and increasing plasma volume. The defects are then corrected, and ADH secretion is shut off. The feedback control system thus operates to maintain plasma osmolality and volume in the face of such things as the hot, dry desert at 102°F and the prankster who drinks a gallon of water all at once. The thirst mechanism is somewhat sluggish in man; it takes up to 72 hours for replenishment of a given water loss. ADH is therefore all the more important in retaining as much water as possible.

In addition, one should note that a decrease in blood volume can cause a higher rise in plasma ADH than an increase in osmolality. ADH may then help maintain an effective circulating plasma volume by a direct constrictive influence on, for example, the renal or other vascular beds whenever the plasma ADH rises to 20 μU/ml or more.

Areas of the brain above the hypothalamus also influence ADH secretion. As a whole, they seem to exert a tonic inhibitory effect on the hypothalamus to inhibit ADH secretion. Various stimuli other than changes in osmolality or plasma volume are able to increase ADH secretion and probably act on these higher areas of the brain; they include pain, anxiety, surgical stress, and drugs such as nicotine. None are involved in the negative feedback control of ADH. All such stimuli probably impinge on the hypothalamus via cholinergic nerve endings although the release of ADH itself is probably not mediated by acetylcholine.

Decreased ADH secretion even in the presence of a low water intake is consistently seen after alcohol intake and results in a large volume of urine. The fact that psychologic conditioning can also decrease ADH secretion points out once again the importance of suprahypothalamic centers of the nervous system.

## OXYTOCIN

The plasma level of oxytocin in man is about 1 to 5 $\mu U/ml$, and the plasma half-life is 1 to 4 minutes. It is metabolized mainly by the kidney and rapidly excreted into the urine.

In women the role played by secreted oxytocin in the delivery of the fetus under natural conditions is not quite clear. The best evidence to date comes from experiments done with goats and cows. The plasma levels were low or undetectable until midway through labor, when there was a sharp rise to about 200 $\mu U/ml$. It would seem that oxytocin has no part in initiating labor but may well help deliver the fetus once labor has begun.

There is little question that it plays a role in lactation. It mediates the milk "let-down" phenomenon whereby suckling, via sensory pathways, causes oxytocin release. The oxytocin in turn causes contraction of the myoepithelium in the breast and is followed by the ejection of milk already secreted but still contained within the breast.

In the male, oxytocin may be instrumental in the ejaculation of semen, but there is little good information other than that men have about the same amount of oxytocin in plasma as women. It may, however, increase the transport of spermatozoa in the uterus and thus help in fertilization of the ovum. Some recent data suggest that in males (and females?) oxytocin regulates blood flow to certain tissues, increasing the blood flow to, for example, the kidney.

## FAT MOBILIZERS

The posterior pituitary as well as the anterior contains fat-mobilizing substances that may be hormonal. Their place in normal physiology is still uncertain.

## CLINICAL NOTE

Clinically, ADH is used to control diabetes insipidus. The usual preparation is a posterior pituitary extract (Pitressin). Synthetic 8-LYS-vasopressin is equally effective and when it becomes more widely available will be a better treatment since it avoids the reactions to other proteins found in the pituitary extract. These preparations must be either injected or sprayed into the nose; they cannot be given by mouth because they are destroyed in the gut.

The opposite of diabetes insipidus, excessive secretion of ADH, is occasionally seen. Often called the "inappropriate ADH syndrome," it may occur with brain injuries or certain infections or may even be due to a cancer secreting ADH, such as carcinoma of the lung. Treatment consists in water restriction (since the body has too much water) or correction of the underlying cause.

Oxytocin's main clinical use is in obstetrics. Labor is induced or speeded up by preparations of oxytocin given intravenously.

## BIBLIOGRAPHY

Czaczkes, J. W., Kleeman, C. R., Koenig, M., and Boston, R.   Physiologic studies of antidiuretic hormone by its direct measurement in human plasma. *J. Clin. Invest.* 43:1625, 1964.

Friesen, H. G., and Astwood, E. B.   Changes in neurohypophysial proteins induced by dehydration and ingestion of saline. *Endocrinology* 80:278, 1967.

Gaitan, E., Cobo, E., and Mizrachi, M.   Evidence for the differential secretion of oxytocin and vasopressin in man. *J. Clin. Invest.* 43:2310, 1964.

Ganote, C. E., Grantham, J. J., Moses, H. L., Burg, M. B., and Orloff, J.   Ultrastructural studies of vasopressin effect on isolated perfused renal collecting tubules of the rabbit. *J. Cell Biol.* 36:355, 1968.

Grantham, J. J., and Orloff, J.   Effect of prostaglandin $E_1$ on the permeability response of the isolated collecting tubule to vasopressin, adenosine 3',5'-monophosphate, and theophylline. *J. Clin. Invest.* 47:1154, 1968.

Hays, R. M.   A new proposal for the action of vasopressin, based on studies of a complex synthetic membrane. *J. Gen. Physiol.* 51:385, 1968.

Kleeman, C. R., and Fichman, M. P.   The clinical physiology of water metabolism. *New Eng. J. Med.* 277:1300, 1967.

Leaf, A.   Transepithelial transport and its hormonal control in toad bladder. *Ergebn. Physiol.* 56:216, 1965.

Moses, A. M., Miller, M., and Streeten, D. H. P.   Quantitative influence of blood volume expansion on the osmotic threshold for vasopressin release. *J. Clin. Endocr.* 27:655, 1967.

Orloff, J., and Handler, J.   The role of adenosine 3', 5'-phosphate in the action of antidiuretic hormone. *Amer. J. Med.* 42:757, 1967.

Sachs, H.   Biosynthesis and release of vasopressin. *Amer. J. Med.* 42:687, 1967.

Senft, G., Hoffman, M., Munske, K., and Schultz, G.   Effects of hydration and dehydration on cyclic adenosine 3',5'-monophosphate concentration in the rat kidney. *Pflueger. Arch. Ges. Physiol.* 298:348, 1968.

# 5. The Adrenal Cortex

There are still, however, certain organs of the body, the actual functions and influence of which have hitherto entirely eluded the researches and bid defiance to the united efforts of both physiologist and pathologist. Of these not the least remarkable are the "Supra-Renal Capsules" . . .

—THOMAS ADDISON,
*On the Constitutional and Local Effects of Disease of the Supra-renal Capsules* (1855)

THE adrenal was first described in 1563 by Eustachius (of eustachian tube fame). Although the adrenal glands are not small, weighing about 5 g each, they escaped notice until then because little surgery was performed in the area and because at autopsy they appear rather nondescript unless the autopsy is performed soon after death. Once they were described, just what the adrenals did was not clear for a long time thereafter. Even though Addison described Addison's disease and the associated adrenal destruction in 1849 and 1855, another half-century passed before it was generally accepted that the adrenal was of some importance. At the beginning of the twentieth century, with the discovery of "the adrenal hormone," epinephrine, in adrenal extracts, the function of the adrenal cortex, as opposed to the medulla, was further obscured. By the 1920's it finally became reasonably plain that the adrenal was functionally as well as anatomically a double gland. The medulla was not the part essential to life, as had been thought. The reason animals died upon removal of the adrenal was the lack of the adrenal cortex. The hormone involved was something other than epinephrine, which had naturally been the focus of attention since it was the only known hormone of the adrenal gland at the time.

## THE ADRENAL CORTICAL HORMONES

Many substances were isolated from the adrenal cortex. Some extracts were clinically useful; others were not. With the steroid chemists working hand in hand with the physiologists and clinicians, three of the fifty different steroids isolated from the adrenal in the last 30 years have been shown to be important and are probably the naturally secreted hormones in man. These are *hydrocortisone* (compound F or cortisol), *corticosterone* (compound B), and *aldosterone*. A convenient neologism for all of them is *corticoid*, a contraction of *corticosteroid*. This term can be applied to any steroid found in the adrenal cortex but usually is applied to the secreted hormone. It has the further advantage of being applicable to synthetic steroids having similar actions.

Other compounds are found in the adrenal vein, mainly *progesterone, estrogens, and androgens*. They probably have relatively little function under normal circumstances, since they will not replace the function of missing ovaries or testes. However, in women at puberty adrenal androgen (probably testosterone) may well account for part of the pubertal growth of body hair and development of normal libido. That the adrenal secretes these hormones serves to illustrate the close relationship between the ovaries, testes, and adrenals both functionally and embryologically. Note that most of the steroids secreted by the adrenal which are androgenic in some species are at best minimally androgenic in man.

Histologically, in most species the adrenal cortex can be divided into three layers. The outer layer, the zona glomerulosa, is not always a discrete one in humans. It is the principal site of aldosterone synthesis. Although the inner reticularis and middle fasciculata layers are often said to make androgens and glucocorticoids, respectively, in fact both of these layers make hydrocortisone and both make "androgens."

*Biosynthesis*

Before looking at the biosynthetic pathways, it would be well to refresh the memory with Figure 19, which reviews the arbitrary numbering system for steroids and some of the other conventions. The

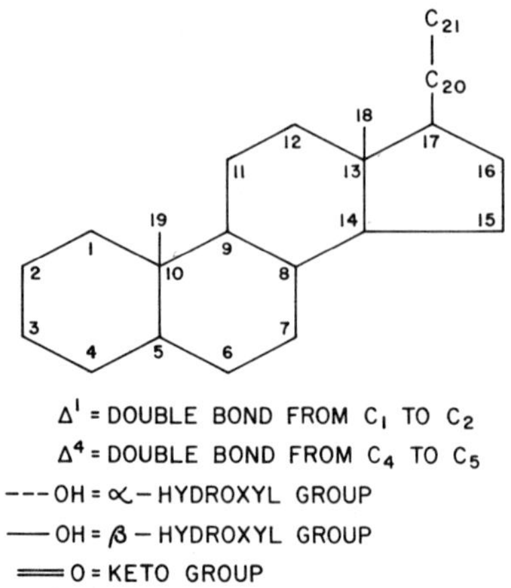
C21
C20
18
12
17
11
13
16
19
14
15
1
9
2
10
8
3
7
4
5
6
Δ1 = DOUBLE BOND FROM C1 TO C2
Δ4 = DOUBLE BOND FROM C4 TO C5
---OH = α-HYDROXYL GROUP
—OH = β-HYDROXYL GROUP
═O = KETO GROUP

FIG. 19. Numbering system for carbon atoms in a steroid and some other commonly used conventions.

biosynthesis of the corticoids is outlined in Figure 20, which will be committed to memory only by the more compulsive. Some important points are:

1. Hydrocortisone is the main secreted glucocorticoid in man whereas only a relatively small amount of corticosterone is made. In the rat, corticosterone is the principal glucocorticoid.

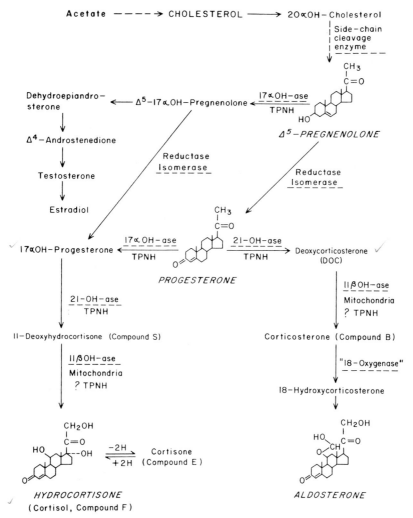

FIG. 20.   Predominant biosynthetic pathways in the adrenal cortex. Reactions involving uncertain steps or two or more steps are indicated by broken arrows. Enzymes, or enzyme activities, are underlined with broken lines.

2. The cleavage of the side chain of cholesterol to give $\Delta^5$-pregnenolone is catalyzed by the appropriately named "side-chain cleavage enzyme." This enzyme system is found in the adrenal mitochondria. Hydroxylation of cholesterol at carbons 20 and 22 precedes cleavage and may, in fact, be an intrinsic part of the whole reaction. The mitochondrial enzyme system includes at least three components: cytochrome P-450, a nonheme iron-protein, and a flavoprotein specific for TPNH.
3. Although progesterone was originally thought to be an obligatory intermediate, this is not the case.
4. The predominant hydroxylation sequence for hydrocortisone is the addition, in order, of 17α-OH, 21-OH, and, finally, 11β-OH. The hydroxylation sequence is of clinical importance since deficiencies in the enzymes involved, even though partial, can cause disease.
5. All the hydroxylations, including that of cholesterol, except possibly the 11β-hydroxylation, require reduced triphosphopyridine nucleotide (TPNH) (NADPH).
6. In the hydrocortisone sequence, the 11β-hydroxylation occurs in mitochondria. It may involve the same components as noted above for side-chain cleavage of cholesterol. The source of the hydrogen may be the Krebs cycle rather than TPNH.
7. The principal difference between the hydrocortisone sequence and the corticosterone-aldosterone sequence is the absence of a 17α-OH in the latter.
8. The reactions converting deoxycorticosterone (DOC) to corticosterone and thence to aldosterone probably occur in the adrenal mitochondria and require calcium. As with hydrocortisone, the 11β-hydroxylation may not require TPNH. Corticosterone is first converted to 18-hydroxycorticosterone and then to aldosterone with its unusual hemiacetal form.

### Secretion and Metabolism

The normal *secretion rates* of several compounds found in the human adrenal vein are:

> Hydrocortisone, 20 mg per day
> Corticosterone, 2 to 5 mg per day
> Aldosterone, 75 to 150 μg per day
>
> Dehydroepiandrosterone (DHEA), 20 mg per day
> $\Delta^4$-Androstenedione-3,17,  5 mg per day
> Progesterone, 0.5 mg per day

In the blood all corticoids are transported bound in some way to protein. Most is known about hydrocortisone (F). F is bound tightly to *transcortin*, an α-glycoprotein (43,000 mol. wt.), with one molecule of F bound to one of globulin. F is also bound to albumin, though not as tightly.

An indication of the tightness of binding is given by the *association constant* (in liters per mole):

$$K_A = \frac{[CP]}{[C]\ [P]}$$

where

$K_A$ is the association constant
C is the unbound ("free") corticoid
P is a protein binding site without corticoid
CP is a protein binding site with corticoid.

The $K_A$ for F and transcortin is 2–3 × 10⁷ at body temperature; for F and albumin it is 5 × 10³.

At body temperature about 60% of F is bound to transcortin and 30% to albumin. Despite the weakness of albumin binding, it is significant because there is so much more albumin than transcortin. Only about 10% of F is unbound or free. Corticosterone is also bound to transcortin but somewhat less tightly. Only a small amount of aldosterone is bound to transcortin; about 60% of plasma aldosterone is bound to albumin.

Using elaborate techniques one can measure the average *plasma levels* in humans of the specific compounds:

F, 12.0 µg/100 ml (in the morning)
B, 0.6 µg/100 ml
Aldosterone, 7 mµg/100 ml (when sodium intake is normal)

Because of the protein binding, the amounts of free corticoids are estimated as follows:

F, 1.2 µg/100 ml
B, 0.06 µg/100 ml
Aldosterone, 3.0 mµg/100 ml

The amounts of *free hormone* are probably the *truly significant ones* in the *physiologic actions* on the various body tissues.

The plasma half-lives are:

F, 1 to 2 hours
B, 30 minutes
Aldosterone, 35 minutes

At the *tissue level* there is some interconversion of the physiologically active F and the inactive cortisone (compound E). This is particularly the case for the adrenals and liver, which last explains why cortisone taken by mouth is physiologically active. Most peripheral tissues convert F to E, with not much going the other way. A small amount of hydrocortisone gets through the choroid plexus to the cerebrospinal fluid, which contains 0.4 µg/100 ml.

The kidney resorbs 80% to 90% of free hydrocortisone and an indeterminate amount of free aldosterone. The gut absorbs almost 100% of these hormones, accounting in part for their effectiveness when given by mouth.

*Inactivation* of hydrocortisone occurs in part by conversion to cortisone. Then both compounds are subjected to reduction and conjugation, principally in the liver, though the kidney and gut play some role. Note that the steroid ring structure is not broken. Hydrocortisone, for example, is reduced at the $\Delta^4$, forming *dihydrohydrocortisone* (DHF). This action requires TPNH. Then the 3-keto group is reduced, forming *tetrahydrohydrocortisone* (THF). THF is then conjugated, and THF-glucuronide is excreted into the urine. A good deal of THF is further reduced at the 20-keto group, forming 20-hydroxylated compounds, called cortols (or cortolones when derived from E rather than F). Cortisone (E) is metabolized like hydrocortisone. Figure 21 shows the changes that take place in the catabolism of hydrocortisone and Figure 22 lists some of the main urinary metabolites of the adrenal steroids.

The urine contains, for example, the following in approximate amounts:

> THF, 3 mg per day
> THE, 5 mg per day
> β-cortol, 3 mg per day
> β-cortolone, 3 mg per day

There is also some *free hydrocortisone* in the urine: about 40 to 80 µg per day or about 0.2% of the daily secretion. Other unknown metabolites of F in the urine make up as much as one-third of the daily F

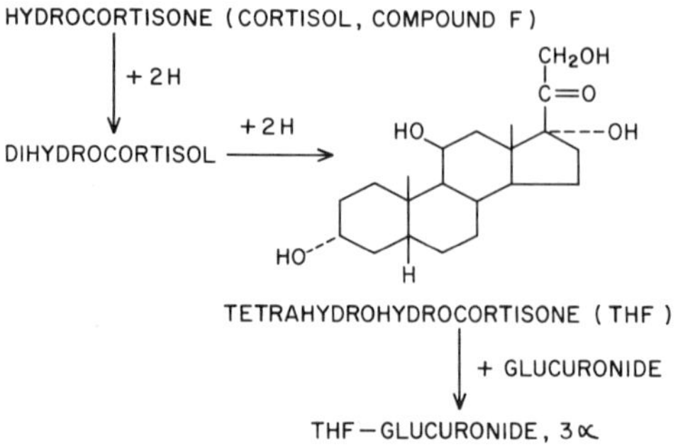

FIG. 21.    Catabolism of hydrocortisone.

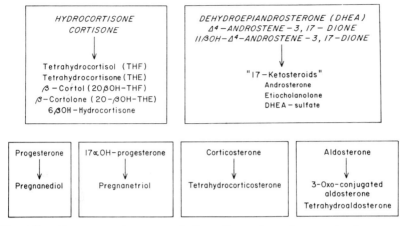

FIG. 22. Common urinary metabolites (beneath each arrow) of common adrenal steroids.

secretion rate. A certain amount (15%) finds its way into the stool. None of the F metabolites (or inactivation products) have any biologic activity.

The inactivation of aldosterone goes partly along a similar pathway to form tetrahydroaldosterone; most of the secreted aldosterone (60% to 75%) appears in the urine as other breakdown products (see p. 52).

## Clinical Assay

The clinical assay of adrenal corticoids in patients is usually done by testing urine or blood. The ideal would be to measure the actual secretion rate, a procedure which, though possible, is technically too difficult to perform as a routine test. A common method for estimating *hydrocortisone* or its metabolites in blood or urine is the measurement of Porter-Silber chromogens. This reaction depends on the dihydroxy-acetone group (Fig. 23) and will therefore measure F and E as well as most of their reduced or conjugated metabolites. It will not measure

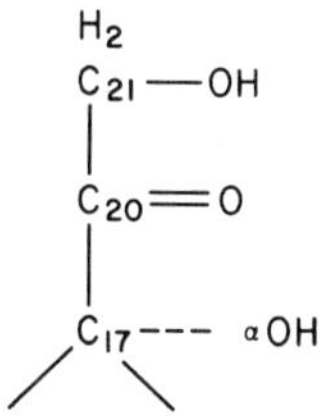

$$
\begin{array}{l}
H_2 \\
C_{21}\!-\!OH \\
| \\
C_{20}\!=\!O \\
| \\
C_{17}\,\text{---}\,\alpha OH
\end{array}
$$

FIG. 23. Reactive group for Porter-Silber reaction.

corticosterone (B), which lacks the 17α-OH, nor will it measure the cortols and cortolones, which have a 20-OH. By convention this test is called *17-hydroxycorticosteroids* (17-OHCS). The normal range for plasma is 5 to 25 μg/100 ml (most of which is hydrocortisone); for urine it is 3 to 10 mg per day (most of which consists of reduced and conjugated metabolites). Plasma F may also be measured fluorimetrically, a technically easier method, or by a more difficult but precise double-isotope method, or by a competitive protein-binding assay, as noted before (see Chap. 1, under Assay of Hormones). The urinary *17-ketosteroids* are often measured but are of little value in testing adrenal function except in a few instances (as in cancer or congenital enzymatic defects).

The measurement of aldosterone or its metabolites is difficult no matter what method is used. Values found in normal people are noted on page 52.

## Actions of Adrenal Cortical Hormones

Loss or removal of the adrenal cortex has many deleterious effects. Not all of them can be explained, but they are reversed by giving the appropriate adrenal hormones. Thus the physiologic actions of the adrenal cortical hormones are those which correct these deficiencies. Adrenalectomy causes:

1. *Sodium loss into the urine.* Effects secondary to this are decreased blood volume, increased hematocrit, decreased renal plasma flow and glomerular filtration rate. Other effects thought by some to be secondary to sodium loss but more probably due to some ill-defined effect of hydrocortisone lack are hypotension, part of the decreased blood volume, weakness, vomiting, and poor growth.
2. *Tendency to hypoglycemia* with at least an increased insulin sensitivity and sometimes actual low blood glucose values.
3. *Poor resistance to infection or shock* (hypotension), often generalized as poor resistance to stress, along with *poor stamina* in that the ability of skeletal muscle to work for a prolonged time is diminished.
4. *Poor water excretion* and *sodium handling* by the kidneys.
5. *Poor fat mobilization* and *utilization.*
6. *Psychic changes* such as depression, mild psychosis, lack of alertness, decreased memory.

All these effects are reversed by giving *hydrocortisone* and *aldosterone. Both* must be given since hydrocortisone has little sodium-retaining power and aldosterone at levels effective on sodium retention has little influence on the other deficiencies. Thus, aldosterone (or steroids with similar action) is called a *mineralocorticoid* and hydrocortisone (because of 2 above) a *glucocorticoid*. Keep in mind, though, that effects on glucose metabolism are only one facet of hydrocortisone's action; i.e., remember items 3 to 6 above. Further, this separation of activities is not absolute; all corticoids have both types of action, but the ratio of mineralocorticoid action to glucocorticoid action varies widely. For example, a milligram of aldosterone causes 500 times as much sodium retention but only one-fifth as much glycogen deposition as a milligram of hydrocortisone.

The actual effect, then, of a corticoid can be assessed only by multiplying its actual amount by its relative potency. Thus, corticosterone, which has good glucocorticoid activity, contributes comparatively little in this regard because there is only a small amount in the blood.

Note here that aldosterone and hydrocortisone are not widely used clinically in Addison's disease or adrenal insufficiency. It is cheaper to use synthetic steroids, which have similar actions and are easier to make.

### Sodium Loss into the Urine

It is no exaggeration to say that the composition of the blood is determined not by what the mouth takes in but by what the kidneys keep.
—HOMER W. SMITH,
*From Fish to Philosopher*

The sodium loss is reversed by *aldosterone,* discovered in 1953 by Simpson and Tait. In Addison's disease (adrenal insufficiency) there is, besides the salt loss, an increased sensitivity to the taste and (believe it or not) the smell of salt. The latter is apparently due to an increased ability to detect the minute amounts of chlorine gas given off by sodium chloride solutions. The sensitivity effects are not, however, aldosterone dependent but are due to hydrocortisone deficiency. In addition, there is an increased appetite, or craving, for salty foods, an effect mediated by the ventromedial nucleus of the hypothalamus. Presumably these effects tend to direct the patient or animal with adrenal insufficiency to sources of salt that might otherwise be missed.

In man aldosterone accounts for 70% of the distal tubular sodium retention due to the adrenal cortex. The other 30% is due to F and B, which are much less potent but are present in much larger amounts. Although 75 to 150 µg of aldosterone are secreted per day, the secretion rate varies inversely with the amount of salt in the diet and can drop as low as 25 µg per day or rise as high as 500 to 1000 µg per day. The liver is the main site of aldosterone inactivation; it extracts 90%

of the aldosterone in blood. The urine contains 1 to 7 µg per day of aldosterone in the form of a labile conjugate, possibly a glucuronide, and at least 12 other metabolites. One of these, TH-aldosterone, amounts to 12 to 50 µg per day and can be measured as a clinical assay, though not easily.

ACTION OF ALDOSTERONE ON THE KIDNEY.    Aldosterone is taken up by the renal tubular cell and acts on the distal tubule to increase sodium resorption. Much evidence suggests that it stimulates the operation of an exchange mechanism whereby sodium is retained while potassium and hydrogen ions are lost into the urine (Fig. 24). There is also an ill-defined effect on magnesium, causing magnesium to be treated like potassium and excreted into the urine.

How does aldosterone increase sodium resorption? Not all the steps involved are clear, but a good deal is known. The effect on sodium transport is not a direct one, for there is always a time lag of 10 to 40 minutes between the administration of aldosterone and increased resorption of sodium. As with ADH, much of the evidence is based on work done with the toad bladder, though the results seem generally applicable to intact mammals.

Recent experiments have shown that actinomycin blocks ribonucleic acid (RNA) synthesis and aldosterone-stimulated sodium resorption in the intact rat; that both actinomycin and puromycin block aldosterone-stimulated sodium transfer in the toad bladder; and that aldosterone localizes in the cell nucleus before stimulating sodium resorption. DNA synthesis, however, is not required. Along with a number of other observations, a reasonable explanation can then be proposed: While aldosterone may freely diffuse into many body cells, it *binds* immediately and strongly to the cell membrane or nucleus of the toad bladder. The initial binding may be to a high-molecular-weight protein with $K_A$'s of $2.1 \times 10^8$ and $5.4 \times 10^{10}$. Eventually it stimulates the synthesis of mRNA of a specific type, and perhaps that of ribosome RNA as well.

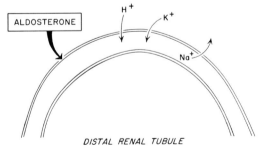

FIG. 24.    Effect of aldosterone on distal tubular movement of electrolytes.

The changes in RNA in turn stimulate the synthesis of specific proteins necessary for sodium transport.

These specific proteins may be somehow directly involved in changing the permeability of the cell to sodium, much as ADH is. There could, for example, be an enzymatic sodium permease. This is a controversial point; some have shown that aldosterone increases permeability to sodium while others have shown that it does not. Or the proteins may be enzymes involved in supplying energy to the cell. Aldosterone has effects on the conversion of glycogen to pyruvate, on pyruvate decarboxylase, and on the Krebs cycle. Since sodium transport accounts for most of the kidney's metabolic activity, aldosterone may enhance sodium transport indirectly simply by supplying more energy for the process. Perhaps the proteins are enzymes involved in directing the use of the available energy, and act to funnel a higher fraction of the cell's energy toward sodium transport. Or, finally, aldosterone may stimulate the formation of a specific enzyme which directly increases the pumping of sodium out of the nonluminal side of the cell. It is possible, of course, that more than one of these mechanisms are at work. Whether cAMP takes part in any of this is not clear; some new work suggests it may.

The end result is probably both an increase in sodium transport activity (the "sodium pump") and an increased permeability to sodium, both enhancing the removal of sodium from the lumen of the renal tubule. The actual sodium transporter in the cell membrane may be a phospholipid or a phosphoprotein.

The *"exchange mechanism"* in the distal tubule is probably not simple exchange of sodium for potassium and hydrogen ion. Although this idea explains generally the main experimental findings, some awkward observations have been made recently:

1. Some sodium may be resorbed under the influence of aldosterone associated with anion resorption rather than cation exchange.
2. There may be a proximal tubule effect of aldosterone which, depending on conditions, may increase or even decrease sodium resorption.
3. Under some conditions aldosterone will increase sodium resorption before potassium excretion is increased.
4. In vivo, actinomycin will block the sodium resorption effect of aldosterone but will not block the potassium loss.
5. In a few normal humans fairly large parenteral doses of aldosterone failed to increase potassium loss.

So, although no better explanation has been proposed, the "exchange mechanism" idea may soon require extensive revision.

Practically nothing is certain about the effect of aldosterone on magnesium except that there is an increased magnesium output into the urine.

ACTIONS OF ALDOSTERONE ON OTHER TISSUES.   Aldosterone acts in other ways to keep sodium in the body. It increases sodium resorption by the sweat glands although it causes only an erratic potassium loss in sweat. It acts on the salivary glands and on the colon to retain sodium. A similar action on the small intestine is controversial at present; there is probably some effect on sodium resorption.

In addition to keeping sodium in the body, aldosterone quite possibly has a major part in determining where the body's sodium goes. As alluded to above (see Chap. 4, under Antidiuretic Hormone), aldosterone, in concert with ADH, seems to maintain at an optimum the sodium and water content of the cells in muscle, liver, and brain. Aldosterone acts to keep too much sodium from entering these cells by pumping the excess back outside the cell. Strictly speaking, since the sodium pump mechanism could be bidirectional, aldosterone could also act by cutting down on the active transport of sodium into the cell. In any case, the net effect is to keep unwanted sodium out. For example, when aldosterone retains sodium in the body, the sodium is not allowed into cells but remains in the extracellular fluid.

Although the idea is largely speculative at present, aldosterone may also help keep potassium and magnesium where they ought to be: inside the cell. This may seem strange, at least with regard to potassium, because one of the features of excessive aldosterone is a loss of potassium from body tissues. However, the latter may be only a response of the body to a loss of potassium by the kidney. Under the same circumstances of excessive aldosterone, one can show that the extra aldosterone helps the tissues take up potassium when it is available.

In muscle, as in the kidney tubule, aldosterone may affect the sodium pump via mRNA-stimulated synthesis of a specific enzyme for sodium transport. Overall, the sodium pump of muscle increases its activity when there is a drop in the osmotic gradient of sodium ($Na_O/Na_I$) or a drop in the transmembrane electric potential; aldosterone seems to help the muscle cell respond better to both stimuli.

CONTROL OF ALDOSTERONE SECRETION.   From what has been said so far, one would logically expect sodium depletion to stimulate aldosterone secretion, which in turn would be shut off by the resulting sodium retention. This in fact occurs, but the major determinant of aldosterone secretion is probably not sodium balance itself but the state of the *intravascular fluid volume.*

Simply stated, a drop in intravascular volume causes a rise in aldosterone secretion. Aldosterone then increases sodium retention. This effect, plus an increase in thirst, sodium appetite, and ADH secretion —all stimulated by a low plasma volume—results in fluid retention by the body and so repairs the volume deficit. When the intravascular volume returns to normal, aldosterone secretion drops.

The mechanism by which changes in plasma volume affect aldosterone secretion is not so simply stated and is still a subject of much investigation. To begin with, in some diseases, as far as we can tell, there is an increased aldosterone secretion without a decreased intravascular volume. So the idea of an *effective* intravascular volume was suggested; by this is meant an intravascular volume which gives effective perfusion of critical tissues with blood. Both the kidney and the brain in some way sense the deficit in effective volume. At the moment, the best evidence is that the immediate stimulus to increased secretion of aldosterone is a decreased effective blood flow to, or a perception of decreased effective intravascular volume by, the kidney, the brain, or both.

*The Kidney and Aldosterone Secretion.*   Decreased blood flow to the kidney stimulates the juxtaglomerular apparatus to secrete *renin* (see p. 19). Perhaps the actual stimulus is decreased stretching of the juxtaglomerular body or decreased sodium arriving at the macula densa —or both. Renin in turn acts on *renin substrate* in the blood stream, forming *angiotensin I*. A converting enzyme then converts angiotensin I to *angiotensin II* (this process occurs in the blood stream in general but may be faster in the circulation of the lungs). Finally, angiotensin II stimulates the adrenal cortex to increase aldosterone synthesis and secretion (mediated by cAMP). In addition, renin may enhance the response of the adrenal cortex to angiotensin II. Then begins the attempt to raise the intravascular volume back to normal. Confirming this whole idea is the fact that sodium depletion causes a rise in plasma renin as well as in the secretion of aldosterone.

Angiotensin II and renin may also directly influence the kidney so as to cause an increase in both sodium and water resorption; the effect is similar to the general action of ADH but is in fact different since patients with a peculiar kind of diabetes insipidus will not respond to ADH but will respond to angiotensin II. In their direct effects on the kidney, angiotensin and renin may act on the kidney tubule or they may instead act as intrarenal vasoconstrictors and affect sodium and water resorption through their power to regulate intrarenal blood flow.

A recent report suggests that the substance we call renin is still present in the blood even in patients who have had both kidneys removed, but this finding is contrary to what most other studies assert.

The chemistry of angiotensin I and II is known, and renin substrate is a 14 amino acid peptide linked to a glycoprotein (58,000 mol. wt.).

*Renin substrate peptide* (made in liver):

ASP–ARG–VAL–TYR–ILE–HIS–PRO–PHE–
HIS–LEU–LEU–VAL–TYR–SER

*Angiotensin I* (human):

ASP–ARG–VAL–TYR–ILE–HIS–PRO–PHE–HIS–LEU

*Angiotensin II:*

ASP–ARG–VAL–TYR–ILE–HIS–PRO–PHE

Angiotensin I and II are formed by sequential removal of amino acids. Angiotensin II is rapidly metabolized, with a half-life in plasma of less than two minutes and disappearing completely from the blood in 30 minutes. It can be immunoassayed, but the values determined range widely from laboratory to laboratory. Normal adults eating a diet of moderate sodium content have somewhere between 10 and 300 picograms per milliliter of plasma (10 to 300 pg/ml).

*The Brain, the Nervous System, and Aldosterone Secretion.*   A drop in blood volume results not only in a rise in plasma renin but also in an increased activity of the sympathetic nervous system. Furthermore, adrenergic stimuli and greater sympathetic nervous activity cause more renin secretion. Since trauma or anxiety can increase aldosterone secretion, it is reasonable to suppose that somewhere in the head is a receptor mechanism for translating a drop in intravascular volume into an increased aldosterone secretion acting via the sympathetic nervous system.

That the brain may be important in stimulating aldosterone secretion is not a new idea. Some years ago it was proposed that the pineal, or a nearby area of the midbrain, secretes a hormone, called glomerulotropin, which stimulates aldosterone secretion. The proposal has not been confirmed, but the possibility still exists. Other work indicates that the pineal, if anything, inhibits aldosterone secretion. Confusion on this point obviously awaits resolution.

The sympathetic nervous system, like angiotensin, may also directly affect sodium resorption by the kidney by acting on renal arterioles and thereby shifting intrarenal blood flow or affecting the countercurrent mechanism.

Overall, then, the functional activity of the sympathetic nervous system, in conjunction with changes in effective blood volume, plays an important role in stimulating renin and aldosterone secretion (Fig. 25)

*Other Factors Stimulating Aldosterone Secretion.*   As we have said, a change in the effective intravascular volume is the major determinant of aldosterone secretion. It is not necessarily the only determinant. Other stimuli, of uncertain relative importance, increase aldosterone secretion:

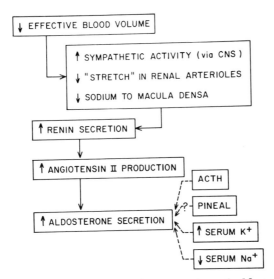

Fig. 25.    Factors that stimulate secretion of aldosterone.

1. *ACTH* may play a supportive role in maintaining the adrenal cortex at a proper size but does not itself directly stimulate much aldosterone secretion at the levels of ACTH found in blood. ACTH also supports aldosterone secretion by enhancing the sensitivity of the adrenal gland to angiotensin II.

2. *Erect posture* probably decreases effective blood volume and increases renin secretion.

3. *Low sodium or high potassium* concentration in plasma is a factor, although the magnitude of change required is rarely encountered in man. One can show, for example, that a high concentration of potassium directly stimulates aldosterone synthesis in vitro.

4. *Low sodium or high potassium diet,* i.e., sodium depletion or potassium excess without any necessary changes in plasma concentration, may play a *direct* role in stimulating aldosterone secretion in addition to the stimulation mediated by changes in vascular volume or by angiotensin II. This is, however, difficult to prove. During sodium depletion, it is not clear precisely what happens in the adrenal cortex; some work suggests an increase in the synthesis of DOC with a resulting rise in aldosterone synthesis, while other work indicates an increased conversion of corticosterone to aldosterone in the adrenal mitochondria.

*Shutting Off Aldosterone Secretion.*    Although the general presumption is that aldosterone secretion is shut off by a reversal of any or all of the above stimulatory mechanisms, only a small amount of evidence bears directly on this point. Sodium loading decreases aldosterone secretion and depresses plasma renin levels from 7 m$\mu$g/100 ml to < 1 m$\mu$g/ml. That seems conclusive enough, but here the level of sodium in the body or in the plasma may play as important a part as effective plasma volume, perhaps more so.

OTHER ASPECTS OF SODIUM REGULATION. There are still problems. Aldosterone is not the whole answer to sodium metabolism. It controls only a small fraction of the total sodium resorbed by the kidney. Most sodium resorption occurs in the proximal tubule and the ascending loop of Henle while aldosterone acts principally on the distal tubule. In the proximal tubule sodium resorption is increased when the cross-sectional area is increased and when there is an increase in the ATPase activated by sodium and potassium. Sodium resorption by the ascending loop of Henle increases when less sodium is resorbed by the proximal tubule. Even if extra sodium gets through to the macula densa in the distal tubule, the latter may sense the increased sodium, cause a decrease in the glomerular filtrate to that tubule, and therefore shunt sodium to other nephrons that have better resorption of sodium in their proximal tubules. All these mechanisms increase sodium resorption by the kidney but do not appear to depend on aldosterone.

Furthermore, in disease states associated with fluid retention, such as ascites or edema, there is a great deal of sodium retention and it is associated with a high secretion rate of aldosterone. The initial reaction is to attribute all the sodium retention to the aldosterone. Unfortunately, some diseases have sodium retention with no excess of aldosterone; more important, in the absence of disease, injected aldosterone will cause retention of only 400 to 500 mEq of sodium no matter how much is given. This is not enough sodium to cause edema or ascites. Another factor, perhaps humoral, must be present. Some workers have suggested that there is an unknown *sodium-retaining hormone*, perhaps originating in the liver, which acts on the proximal tubule to increase sodium resorption. Others feel that this may all be due to decreased arterial pressure or flow to the kidney with resulting shifts in intrarenal blood flow that enhance sodium resorption. The problem is not really solved.

How is it that aldosterone cannot cause more sodium retention in the normal individual? Again, this is an unsolved problem. No matter how much aldosterone is given, the normal response, after retention of the 400 to 500 mEq of sodium noted above, is to retain no more sodium and to excrete promptly into the urine any extra sodium that is given. Although no completely convincing evidence has been presented, there may be a *salt-losing hormone*. Candidates have included ADH, prostaglandin $E_1$ or $E_2$, hydrocortisone (in small doses it will cause sodium loss), estradiol (in small doses), progesterone (in such large amounts it would be physiologically significant only in pregnancy), an unknown adrenal hormone, an unidentified pineal factor, and some humoral factor from the liver. Whatever this hormone is, it is stimulated by the expansion (or rate of expansion) of the extracellular fluid volume (ECF) and it acts on the proximal renal tubule to decrease sodium resorption. Some researchers, however, feel that there is no hormone involved and that the increase in ECF lowers sodium resorption by other means such as decreasing the concentration of plasma protein, increasing renal perfusion pressure, dilating renal blood vessels, or speeding up the flow of the glomerular filtrate through the proximal tubule.

Here is another unresolved problem requiring more research. About all that is really known is that a mechanism exists which can cause sodium loss in the urine even in the absence of a drop in aldosterone secretion.

Summing up: Aldosterone, acting on the distal renal tubule, is a major but not the only regulator of sodium metabolism. Effective blood volume, dietary potassium, renin-angiotensin, and the sympathetic nervous system, all working together, are important in regulating aldosterone secretion. Other factors affect sodium resorption by the proximal tubule and ascending loop of Henle but are not well understood. Even today, many questions about sodium balance are unanswered.

### Hypoglycemia and Increased Sensitivity to Insulin

All changes, except sodium loss, resulting from the loss of the adrenal cortex are due principally to hydrocortisone (F) deficiency. Since hypoglycemia and increased insulin sensitivity are reversed with hydrocortisone, it is called a *glucocorticoid*. Hydrocortisone corrects the deficit in carbohydrate metabolism mainly by *increasing gluconeogenesis* in the liver, i.e., increasing the conversion of amino acids to glucose, with a resulting rise in glucose output to the blood. Hydrocortisone can cause a temporary short-term decrease in hepatic glucose output, but the predominant long-term effect is an increase.

The greater gluconeogenesis due to hydrocortisone is associated with:

1. An increase in the net flow of amino acids from other tissues to the liver. For example, F decreases amino acid uptake and incorporation into protein in muscle. This is the so-called antianabolic or catabolic effect of hydrocortisone. With excess hydrocortisone (*Cushing's syndrome*) one sees a net nitrogen loss from the body, osteoporosis, and muscle wasting.
2. An increase in the uptake of amino acids by liver cells and a rise in the conversion of amino acids to glucose by them.

3. An increase in the removal of glucose at the end of the gluco-neogenetic pathway by its return to the blood or its conversion to glycogen, depending on the body's needs. Hydrocortisone can increase glycogen synthesis in both liver and muscle, but perhaps only in the liver and cardiac muscle does it cause a net increase in glycogen. Insulin is required for the increase in glycogen synthesis, since in this instance the latter depends not only on higher gluconeogenesis but also on an increase in the active form of glycogen synthetase. This enzyme needs insulin for conversion from its less active to its more active form (the D to I transformation). Although increased enzyme activity occurs, no mRNA synthesis is needed. The increase in the amount of glycogen in the liver is a classic assay for glucocorticoid activity.

The hepatic action of hydrocortisone on gluconeogenesis, insofar as we know it, takes place something like this:

1. Although most of the hydrocortisone that comes to the liver is metabolized and inactivated, a small amount remains free and is bound to liver cells. The binding is probably not to the nucleus but rather to cellular protein, although this point is controversial and F in fact may bind to nuclear histones. The free but bound hydrocortisone is probably the active hormone.
2. Although there is no immediate increase in total protein synthesis, some specific protein synthesis is stimulated at an early time by F.
3. One then can detect an increased activity of nuclear RNA polymerase, and an increase in RNA synthesis, both of transfer RNA and of messenger RNA.
4. Total protein synthesis in the liver is then increased, probably secondarily in part to increased mRNA synthesis.
5. Many different enzymes show heightened activity and probably greater synthesis. Some of these enzymes are involved in converting pyruvate to glucose-6-phosphate and beyond while others metabolize specific amino acids such as TYR, GLY, and TRP. With the latter group, the increase has been shown to be due to actual synthesis of the enzyme and occurs in 30 to 60 minutes.
6. The changes in various enzymes then result in increased deamination of amino acids and conversion of the products to glucose. It may be that not all amino acids are treated in this way, but hydrocortisone has been shown specifically to increase the conversion of VAL, PHE, and ALA to glucose.
7. cAMP may somehow be involved in all this. Hydrocortisone lowers hepatic phosphodiesterase, an enzymatic change differing from the changes just noted. The process takes a while but results

in more cAMP (see Fig. 4). Conceivably, the cAMP then may be involved in gluconeogenesis.

All gluconeogenesis need not, however, be from amino acids. Pyruvate, lactate, and glycerol, for example, can be substrates. Nevertheless, amino acids are probably the preferred substrates since tryptophan tends to inhibit the conversion of pyruvate to glucose by blocking the activity of phosphoenol-pyruvate carboxykinase. Furthermore, in vivo, amino acids are quantitatively much more important, accounting for about 80% to 90% of gluconeogenesis in humans. Figure 26, outlining gluconeogenesis, will refresh the memory; the enzyme activities stimulated by hydrocortisone are underlined.

The mechanism just described for the stimulation of gluconeogenesis by hydrocortisone is a reasonable one, but it is not the only one. For example, hydrocortisone can stimulate pyruvate conversion to glucose (and decrease conversion to acetyl-CoA) without increasing

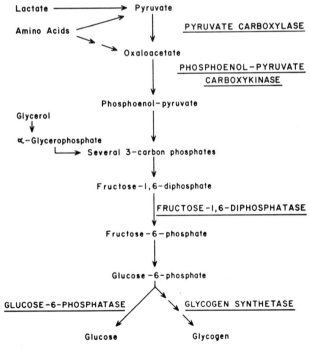

Fig. 26.   Gluconeogenesis. Enzyme activities stimulated by hydrocortisone are underlined.

any of the enzymes involved. For that matter, it is possible that hydrocortisone stimulates gluconeogenesis by the liver without acting on the liver at all; some recent work suggests that it might result from effects on peripheral amino acids. All the changes in the liver may simply be caused by an increased influx of amino acids, any changes in enzymes being due to induction by substrate.

Hydrocortisone, then, may act to increase gluconeogenesis by increasing the amount of substrate, by redirecting the activity of existing enzymes in some way, by somehow increasing enzyme activity, or by actually increasing enzyme synthesis. No one knows which of these, if any, is the most important.

In addition to the effects on hepatic glucose metabolism, hydrocortisone probably causes inhibition of glucose uptake by muscle and adipose tissue, possibly by inhibiting glucose conversion to glucose-6-phosphate. This action is separate from the inhibition of amino acid conversion to protein. Whether other tissues are affected has not been investigated.

It is fair to say that hydrocortisone plays a major role in glucose metabolism. Overall, one can see how hydrocortisone reverses the tendency to hypoglycemia that occurs in adrenal insufficiency and, in times of glucose shortage, both maintains the level of blood sugar and directs glucose to those tissues requiring it most, particularly the brain. The effects of hydrocortisone on the liver and peripheral tissues may even cause hyperglycemia (elevated blood glucose). Normally, however, a high blood glucose does not occur because a slight rise in blood glucose stimulates insulin secretion, which keeps the blood glucose down. In addition, hydrocortisone itself may directly stimulate insulin secretion by the pancreas. With high or prolonged doses of hydrocortisone, the effects on insulin may be overwhelmed and hyperglycemia then occurs.

### Poor Resistance to Infection and Shock and Poor Stamina

Resistance to infection and shock is difficult to deal with because it is hard to define in quantitative physiologic terms. Nevertheless, hydrocortisone seems necessary for the animal to respond appropriately to these "stresses"—another ill-defined term. Whatever hydrocortisone does, its actions here are probably closest to the problem of how hydrocortisone prevents death.

There are a number of effects of hydrocortisone which make at least its ability to enhance resistance to shock more understandable. First, hydrocortisone is needed to maintain plasma volume; aldosterone is not enough. It will increase plasma volume even at the expense of the remaining extracellular fluid volume. Second, hydrocortisone inhibits the inappropriate dilation of small arterioles, closes capillary sphincters, and enhances the constrictive response of arterioles and small veins to norepinephrine. In these cases it probably acts directly on vascular smooth muscle to increase its contractibility. Finally, the fact that glucocorticoids stimulate the heart to contract more strongly obviously helps in maintaining blood pressure and in perfusing tissues with blood.

### Poor Handling of Water and Sodium by the Kidneys

The adrenalectomized patient cannot get rid of excess water as fast as the normal person. This phenomenon can be used as a test for adrenal insufficiency. F corrects the condition, probably by a direct effect on the renal tubule. There is evidence, however, that F may inhibit ADH secretion, thus allowing more water excretion. The renal effect of hydrocortisone may be due to an increased sodium resorption in the distal loop of Henle, thus increasing free water formation. Under conditions of a water load, the excess would be lost more rapidly. Further, if there is water deprivation, less water might be lost than if hydrocortisone were not present. Whether this is the mechanism or not, F seems to enable the kidney to handle water more efficiently, making it easier for the kidney both to keep and to get rid of water as the situation demands.

As for sodium, it should be noted that, although most of the sodium retention due to the adrenal is secondary to aldosterone, the presence of some F is necessary for the sodium retention to occur. Hydrocortisone also has an important effect on sodium resorption by the proximal tubule which is probably mediated by an increase in the sodium-potassium activated ATPase. In addition, F seems necessary for the body to get rid of excess sodium. F is thus required for the optimum handling of sodium, whether too much or too little.

### Poor Mobilization and Utilization of Fat

F is required for the mobilization of free fatty acids (lipolysis) from *adipose tissue* that occurs with epinephrine and growth hormone and probably can act as a free fatty acid mobilizer itself if the insulin level is low. When acting as a mobilizer of free fatty acids, i.e., as a lipolytic agent, F may decrease fatty acid conversion to triglycerides (reesterification) rather than directly increasing the breakdown of triglycerides. Either way, the net release of free fatty acids is higher. Recent work suggests that, although the effect is somewhat delayed, hydrocortisone *does* directly stimulate triglyceride breakdown (lipolysis). Here F's decreasing of phosphodiesterase results in more cAMP (see Fig. 4) and then more lipolysis (see Fig. 31). In the *liver* F increases the conversion of glucose to fatty acids (lipogenesis), increases ketone body formation, and increases the mobilization of triglycerides from the liver.

The overall effect on the body is greater fatty acid oxidation, which may be both a direct effect and also secondary to the increased mobilization of fatty acids from adipose tissue.

Nevertheless, in vivo, the gluconeogenic effect of hydrocortisone seems more important than the lipolytic effect. For example, with an excess of hydrocortisone, as in Cushing's syndrome, there is a rise in total body fat rather than a decline because the hyperglycemia resulting from excessive hydrocortisone stimulates insulin secretion; the insulin here has an antilipolytic effect that apparently outweighs the lipolytic effect of hydrocortisone and the outcome is more, not less, fat.

### Psychic Changes

In adrenal insufficiency there may be depression and even psychosis. These changes are reversed by hydrocortisone, but what really happens is a complete mystery.

## Permissive Actions of Hydrocortisone

Hydrocortisone is the classic hormone said to have permissive actions (see p. 10). For example, as just noted, it is needed so that epinephrine and growth hormone can cause lipolysis in adipose tissue. While this particular action may be related to cAMP, just what happens is not known.

## Pharmacologic Actions of Hydrocortisone

Hydrocortisone has other actions which are for the most part seen only when an excessive amount of it is given. They are consequently called pharmacologic actions. This distinction may be artificial; perhaps the observed action *does* occur with the usual amount of hydrocortisone found in the body but is too subtle to be measured without first being exaggerated. Many of the effects of large amounts of glucocorticoids are harmful to patients and cause serious complications; they are the limiting factors in using glucocorticoids as therapy, and many are the presenting signs of Cushing's syndrome. One, the *anti-inflammatory* action, was so striking when in 1948 cortisone was first given to patients with rheumatoid arthritis that a Nobel Prize was awarded for the discovery.

Actions of excessive hydrocortisone include:

1. Inhibition of *thyroxine secretion*, although the usual amounts of hydrocortisone may be necessary for normal thyroxine secretion.

2. Increase in *calcium excretion*. One can show that there is decreased RNA and protein synthesis in bone, the so-called anti-anabolic effect, and that ultimately the bone loses calcium; the result is *osteoporosis*. The effect on bone, plus the fact that glucocorticoids can decrease calcium absorption from the gut, results in a net loss of calcium from the body.

3. Increase in *gastric acid* and *pepsin* production, which may be related to the gastric ulcers that occur in some patients.

4. Several effects on the *blood cells*. There is a decrease in the number of eosinophils and in the motility of neutrophils. The number of lymphocytes drops on account of increased maturation and decreased differentiation. Lymphocyte-containing tissue (the lymph nodes and the thymus) shrinks. A number of things happen in these tissues when they are exposed to hydrocortisone: The hydrocortisone binds to histones in the cell nuclei, and then in the cell as a whole there is a drop in DNA synthesis, nuclear RNA polymerase activity, protein synthesis, glucose uptake, and glucose utilization. Some of the latter effects may, however, be due simply to a decrease in the total number of cells in the preparation studied. In the bone marrow, red cell production increases, as does the growth of fibroblasts.

5. The *anti-inflammatory action*. Histologically, inflammation occurs in connective tissue and involves dilation of small vessels and capillaries, proliferation of fibroblasts, and increased deposition of collagen. Often the patient or animal will have a fever as well. Hydrocortisone inhibits the dilation of blood vessels and the proliferation of fibroblasts and actively reverses the increased collagen deposition. The effect on collagen is twofold; there is less synthesis of collagen, perhaps by interference with activation of mRNA and ribosomal aggregation, and more breakdown of collagen. These actions may be related to the inhibitory effect of hydrocortisone on nonliver protein synthesis (noted above in discussion of gluconeogenesis).

Another attractive hypothesis has been recently proposed to explain this general effect of glucocorticoids. Inflammation as we know it may be largely a result of hydrolytic enzymes released from the lysosomes. Hydrocortisone stabilizes the lysosomes, prevents their breakdown and the release of their enzymes, and therefore prevents inflammation. The evidence to bolster this idea is still coming in but it certainly seems reasonable on the basis of what is now known. Here the action may be due to a direct insertion of hydrocortisone into the structure of the lysosomal membrane.

The fever of inflammation is rapidly dissipated by hydrocortisone. In many instances, probably including this one, the actual temperature elevation results from the action on the hypothalamus of a pyrogen released from circulating granulocytes. Analogous to the effect on lysosomes, hydrocortisone prevents fever by inhibiting the release of pyrogen from the granulocytes.

## GENERAL COMMENT ON THE ACTION OF GLUCOCORTICOIDS

On the whole, it is difficult to grasp just what hydrocortisone does. The multiplicity of actions just noted, the ignorance that underlies the words *permissive action*, and the uncertainty as to whether the pharmacologic actions are truly physiologic—all these factors together indicate that an answer to the basic question of how hydrocortisone works remains elusive. Present information is extensive but, although several authors have made the attempt, no one has yet put it together so that a single, precise action of hydrocortisone can be discerned. It may be that hydrocortisone has several different actions relatively independent of one another, but at the moment that is speculative. The problem continues to be one for intensive investigation.

## CONTROL OF HYDROCORTISONE SECRETION

### ACTH and the Adrenal Cortex

The basic facts are simple. Over the short term, in seconds to minutes, ACTH increases hydrocortisone and corticosterone secretion with only minimal effects on aldosterone secretion. The gland responds both to the absolute amount of ACTH and to the rate of increase in ACTH concentration. When ACTH is removed, the secretion of corticoids returns to normal in an equally short time. Over the long term, in hours to days, ACTH stimulates the growth of the adrenal cortex.

The relationship between short-term and long-term actions is elusive. Some have postulated the existence of two separate ACTH's, but this idea is not popular. The twofold action of ACTH may be explained in part as follows.

Since the adrenal gland contains only small amounts of corticoids compared to the amount of secretion, whatever ACTH does to increase corticoid output must be concerned primarily with corticoid synthesis and not simply release. A glance at Figure 20 shows that there are many possibilities for action, e.g., on substrate availability, cofactor synthesis, enzyme synthesis, and structural alterations. If one could somehow tie together the effects on protein synthesis with those on corticoid synthesis, he would have a link between the effects on corticoid secretion and adrenal growth. Most of the recent research activity in this area has in fact been aimed in this direction.

ACTH does have many effects on the overall mechanism for protein synthesis. It (1) increases mRNA synthesis; (2) increases total adrenal RNA content with a greater number of polysomes (though most of the increased RNA seems to be in mitochondria rather than ribosomes); (3) raises the number of mitoses, the number of mitochondria, and the amount of endoplasmic reticulum; and (4) increases the total amount of protein synthesis. All these actions of ACTH are specific for the adrenal gland. However, they are by and large long-term effects. While they account adequately for the growth of the gland, over the short term an increase in total amino acid incorporation into protein has not been consistently demonstrated under conditions in which corticoid synthesis was definitely increased. Indeed, some workers have shown that ACTH actually can decrease amino acid incorporation into adrenal protein under appropriate circumstances.

Nevertheless, other critical experiments strongly suggest a close relationship between protein and corticoid synthesis. Puromycin blocks protein synthesis in the adrenal cortex; it also blocks corticoid synthesis at the same time. Actinomycin, which blocks RNA synthesis, does not inhibit either protein synthesis or corticoid synthesis. Reasonable conclusions then are that:

1. The short-term effect of ACTH on corticoid synthesis is not mediated by mRNA synthesis. The mRNA involved must be relatively stable.
2. Some protein synthesis is required for an increase in corticoid synthesis.
3. The protein involved is synthesized in small amounts (since it is hard to show an increase in total protein synthesis) and is specific in kind (since insulin will increase adrenal protein synthesis but not corticoid synthesis).

More recent work shows that another inhibitor of protein synthesis, cycloheximide, blocks nuclear RNA synthesis, suggesting that the synthesis of some protein is needed even for RNA synthesis.

The probable locus of the effect of ACTH on protein synthesis is the ribosome or polysome, where it may change the structure or the permeability to substrates. However, the work with cycloheximide intimates that the effect may be on the nucleus, and the question must be investigated further.

All this suggests that an *enzyme* of some kind is the protein whose synthesis is stimulated. Several candidates for this enzyme have been proposed and are discussed below, but which is the most important, i.e., most crucial or rate limiting, has not been settled.

Since cholesterol is the precursor of the corticoids, and adrenal cholesterol is largely esterified, changes in an *adrenal lipase* or *esterase* which hydrolyzes the cholesterol esters may be important. In fact, ACTH does increase the activity of an adrenal lipase. On the other hand, some evidence suggests that the corticoids synthesized under the influence of ACTH are derived from plasma unesterified cholesterol and not from adrenal cholesterol esters at all.

ACTH increases the conversion of cholesterol to pregnenolone. At least two reactions are involved here. The first is the hydroxylation of cholesterol to $20\alpha$-OH-cholesterol and $20\alpha,22$-OH-cholesterol and the other is the conversion of the latter to pregnenolone by cleaving off the side chain at $C_{20}$. The latter is catalyzed by a *side-chain cleavage enzyme*. It may be the rate-limiting reaction in the synthesis of hydrocortisone and may also be the specific reaction ultimately stimulated by ACTH.

Another hypothesis explaining the action of ACTH that involves increased enzyme activity is that pieced together over several years by Haynes and his co-workers, based on the work with cAMP begun by Sutherland. They observed that:

1. ACTH increased adrenal cAMP content.
2. Both ACTH and cAMP increased adrenal phosphorylase activity.
3. cAMP increased adrenal corticoid synthesis.
4. TPNH (NADPH) is required for several steps in corticoid synthesis.

It was then hypothesized that ACTH acts on the adrenal cell membrane to increase the activity of the enzyme *adenyl cyclase* (which it does within one minute) and that the resulting cAMP in turn increases adrenal phosphorylase, leading to increased glycogen breakdown and an increased adrenal glucose-6-phosphate. The glucose-6-phosphate could then be oxidized via the hexose monophosphate pathway to $CO_2$ with a resulting rise in TPNH (NADPH) synthesis. The extra TPNH would stimulate more corticoid synthesis. Unfortunately, a number of observations are not consistent with this entire hypothesis:

1. At physiologic levels of ACTH, there is no increase in adrenal phosphorylase.
2. With appropriate manipulation one can demonstrate increased adrenal phosphorylase without increased corticoid synthesis.
3. ACTH does not increase oxidation of glucose-1-C to $CO_2$, nor is this oxidation required for corticoid synthesis.
4. ACTH does not increase adrenal TPNH content.
5. ACTH probably does not increase conversion of progesterone to hydrocortisone, which requires TPNH.

Nevertheless, the hypothesis is generally valid and must be accepted. In the light of more recent work, it has only to be modified. One cannot avoid the facts that ACTH increases both adenyl cyclase and cAMP in the adrenal and that cAMP increases corticoid synthesis. TPNH added to the adrenal cortex in vitro also increases corticoid synthesis but by a different mechanism from that utilized by cAMP and, in view of 4 and 5 just above, is not likely to play a regulatory role in corticoid synthesis. We now know that cAMP acts on corticoid synthesis very much like ACTH: Both have their predominant action at a point before pregnenolone in the biosynthetic pathway and both can stimulate the 11β-hydroxylation reaction by some sort of direct mitochondrial action. More specifically, both ACTH and cAMP seem to have their main action at the site of the *side-chain cleavage of cholesterol*; in the case of cAMP, this action is blocked by puromycin, suggesting that cAMP stimulates the synthesis of some protein before side-chain cleavage occurs.

The current thought is then as follows: ACTH stimulates adenyl cyclase in the adrenal cell membrane (internal cellular or nuclear membrane?) with a resulting increase in cAMP concentration. The cAMP in turn stimulates the synthesis (mechanism?) of a specific protein (cleavage enzyme?), which in turn increases the side-chain cleavage of cholesterol. Since this is probably the rate-limiting reaction in hydrocortisone synthesis, an increase here causes an increase in the amount of hydrocortisone made and secreted (Fig. 27).

It has been suggested that the ultimate action of ACTH can be better explained if one postulates two sites of action rather than one; the idea is not yet well defined. Another possibility is that ACTH increases adrenal blood flow and that this alone is responsible for increased corticoid synthesis. There is some experimental support for this proposal, but one can also show increased blood flow without increased corticoid synthesis.

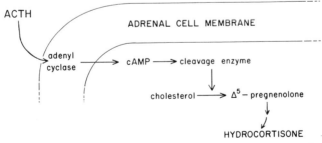

FIG. 27.   Postulated mechanism of the action of ACTH on the adrenal cortex. The question is not settled and other mechanisms are possible.

## Negative Feedback Control Systems

While ACTH stimulates corticoid synthesis, obviously for effective homeostasis and body responses some control is required over the whole ACTH-corticoid system. There may be some intrinsic control in the adrenal cortex itself; thus, pregnenolone can inhibit cholesterol conversion to 20α-OH-cholesterol. However, intrinsic control has little part in the overall pattern.

The *main control system* involves a negative feedback inhibition of ACTH secretion by hydrocortisone, whereby a rise in plasma hydrocortisone tends to shut off ACTH secretion and a drop in hydrocortisone tends to turn on ACTH. Suggested as long ago as 1888, the system was first well defined by Ingle in 1938.

Although it was originally regarded as a pituitary-adrenal system, in fact the central nervous system plays a major role. Selye had shown in 1936 that nonspecific stressful stimuli would increase adrenal size. A more recent observation in man was that plasma hydrocortisone and urine 17-hydroxycorticosteroids show a *diurnal variation*. In humans the peak is about 6 A.M. and the low point about 4 P.M. Urine levels lag slightly behind with a peak at 8 to 12 A.M. Nocturnal animals such as the rat have exactly opposite high and low points. This variation seems closely related to the sleep-activity cycle which, if reversed, is followed 5 to 10 days later by a parallel change in the diurnal variation. Exposure to light also seems to affect its timing. The central nervous system must therefore have a controlling role in the variation through hour-to-hour changes in ACTH secretion, which indeed has been shown to be the case in man. The diurnal variation depends on a mature central nervous system, since it appears only after 1 to 2 years of age.

How then does the central nervous system influence ACTH secretion? The connection is from the hypothalamus to the pituitary via the pituitary portal blood vessels. There is little if any neural connection to the anterior pituitary. A humoral substance elaborated by the median eminence area of the hypothalamus stimulates the pituitary to secrete ACTH. The straightforward negative feedback system now becomes complicated.

The hypothalamic substance is called *corticotropin-releasing factor* (CRF). CRF has been found in hypothalamic extracts, in pituitary portal blood, and in the peripheral blood of hypophysectomized animals. Thus far, three different CRF's have been isolated, but none of these specific compounds has been isolated from the pituitary portal vessels. There is no proof then as to which (if any) of the three isolated CRF's is the principal one. All three are small peptides:

1. $\alpha_1$-CRF has 16 amino acids and is similar to α-MSH.
2. $\alpha_2$-CRF has 13 amino acids and is almost identical with α-MSH.
3. β-CRF has 8 amino acids and is similar to ADH. Note that ADH

itself does not seem to be a significant CRF, although some have suggested this; it may stimulate CRF secretion.

Hydrocortisone, in shutting off the secretion of ACTH, probably acts principally through the hypothalamus rather than the pituitary, since more free F is taken up by the hypothalamus than by the pituitary and corticoids implanted into the median eminence will decrease ACTH secretion whereas similar implants in the pituitary have no such effect (Fig. 28).

While the shutoff of ACTH by hydrocortisone is fairly quick (seconds to minutes), the reverse, a decreased level of hydrocortisone leading to an increased ACTH output, takes a bit longer. This last effect is also largely mediated by the hypothalamus in humans, since hypothalamic tumors that do not involve the pituitary can abolish the expected increase in ACTH secretion when the level of hydrocortisone drops.

### Stress and Hydrocortisone Secretion

Many types of stress, as suggested above, stimulate F secretion. The term *stress* is vague, and although such things as trauma, surgery, anesthesia, cold, low blood pressure, noise, intense emotion and medical school examinations involve stress, severe exercise, for example, does not. The effects of stresses on the secretion of hydrocortisone are, in the intact animal, mediated by the central nervous system. All there-

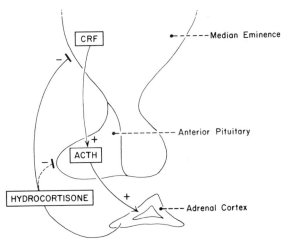

Fig. 28. Inhibition of the secretion of CRF and ACTH by hydrocortisone, an example of negative feedback. Stimulation represented by an arrow and +; inhibition represented by a bar and —.

fore depend on intact sensory pathways leading to the brain, where the signal finally impinges on the median eminence and causes CRF release. Low blood pressure (hypotension) has been studied more carefully than most of these stresses. It stimulates CRF release via nervous impulses originating in carotid and aortic baroreceptors and also by stimulating the production of angiotensin II (see p. 55), which in turn directly stimulates the hypothalamus. There are, incidentally, both stimulatory (amygdaloid and forebrain) and inhibitory (hippocampus) areas of the brain above the hypothalamus, but not much is known of them.

Such stresses are associated with an elevation in both plasma ACTH and plasma hydrocortisone. From what we have said, when hydrocortisone goes up, ACTH should go down. What happened to the negative feedback? Some have postulated a non-CRF pathway from the brain to the pituitary, but what probably happens is that the high plasma F is not enough to shut off CRF release in the presence of intense stimulation of the median eminence by nervous impulses from other areas of the brain. It is also worth noting that the diurnal variation in F secretion, the stress-induced F secretion, and the maintenance of adrenal weight, though all are mediated by the median eminence of the hypothalamus and by ACTH, have different control areas in the upper hypothalamus.

Summing up: Plasma hydrocortisone levels control the basal output of ACTH, mediated in large part by the hypothalamus and to a lesser extent by the pituitary. An acute stress overwhelms this basal secretion and causes a sudden CNS-mediated outpouring of ACTH, without regard for the plasma hydrocortisone level.

An important point to keep in mind is that, logically, control of a hormone secretion should be related to its biologic activity. Yet here we have been concerned with plasma levels. The assumption is that the plasma level affects the central nervous system control areas in parallel with its biologic activity. Partial support for this is seen in the fact that a drop in plasma F is associated with somewhat of a lag in increased ACTH output. Thus there may be a prolonged nervous system effect of the previously elevated plasma F similar to that known to exist in other tissues, e.g., the liver. Perhaps the immediate determinant of control is the amount of cortisol in the cells of the hypothalamus rather than the amount in the plasma.

There are also some as yet unexplained findings. Removal of the entire central nervous system including the spinal cord, but with the pituitary left in situ, apparently does not stop the stress response in a dog in which a burn causes increased F secretion. An isolated pituitary then seems capable of responding, but no one knows why.

Other influences on ACTH production, of uncertain significance, are the following:

1. Thyroxine increases ACTH output and exaggerates diurnal rhythm, and increases both secretion and inactivation of hydrocortisone.
2. Testosterone or progesterone can decrease ACTH secretion, even while directly stimulating the adrenal cortex.
3. Estrogens may increase ACTH secretion directly or indirectly by inhibiting adrenal corticoid synthesis.
4. Hydrocortisone itself may directly suppress adrenal F synthesis and increase the liver metabolism of F, the two together causing a lower plasma F. This effect plays a small role in the total picture, as we have said.
5. Liver disease, by decreasing F metabolism, can increase plasma F temporarily, resulting in decreased ACTH secretion.

A brief sidenote on adrenal "androgens" which have been mentioned above (p. 44). There is continual confusion between the 17-keto-steroids and androgens. DHEA (dehydroepiandrosterone) is a 17-ketosteroid made in large amounts by the adrenal (20 to 30 mg per day), yet it has little if any androgenic activity in man. The problem is complicated because, although in many species the three major 17-ketosteroids secreted by the adrenal are androgenic, they are at best only weakly androgenic in man (DHEA, $\Delta^4$-androstenedione, 11β-OH androstenedione). Further, testosterone, which is in all probability the androgen in man and is not a 17-ketosteroid, can be found in the adrenal vein though most of it comes from the testis in the male.

In this regard, one should remember the basic fact that the castrate male may lose or never acquire full androgenic characteristics, a fact that emphasizes the primary importance of the testis and the relative unimportance of the adrenal "androgens." Under normal circumstances the adrenals probably stimulate pubic and axillary hair growth but otherwise have no androgenic function; only in certain diseases such as cancer or the adrenogenital syndrome does the adrenal make significant androgen.

The same general comments apply to the adrenal estrogens.

## CLINICAL DISORDERS OF THE ADRENAL CORTEX

A knowledge of the actions of hydrocortisone and aldosterone now makes it possible to predict many but not all of the findings one sees when too much or too little of these hormones is secreted.

A primary deficit of aldosterone alone is rare but can occur. The expected findings are low blood pressure, low serum sodium, high serum potassium, and sodium loss in the urine. These are in fact what one tends to encounter in the patient. It is not clear whether the adrenal is at fault or whether the defect is in some part of the aldosterone-regulating system.

More common than a deficiency of aldosterone alone, though still unusual, is classic Addison's disease. Here there is a deficiency of both aldosterone and hydrocortisone, and the findings are as one would expect. The effects of the lack of aldosterone have just been described, but the patient with Addison's disease feels much worse because he also lacks hydrocortisone. He is tired, cannot work very long, may be depressed, and may have low blood glucose especially when he goes without eating for a few hours. He craves salt, but if instead he drinks too much water because of thirst, he may get symptoms of hyponatremia, such as drowsiness or even coma. Finally, because he secretes a great deal of ACTH and MSH, his skin is often darkly pigmented although perhaps only in spots. Formerly most often due to tuberculosis, in most of these patients adrenal insufficiency now has no other obvious disease as its cause. Absence of ACTH secretion (pituitary disease) will also cause adrenal insufficiency but the lack is principally in hydrocortisone—again, a predictable finding from what has been learned above.

The treatment of adrenal insufficiency is relatively simple once the diagnosis is made. The patient should receive either a glucocorticoid, such as cortisone or prednisone, or a mineralocorticoid, such as deoxycorticosterone or Florinef, or both, depending on what is needed. Hydrocortisone and aldosterone are not usually used, largely because of cost.

Another group of adrenal diseases is lumped into a class called congenital adrenal hyperplasia. Although presumably congenital, or present at birth, the disease may be so mild that the patient does not see a physician until adulthood. These diseases all show a relative deficiency of hydrocortisone, aldosterone, or both, yet the adrenals are larger than normal, for the actual cause of the disease lies in the metabolic pathways of the adrenal gland itself. One or another of the enzymes that catalyze hydrocortisone synthesis is deficient, the most common being a 21-hydroxylase deficiency. The result is poor hydrocortisone secretion, increased ACTH secretion, and, since the adrenal cells still grow in response to ACTH, adrenal hyperplasia. Because of the enzymatic block, steroid synthesis tends to shift to other pathways; as more testosterone than usual is secreted, the patient may therefore come to the physician either complaining of hirsutism (extra hair) if adult or with pseudohermaphroditism (in this instance, a girl who looks like a boy) if in childhood. Diseases such as this are good arguments for being familiar with the metabolic pathways shown in

Figure 20. The treatment is straightforward and is the same as for adrenal insufficiency; one gives a glucocorticoid, a mineralocorticoid, or both, depending on the needs of the patient.

Too much hydrocortisone results in Cushing's syndrome, first described by Cushing in 1912 and later, more definitively, in 1932. The patient is usually somewhat obese, with a rounded face, and often has a high blood glucose, osteoporosis, calcium stones in the kidney, plethora (a reddish face and neck), high blood pressure, and other conditions. Occasionally the patient is pigmented, which state strongly suggests a pituitary or hypothalamic origin of the disease. Those who have adrenal hyperplasia usually have more ACTH in the plasma than they should; again, the hypothalamus or pituitary is indicated as the true site of disease. The disease may also be due to an adrenal tumor, a specific pituitary tumor, peculiar cancers that secrete ACTH, or, perhaps most commonly an incautious physician's prescribing too much of a good thing.

Treatment of Cushing's syndrome depends on the cause. If it is due to taking too much corticoid as medication, one simply stops doing so. If it is due to an adrenal tumor, surgery often cures the disease. When excessive ACTH secretion is the problem, one may aim heavy-particle radiation at the pituitary area, remove the pituitary, remove both adrenal glands, or give a drug which blocks hydrocortisone synthesis. The last treatment is still experimental, and the first two, though effective, are limited in application for one reason or another. Bilateral total adrenalectomy is the preferred therapy at the moment; however, in the near future this preference may change to drug therapy or heavy-particle radiation of the pituitary.

Other kinds of adrenal tumors, which are often cancerous, may produce too much estrogen or too much testosterone. For obvious reasons, tumors making too much estrogen are usually recognized in males and are associated with loss of the usual man's hair distribution, smaller testes, enlargement of the breasts, and a loss of sexual drive. These are feminizing tumors and are not common. In the same way, tumors secreting too much testosterone are usually discovered in women. The patients have hirsutism (increased hair) and develop more masculine traits (virilization) such as male-pattern balding, increased muscle strength, male distribution of pubic hair, etc. A fair fraction of adrenal cancers, however, are not functional, do not secrete hormones, and therefore are found only when the expanding mass causes symptoms. Treatment of these tumors is essentially surgical at the moment, although some are responsive to certain adrenal blocking agents.

Adrenal tumors secreting testosterone are rare. Hirsutism, on the other hand, is a common complaint in women. Many if not most have no discernible endocrine disease. Of the rest, a few have an adrenal tumor and a few have an ovarian tumor secreting testosterone. A goodly number of hirsute women, perhaps more than we now think, have a partial enzymatic defect of steroid-producing tissue. Hirsutism with an adrenal enzymatic defect has just been mentioned (p. 74). The same thing may happen in the ovary with a block in the conversion of testosterone to estradiol and a resulting excess in testosterone secretion (pp. 154–155).

A primary excess of aldosterone secretion (primary hyperaldosteronism or Conn's syndrome) is usually due to a benign tumor of the adrenal cortex. It should be suspected in anyone with high blood pressure, particularly if hypokalemic alkalosis—low serum potassium and high serum bicarbonate and pH—is also present. Other findings are a slight elevation of serum sodium, a moderate increase in total body sodium and in plasma volume, and wasting of potassium and magnesium in the urine, usually without edema. From our discussion of aldosterone, one would be able to predict all these findings except the one that brought the patient to attention in the first place, the hypertension. The aldosterone seems to be the cause of the hypertension since removal of the tumor is likely to remove the hypertension as well, but how aldosterone causes elevated blood pressure is not clear.

Treatment of primary hyperaldosteronism is straightforward: removal of the offending tumor. Sometimes the tumor is not easy to find, but removal is essential for cure. If one wants to avoid surgery (for whatever reason), medical treatment is worth a try. The actions of aldosterone, including all the abnormalities of primary hyperaldosteronism, can be blocked with spironolactone, a synthetic steroid. The synthesis of aldosterone can be blocked with heparin or one of its analogues; these agents probably act by local binding of calcium which is needed for aldosterone synthesis. None of the heparinoids are yet approved by the FDA for this use.

## BIBLIOGRAPHY

*General*

Eisenstein, A. B. (*Ed.*). *The Adrenal Cortex.* Boston: Little, Brown, 1967.
Soffer, L. J., Dorfman, R. I., and Gabrilove, J. L. *The Human Adrenal Gland.* Philadelphia: Lea & Febiger, 1961.

*Aldosterone and Sodium*

Blair-West, J. R., Coghlan, J. P., Denton, D. A., Goding, J. R., Wintour, M., and Wright, R. D. The control of aldosterone secretion. *Recent Progr. Hormone Res.* 19:311, 1963.
Boyd, G. W., Landon, J., and Peart, W. S. Radioimmunoassay for determining plasma-levels of angiotensin II in man. *Lancet* 2:1002, 1967.

Brodie, A. H., Shimizu, N., Tait, S. A. S., and Tait, J. F. A method for the measurement of aldosterone in peripheral plasma using ³H-acetic anhydride. *J. Clin. Endocr.* 27: 997, 1967.

Fimognari, G. M., Fanestil, D. D., and Edelman, I. S. Induction of RNA and protein synthesis in the action of aldosterone in the rat. *Amer. J. Physiol.* 213:954, 1967.

Johnston, C. I., Davis, J. O., Howards, S. S., and Wright, F. S. Cross-circulation experiments on the mechanism of the natriuresis during saline loading in the dog. *Circ. Res.* 20:1, 1967.

Rector, F. C., Jr., Martinez- Maldonado, M., Kurtzman, N. A., Sellman, J. C., Oerther, F., and Seldin, D. W. Demonstration of a hormonal inhibitor of proximal tubular reabsorption during expansion of extracellular volume with isotonic saline. *J. Clin. Invest.* 47:761, 1968.

Sharp, G. W. G., and Leaf, A. Studies on the mode of action of aldosterone. *Recent Progr. Hormone Res.* 22:431, 1966.

Thurau, K., Schnermann, J., Nagel, W., Horster, M., and Wahl, M. Composition of tubular fluid in the macula densa segment as a factor regulating the function of the juxtaglomerular apparatus. *Circ. Res.* 20, 21 (Suppl. II):79, 1967.

Vallotton, M. B., Page, L. B., and Haber, E. Radioimmunoassay of angiotensin in human plasma. *Nature* (London) 215:714, 1967.

Vander, A. J. Control of renin release. *Physiol. Rev.* 47:359, 1967.

## Hydrocortisone

Dahmus, M. E., and Bonner, J. Increased template activity of liver chromatin, a result of hydrocortisone administration. *Proc. Nat. Acad. Sci. U.S.A.* 54:1370, 1965.

Demura, H., West, C. D., Nugent, C. A., Nakagawa, K., and Tyler, F. H. A sensitive radioimmunoassay for plasma ACTH levels. *J. Clin. Endocr.* 26:1297, 1966.

Estep, H. L., Island, D. P., Ney, R. L., and Liddle, G. W. Pituitary-adrenal dynamics during surgical stress. *J. Clin. Endocr.* 23:419, 1963.

Garren, L. D., Ney, R. L., and Davis, W. W. Studies on the role of protein synthesis in the regulation of corticosterone production by adrenocorticotropic hormone in vivo. *Proc. Nat. Acad. Sci. U.S.A.* 53:1443, 1965.

Karaboyas, G. C., and Koritz, S. B. Identity of the site of action of 3', 5'-adenosine monophosphate and adrenocorticotropic hormone in corticosteroidogenesis in rat adrenal and beef adrenal cortex slices. *Biochemistry* (Washington) 4:462, 1965.

Kenney, F. T., and Kull, F. J. Hydrocortisone-stimulated synthesis of nuclear RNA in enzyme induction. *Proc. Nat. Acad. Sci. U.S.A.* 50:493, 1963.

Lefer, A. M. Influence of corticosteroids on mechanical performance of isolated rat papillary muscles. *Amer. J. Physiol.* 214:518, 1968.

Orth, D. N., Island, D. P., and Liddle, G. W. Experimental alteration of the circadian rhythm in plasma cortisol (17-OHCS) concentration in man. *J. Clin. Endocr.* 27:549, 1967.

Riley, G. A., and Haynes, R. C., Jr. The effect of adenosine 3',5'-phosphate on phosphorylase activity in beef adrenal cortex *J. Biol. Chem.* 238:1563, 1963.

Sandberg, A. A., and Slaunwhite, W. R., Jr.    Transcortin: A corticosteroid-binding protein of plasma: V. In vitro inhibition of cortisol metabolism. *J. Clin. Invest.* 42:51, 1963.

Urquhart, J., and Li, C. C.    The dynamics of adrenocortical secretion. *Amer. J. Physiol.* 214:73, 1968.

Yates, F. E., and Urquhart, J.    Control of plasma concentrations of adrenocortical hormones. *Physiol. Rev.* 42:359, 1962.

# 6. The Sympathetic Nervous System and the Adrenal Medulla

These changes—the more rapid pulse, the deeper breathing, the increase of sugar in the blood, the secretion from the adrenal glands—were very diverse and seemed unrelated. Then, one wakeful night, after a considerable collection of these changes had been disclosed, the idea flashed through my mind, that they could be nicely integrated if conceived as bodily preparations for supreme effort in flight or in fighting.

—WALTER B. CANNON,
*The Way of an Investigator*

WHEN Thomas Addison described adrenal insufficiency in the mid-nineteenth century, the idea that the disease was in fact an adrenal disorder was not immediately popular. However, by the end of the century it had won acceptance; the adrenal gland, moreover, was established as being essential for life. An intensive search for the "adrenal hormone" did not lead directly to the corticoids but nevertheless greatly contributed to our understanding of the adrenal gland.

## HORMONES OF THE ADRENAL MEDULLA AND SYMPATHETIC NERVOUS SYSTEM

In 1894 Oliver and Schafer showed that an adrenal extract raised the blood pressure—the first observed physiologic effect of an adrenal substance. Shortly thereafter, *epinephrine* became the first hormone ever to be isolated (Abel, 1898), crystallized (Takamine, Aldrich, 1901), and synthesized (Stolz, 1904). Since epinephrine raises blood pressure and since patients with Addison's disease have low blood pressure, it seemed logical to attribute the disease to a lack of epinephrine. Many then thought epinephrine to be *the* adrenal hormone and required for life.

Further work on the adrenal gland, particularly studies using extracts of the adrenal cortex, proved this idea wrong. We now know that the adrenal medulla and epinephrine are not that critical. How-

79

ever, a broader viewpoint is needed to avoid thinking that epinephrine and similar substances have no role to play. The adrenal medulla is only part of the entire sympathetic nervous system, the whole of which might be looked upon as one large, extensive, neuroendocrine organ.

Besides epinephrine, the adrenal medulla contains *norepinephrine*. Both substances are *catecholamines*, so called because of the amine side chain and the catechol-like hydroxylated benzene ring. Outside the adrenal medulla, epinephrine is scarce. Norepinephrine, on the other hand, is found wherever there are sympathetic nerve endings and in the central nervous system, or in practically every tissue of the body. Norepinephrine is somewhat of an endocrine anomaly since its structure was known and synthesized 30 years before anyone knew it was a hormone, as finally established in 1946 by von Euler. We may live perfectly well without the adrenal medulla but we would have difficulty in simply standing up if it were not for norepinephrine and the sympathetic nervous system.

The classic work on the physiology of these hormones was done by Walter Cannon beginning in 1911, and his idea that the catecholamine hormones are responsible for emergency reactions ("fright, fight, flight") is still generally accepted.

In the *adrenal medulla*, epinephrine and norepinephrine may be made in different cells, but this is not certain, nor is it clear whether they are secreted separately. The adrenal medulla contains about 10 mg of epinephrine and norepinephrine—80% epinephrine and only 20% norepinephrine. The sympathetic *nerve endings* have little epinephrine and for practical purposes contain only norepinephrine. Consequently, while the adrenal contains mostly epinephrine, in the body as a whole there is much more norepinephrine than epinephrine. The heart, for example, is so rich in sympathetic nerve endings, and therefore in norepinephrine ($0.64\ \mu g/g$), that it might be considered an endocrine organ as well as a pump.

Most of the catecholamines in tissue are located in granulated vesicles. In the adrenal these are called chromaffin granules. Smaller granules or vesicles are found in the sympathetic nerve endings. In addition to the catecholamines, the adrenal granules contain ATP and an RNA-protein, either or both of which may bind the catecholamines in the granules. The nerve vesicles probably have a roughly similar composition with a norepinephrine/ATP ratio of 4/1. Of course, in the nerves there is little epinephrine; one finds instead norepinephrine and dopamine in about equal amounts. The nerve and adrenal vesicles also differ in that the nerve vesicles seem to bind norepinephrine more tightly.

### Biosynthesis of Catecholamines

The granules of the sympathetic nerve endings and the adrenal medulla are essential for the synthesis of the catecholamines. The hydroxylation of dopamine occurs in the granules; without them, neither norepinephrine nor epinephrine could be made. Recent work suggests that the enzyme tyrosine hydroxylase is also largely associated with some cellular particles. If so, while many believe tyrosine hydroxylase to be rate limiting in this synthesis, the actual rate-limiting step may be the ability of tyrosine to get to the site of the enzyme in the particle. The biosynthetic pathway is similar in the adrenal medulla and in the nerve endings with the exception of the last step, which occurs only in the adrenal medulla (Fig. 29).

The last reaction, which completes the synthesis of epinephrine, occurs in the cytoplasm of the adrenal medullary cells. S-Adenosylmethionine acts as the carrier for the methyl group. Hydrocortisone coming from the contiguous adrenal cortex is apparently essential for optimal activity of the N-methyl transferase enzyme; hydrocortisone could therefore act as a regulator of epinephrine synthesis.

### Secretion and Metabolism of Catecholamines

Secretion of the catecholamines from adrenal medulla and sympathetic nerve seems to be almost entirely under nervous control via subcortical and probably nonhypothalamic brain centers and sympathetic preganglionic fibers. Angiotensin II and bradykinin may contribute to adrenal epinephrine secretion. Release and the resulting physiologic effects are *rapid*, consistent with Cannon's hypothesis.

The *mechanism* of secretion in the adrenal, and presumably in the nerve endings, is fairly clear. Acetylcholine released from the preganglionic fiber causes an increased calcium influx into the cell and into the intracellular granules. The calcium influx in turn somehow causes the release of the catecholamines. The entire contents of the granule or vesicle are released, i.e., catecholamines, protein, and ATP. The ATP

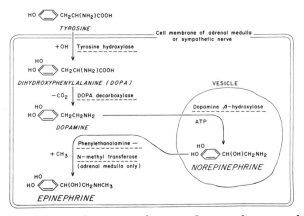

FIG. 29.    Biosynthesis of norepinephrine and epinephrine in the adrenal medulla and sympathetic nerve. Enzymes are underlined by broken lines.

released may actually play a role in the further release of catecholamines from the same or nearby vesicles. While most of the contents of the vesicles wind up outside the cell, the vesicular membrane stays behind as an empty saccule in the cell.

The secretion process is not just that; it is rather a balance between release of catecholamines from the granules and cells and uptake of catecholamines by the same granules. Here there is a significant difference between the adrenal and nerve granules: The release of catecholamines is much faster from the nerve granules than from the adrenal ones; in vitro at body temperature, the former can release half their norepinephrine in 7 minutes while the latter take about 100 minutes to do the same. The rapidity of release by the nerve granules allows a rapid response by the organism to whatever stress has been applied.

The *blood levels* vary widely depending on the state of the individual. The levels usually quoted are in the following range:

epinephrine      0.06 µg/liter (or $4 \times 10^{-10}$ M)
norepinephrine    0.3 µg/liter (or $2 \times 10^{-9}$ M)

More recent measurements are lower, the disagreement being largely due to technical problems. At any rate, there is more norepinephrine than epinephrine. Furthermore, since venous norepinephrine always seems to be greater than arterial norepinephrine (0.4 µg/liter vs. 0.3 µg/liter), some norepinephrine is probably being secreted all the time. Most of it, of course, comes from the sympathetic nerve endings, with those in the heart contributing a fairly large fraction.

Both epinephrine and norepinephrine are *rapidly metabolized*, lasting only a few seconds in the circulating blood. In most tissues, particularly the liver and kidney, the initial step is methylation of the 3-hydroxyl group via the enzyme O-methyl transferase. This results in the formation of *metanephrine* and *normetanephrine* from epinephrine and norepinephrine, respectively. These compounds may then be conjugated and excreted as such, or both may be oxidized by monoamine oxidase to an identical compound, *vanillyl mandelic acid* (3-methoxy-4-hydroxymandelic acid or VMA) (Fig. 30).

In the urine, only 2% to 5% of the secreted catecholamines is found unchanged. This amounts to at most 100 µg per day, of which 80% to 85% is norepinephrine. About 20% to 25% of the catecholamines metabolized each day is found in the urine as metanephrine and normetanephrine while perhaps 30% to 50% is found as VMA. Clinical testing usually depends on the assay of these urinary metabolites or on the measurement of the unchanged catecholamines in the urine.

### Norepinephrine in the Nerve Endings

Because of their peculiar location in nerve endings, the catecholamines released to the blood correlate only roughly with their physio-

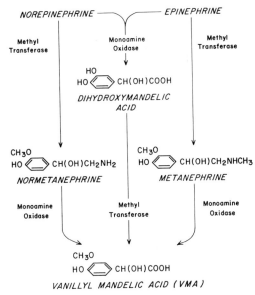

Fig. 30. Breakdown of epinephrine and norepinephrine, the end products appearing in the urine (for amounts, see text).

logic activity. Release to blood and subsequent effects on distant tissues provide an appropriate way of discussing the catecholamines of the adrenal medulla—or, for that matter, any typical hormone. It is not necessarily a good way to describe events occurring in and near the sympathetic nerve endings, where the hormone may reach and stimulate its effector site without ever being in the blood stream.

Here in the nerve endings there seem to be two "pools" of norepinephrine. The smaller consists of the scant amount of cytoplasmic norepinephrine not in the vesicles (no more than 10% to 20%) plus a small amount of that in the vesicles. The latter is probably the norepinephrine most recently synthesized or taken up by the vesicles. This is the *active pool*. It shows a fast turnover and is more easily released on sympathetic nerve stimulation. The bulk of vesicular norepinephrine appears to be in a relatively *inactive pool*, which has a slow turnover, is not easily released after nerve stimulation, and mixes only slowly with the first, more active pool. These pools are of course conceptual and cannot be rigidly located anatomically, but the concept serves to explain the observed physiologic data.

The concentration of norepinephrine in the sympathetic nerve endings is rather high, about 1 mg/g of nerve endings, which is approximately $6 \times 10^{-3}$ M. Perhaps as little as 1% is actually free and outside the vesicles in vivo (the 10% to 20% noted above is based on in vitro studies after the granules have been ground up and possibly altered).

Several things can happen to the norepinephrine in the nerve ending. Most important physiologically is the *active pool*. When its release is stimulated, some of the free norepinephrine of the active pool directly stimulates nearby effector sites without getting into the blood stream at all. Although it is of great importance, probably only a small amount of the synthesized norepinephrine is ever involved in this reaction. The rest of the released active pool norepinephrine is:

Actively taken up again by the vesicles, particularly if the concentration of free norepinephrine in the vesicle is high, *or*

Metabolized to normetanephrine by nearby tissue O-methyl transferase (the nerve ending does not have this enzyme), *or*

Finds its way into the blood unchanged, eventually acting on distant tissues and being metabolized as noted above.

*Note then that the vesicles are not simply storage sites for norepinephrine but are actively involved in its synthesis, release, and uptake.*

The norepinephrine of the larger, *inactive pool* probably plays little physiologic role except under unusual circumstances, such as severe depletion of tissue norepinephrine. This norepinephrine, composing the bulk of that found in the vesicles, is not easily released with sympathetic nerve stimulation. Most is slowly metabolized in the nerve ending without ever being released as free norepinephrine. The nerve endings contain monoamine oxidase in their mitochondria, in contrast to the absence of O-methyl transferase. The monoamine oxidase converts the norepinephrine to dihydroxymandelic acid, which can get into the blood stream directly or be converted to VMA by nearby tissue O-methyl transferase. Ultimately, most of the metabolized norepinephrine appears in the urine as VMA.

It is easy to see that a large amount of norepinephrine can be metabolized without having the blood level rise to any degree, and also that the amount of VMA excreted may have little to do with the actual physiologic activity of norepinephrine.

## ACTIONS OF THE CATECHOLAMINE HORMONES: CONCEPT OF $\alpha$ AND $\beta$ RECEPTORS

The actions of the catecholamines are manifold; it is not clear whether some of them are true physiologic effects of the endogenous hormone or are apparent only at excessive "pharmacologic" levels. Here, we will try to limit the discussion to the former. In general, hydrocortisone and appropriate amounts of thyroid hormone are needed for a good response to the catecholamines by the responding tissues.

In view of Dr. Cannon's idea that these hormones are important in the "fright, flight, fight" types of responses to stressful situations and since they are rapidly released upon sympathetic nerve stimulation, it makes sense teleologically to expect the actions of epinephrine and norepinephrine to be reasonably quick. And indeed this seems to be the case.

One of the main sites of action is the *cardiovascular system. Norepinephrine* will generally increase vascular tone and causes *vasoconstriction* (except in the heart and brain) of arterioles. *Epinephrine* generally causes *arteriolar dilation.* Thus, norepinephrine increases total peripheral resistance and epinephrine decreases it.

Ahlquist proposed two different kinds of receptor sites in the tissues that respond to catecholamines. By definition, in the case of vascular smooth muscle, the *alpha* (α) type responds to norepinephrine and mediates contraction of vascular smooth muscle and the *beta* (β) type responds to epinephrine and mediates relaxation of vascular smooth muscle. There are drugs which specifically block the norepinephrine-induced vasoconstriction and are thus α-adrenergic blocking agents; other drugs, which prevent vasodilation after epinephrine, are the β-adrenergic blocking agents. By extension, various other nonvascular actions of epinephrine and norepinephrine have been classified as α or β in type, largely by determining which type of blocking agent inhibits the action. For example, both epinephrine and norepinephrine cause a faster heart rate by increasing the automaticity of the pacemaker cells. This is neither vasoconstriction nor relaxation. Epinephrine is more potent in this action, but both epinephrine and norepinephrine are blocked by a β-adrenergic blocking agent. The α-adrenergic blocking agent has no effect. Thus catecholamine-induced tachycardia is classed as a β-adrenergic response. In such an instance norepinephrine acts as a weak β-adrenergic stimulant rather than as an α-adrenergic stimulant.

Under some circumstances epinephrine is apparently both an α- and a β-stimulator—obviously a cause for confusion if one is trying to classify a particular response. A synthetic catecholamine, isoproterenol, is a β-stimulator with practically no α-adrenergic action; it is therefore a better agent for typing a response as α or β. The same problem exists to a lesser degree with norepinephrine, and other synthetic catecholamines are purer α-stimulators. Even with the synthetic agents, however, a lengthy review by Himms-Hagen recently concluded that some adrenergic responses cannot be confidently classified. Perhaps the classification scheme is too rigid; nevertheless, it does help in understanding many of the major effects of the catecholamines.

It has been shown lately that, in many instances not involving the blood vessels, an α-adrenergic response is ultimately an inhibitory one and associated with lower cyclic AMP synthesis, while β-adrenergic responses are stimulatory and the tissues show evidence of increased cAMP synthesis. Once again, cAMP acts as an intracellular mediator of hormonal stimulation. As noted above, the effects of catecholamines are optimal only in the presence of hydrocortisone and thyroid hormone. It seems likely that thyroid hormone enhances the ability of catecholamines to stimulate cAMP synthesis (in β-adrenergic responses) while hydrocortisone somehow allows the cAMP to act as a stimulant. However, since these particular details are known for only a few adrenergic responses, it is perhaps a bit early to generalize.

The catecholamines have other pertinent actions. Both epinephrine and norepinephrine increase blood pressure, venous tone, and strength of muscular contraction. Epinephrine raises systolic blood pressure despite the fact that it lowers total peripheral resistance because of the associated tachycardia and increased cardiac output. Norepinephrine, of course, is a vasoconstrictor and would be expected to increase blood pressure; this effect may be enhanced by a simultaneous drop in plasma bradykinin since the latter generally acts as a vasodilator. Epinephrine also causes increased sweating. Putting all these actions together, one can see how the catecholamines mediate the rapid changes seen in anybody when exposed to an acute stress.

During an acute stress there is an increase in ACTH secretion; some have thought this to be due to epinephrine, but it is probably an associative rather than a causal relationship.

There are several *metabolic effects*, which are partly interrelated. Two of the oldest observations are that injections of epinephrine and norepinephrine stimulate an *increase in oxygen consumption* (Barcroft and Dixon, 1906) and that epinephrine in particular *increases the blood glucose* (Zuelzer, 1901).

The latter *hyperglycemic response* is due to a β-adrenergic effect on the liver, although there is some doubt whether this is the case in humans. This was, in fact, the first hormonal response shown to be mediated by cAMP (Rall, Sutherland, Berthet, 1957). The catecholamines first cause a rise in cAMP, which activates phosphorylase. The phosphorylase then enhances the breakdown of glycogen and the ultimate result is that glucose is sent by the liver into the blood (Fig. 31).

For some years now the general thought was that epinephrine causes hyperglycemia, which in turn increases glucose oxidation, and that higher glucose oxidation causes the increase in oxygen consumption. Unfortunately, epinephrine, at the levels found in the plasma, does not seem to increase glycogenolysis or the glucose output by the liver. This makes it more difficult to explain the greater oxygen consumption in an acutely stressed animal or patient on the basis of an epinephrine-mediated rise in blood glucose. It does not necessarily mean that the sympathetic nervous system has nothing to do with glycogenolysis in

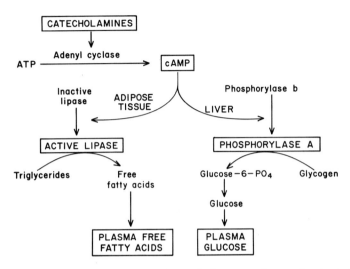

Fɪɢ. 31. Some metabolic effects of catecholamines: the mechanism of stimulation of lipolysis and glycogenolysis.

vivo; impulses from the central nervous system could travel down through the sympathetic nervous system to the liver, there causing glycogen breakdown and glucose release (this was suggested over 100 years ago by the work of Claude Bernard). Furthermore, the catecholamines can raise the blood glucose by other means. Both epinephrine and norepinephrine can increase glucose absorption from the gut; epinephrine inhibits insulin secretion (the inhibition is an α-response by the pancreatic islet); and it may inhibit net glucose uptake by skeletal muscle under some circumstances. The outcome of these actions would be a rise in blood glucose. So, by one means or another, the catecholamines and the sympathetic nervous system raise the blood glucose in a stressful situation, but it may not be via an epinephrine-enhanced hepatic glycogenolysis.

The heart, skeletal muscle under certain conditions other than those just noted, adipose tissue, and probably the brain show an increased glucose uptake with epinephrine which again makes sense teleologically since these are essential tissues to an emergency response and the brain at least has a relatively specific requirement for glucose. Furthermore, some evidence supports the idea that increased glucose oxidation is indeed the reason why oxygen consumption rises with the catecholamines. Nevertheless, because of the difficulties with glycogenolysis already mentioned and because of some discrepancies in the action of different catecholamines on oxygen consumption and blood glucose, many have searched for another explanation for the increased use of oxygen.

A likely answer lies in the adipose tissue. Epinephrine and norepinephrine *increase lipolysis* or the release of free fatty acids (FFA) from adipose tissue. The effect is a β-adrenergic response mediated by an increase in cAMP which in turn increases the lipase activity of the adipose cell (Fig. 31). Since the sensitivity of adipose tissue is probably greater than that of liver, the effect on lipolysis is more likely to be a physiologic one. Moreover, the response is apparently not present only with stress, for the sympathetic nervous system seems to exert a tonic, constant, stimulating effect on FFA release. There is a need for both hydrocortisone and thyroid hormone for lipolysis to be optimal. Thyroid hormone, for example, specifically enhances adenyl cyclase— not the activity of lipase—and therefore increases the amount of cAMP. The effect on lipolysis can be modulated and diminished by prostaglandin E (PGE); PGE probably lowers the concentration of cAMP by inhibiting adenyl cyclase.

Once the FFA are in the plasma after the catecholamines have acted, they are to a very considerable extent taken up and oxidized by those tissues capable of doing so, e.g., skeletal muscle and heart muscle. Within a few minutes one finds an increased oxygen consumption and a decreased respiratory quotient (which last could not be explained by greater glucose oxidation). Thus, the calorigenic effect of epinephrine and norepinephrine may be largely indirect (calorigenic = causing increased oxygen consumption) and secondary to a rise in fatty acid consumption.

Even here, however, the answers are not complete. Recent experiments with rats have shown that catecholamines may cause a small increase in oxygen consumption without a rise in plasma FFA, that an infusion of FFA need not be calorigenic, and that catecholamines may increase oxygen consumption without lowering the respiratory quotient. Furthermore, in humans there is good evidence that only part of the calorigenic effect of catecholamines can be explained by the effect on lipolysis.

So the old observation remains incompletely explained more than 60 years after it was made. Perhaps the effect of catecholamines on oxygen consumption is due to a combination of factors, namely, (1) an increase in glucose oxidation, (2) a larger increase in fatty acid oxidation, and (3) some other effect, perhaps a direct effect on mitochondrial oxidation. Since practically nothing is known about the last possibility, it is at least worth investigating.

In some unknown way mental alertness is also increased, as seen in anyone who has been frightened. This might possibly be related to an increased glucose utilization by the brain.

## CONTROL OF CATECHOLAMINE SECRETION

Control of epinephrine and norepinephrine secretion does not exist in the usual "negative feedback" sense. The response to the catecholamines, e.g., a rise in plasma FFA, does not inhibit the secretion of the hormones, partly, no doubt, because these hormones are almost an intrinsic part of the nervous system and so are more likely to be controlled by nervous impulses rather than by responses of receptors. Another reason secretion is not inhibited is the transient nature of the response to an emergency; secretion would cease after a short time with no need for any negative feedback if the stimulus or stress were present only briefly. There is probably some basal secretion of epinephrine and norepinephrine from the nerve endings and adrenal medulla, but most of the secretion is stimulated by various stresses, including noise, pain, fright, apprehension, new environment, exercise, cold, hypoglycemia, fasting, blood loss, and physiology exams, which have all been shown to increase epinephrine and norepinephrine secretion. In a sense, then, almost any change in the external or internal environment, unless the brain recognizes it as completely usual and not out of the ordinary, can increase epinephrine and norepinephrine output. If one includes all such stimuli in a feedback scheme, then one can speak of a negative feedback control mechanism.

There are, however, what might be termed internal negative feedback control mechanisms which are examples of end-product inhibition; that is, the biosynthesis of the catecholamine hormones in the nerve endings and adrenal medulla is inhibited by higher concentrations of the hormones themselves. For instance, a slight excess of norepinephrine inhibits the activity of tyrosine hydroxylase in the sympathetic nerves of tissues such as the heart, thus cutting down the synthesis of norepinephrine until its concentration drops. In the adrenal medulla both epinephrine and norepinephrine inhibit tyrosine hydroxylase. Since the activity of tyrosine hydroxylase is probably the limiting factor in the biosynthesis of these hormones, anything that regulates its activity will in turn regulate the biosynthesis.

This mechanism of biosynthetic control may be directly involved in permitting a relatively prolonged secretion of norepinephrine, at least in some tissues. Stimulation of the sympathetic nerves supplying the heart and adrenal medulla results in an increased activity of tyrosine hydroxylase; the effect, however, may be indirect. Stimulation of the nerve releases catecholamines from the nerve ending or adrenal medulla; the lower concentration of catecholamines removes the end-product inhibition. The result is an increase in the activity of tyrosine hydroxylase and in the synthesis of catecholamines. The effect is not universal, since stimulation of the sympathetic nerves to the spleen does not increase norepinephrine synthesis. But in those nerve endings (and in the adrenal medulla) where the phenomenon occurs, it seems to be a useful mechanism for maintaining the supply of catecholamines at least as long as the nerve is being stimulated.

Another example of end-product inhibition, applicable only to the adrenal medulla, is the inhibition of N-methyl transferase by epinephrine. Thus, epinephrine itself, as well as hydrocortisone, regulates the activity of this enzyme, the one inhibiting it and the other enhancing it.

## CLINICAL NOTE

The catecholamines are most commonly used to raise the blood pressure of patients in shock. Some controversy prevails at present as to which catecholamine is best; norepinephrine has been used for years, but others may be better and safer in certain circumstances. This treatment is pharmacologic, however, and is utilized not because the patient lacks catecholamines but because it just happens to make him better (we hope).

The abnormality most likely to be seen in catecholamine secretion, though still uncommon, is the increased secretion from a *pheochromocytoma*. This tumor, usually though not always found in the adrenal gland, may secrete either norepinephrine or both epinephrine and norepinephrine. It is suspected most often because of hypertension. The best test for the tumor is a measurement of urinary catecholamines, urinary VMA, urinary metanephrines, or any combination of these. Surgery is the treatment for most patients although some drugs will also work, such as α-methyl paratyrosine, an inhibitor of tyrosine hydroxylase.

Rather rarely one sees a patient with a defect of the sympathetic nervous system who is unable to make or secrete sufficient catecholamines. He complains of dizziness, light-headedness, or actual fainting on standing up. The trouble is that there is a sharp drop in blood pressure on standing, and the patient is said to have orthostatic hypotension. The diagnosis depends on showing in some way poor secretion of catecholamines; one treatment is to give catecholamine-like drugs with longer durations of action than the catecholamine hormones themselves, such as ephedrine.

## BIBLIOGRAPHY

Ahlquist, R. P. Development of the concept of alpha and beta adrenotropic receptors. *Ann. N.Y. Acad. Sci.* 139:549, 1967.

Himms-Hagen, J.    Sympathetic regulation of metabolism. *Pharmacol. Rev.* 19:367, 1967.

Opitz, K., and Chu, H.    Zur stoffwechselsteigernden Wirkung der Brenz-catechinamine. (A study of the calorigenic action of catecholamines.) *Naunyn Schmiedeberg. Arch. Pharm. Exp. Path.* 259:329, 1968.

Potter, L. T.    Role of intraneuronal vesicles in the synthesis, storage, and release of noradrenaline. *Circ. Res.* 20, 21 (Suppl. III):13, 1967.

Spector, S., Gordon, R., Sjoerdsma, A., and Udenfriend, S.    End-product inhibition of tyrosine hydroxylase as a possible mechanism for regulation of norepinephrine synthesis. *Molec. Pharmacol.* 3:549, 1967.

von Euler, U. S.    Some factors affecting catecholamine uptake, storage, and release in adrenergic nerve granules. *Circ. Res.* 20, 21 (Suppl. III):5, 1967.

# 7. The Thyroid Gland

> Yet we may one day be able to
> shew, that a particular material
> principle is slowly formed [by
> the thyroid gland], and par-
> tially kept in reserve; and that
> this principle is also supple-
> mentary, when poured into the
> descending cava, to important
> subsequent functions.
> —T. W. KING,
> *Observations on the Thyroid
> Gland* (*1836*)

A GOITER, or enlarged thyroid, has probably been recognized as a human disease for thousands of years. The patient may at the same time
be short and of low intelligence, a cretin or hypothyroid dwarf. It was
some time, however, before the connection was made between the
clinical diseases we now recognize as forms of hypothyroidism and the
fact that in these diseases the thyroid gland is deficient in hormonal
secretion.

Although the gland is prominent enough to have been recognized
no doubt as a separate structure from early times, the word *thyroid,*
or "shield-shaped," was not used to name it until 1656 (Thomas Whar-
ton) and originally described the cartilage, only later being applied to
the gland. A suspicion that the thyroid might secrete something existed
as long ago as 1836 (King), and in 1850 Curling described probably the
first cases of proved thyroid deficiency associated with signs such as
poor cerebral development and excessive fat deposits. However, the
times were not yet ripe for the idea. In 1873 Gull noted a disease in
adults very similar to cretinism in children; the disease was called
myxedema by Ord in 1877. A few years later, in 1882 and 1883, the
Reverdins and Kocher described the changes that occurred in patients
after total thyroidectomy. Even so, when Semon proposed in 1883 that
the signs and symptoms seen in cretinism and myxedema and after
thyroidectomy were similar and all due to thyroid deficiency, he was
ridiculed.

That same year, 1883, the Clinical Society of London appointed a
committee, with Ord as its chairman, to investigate the problem. Their
now classic report, published in 1888, fully confirmed Semon's proposal
and firmly established thyroid deficiency or hypothyroidism as a clinical
entity. Three years later, when Murray successfully treated hypothyroidism with extracts of the thyroid glands of sheep, the importance of
the thyroid hormones was universally recognized. Ever since then, the
thyroid gland and its hormones have held the interest of both physicians and laboratory investigators.

## Hormones of the Thyroid Gland

In 1895, while looking for phosphorus in thyroid extracts, Baumann accidentally found iodine. Magnus-Levy showed the same year that thyroid extracts increased oxygen consumption, or metabolic rate. Knowing that the thyroid gland makes a hormone (or hormones) and that in all likelihood iodine is somehow involved (because of the large amount found in the gland relative to other tissues), many workers spent almost the next 60 years before the hormones we know as *thyroxine* and *triiodothyronine* were chemically defined with certainty. The metabolic effect is still being investigated to this day.

On Christmas day, 1914, Kendall first isolated thyroxine. However, the structure he proposed was wrong and was corrected by Harington in 1926. Dakin had also deduced the correct structure but withdrew his work in favor of Harington, who with Barger synthesized the hormone the following year. Kendall (1928) realized, however, that the thyroid gland might contain a more active substance in addition to thyroxine; the search for another thyroid hormone ended in 1952, when triiodothyronine was isolated (Gross and Pitt-Rivers, Roche) and shortly thereafter synthesized. It is three to five times as active as thyroxine but is secreted in smaller amounts.

Thyroxine is abbreviated as $T_4$ because of the four iodine atoms on the thyronine nucleus. In like manner, triiodothyronine is called $T_3$. The three iodine atoms are specifically located at the 3, 5, 3' positions in $T_3$; because of a three-dimensional structure, not shown in the chemical formula in Figure 32, the 3' and 5' positions are not equivalent and any change in the location of the iodine atoms in $T_3$ will cause a marked decrease in activity. In both $T_3$ and $T_4$ the alkyl group, as well as the iodine, is important for proper hormonal activity.

The thyroid gland also contains *thyrocalcitonin*, a hormone that lowers serum calcium. It is made by cells located in the thyroid but

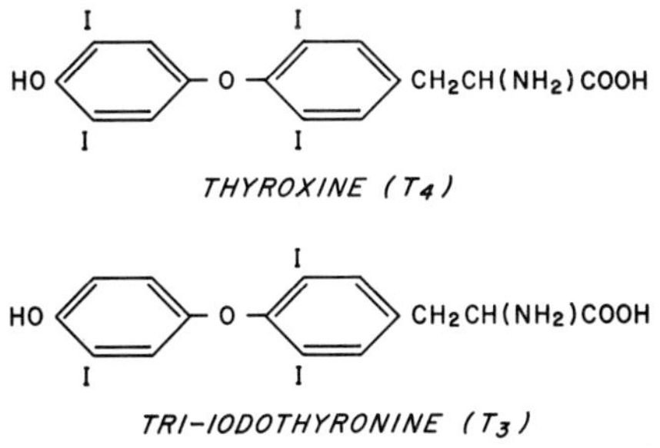

FIG. 32.    Two-dimensional diagram of thyroxine and triiodothyronine. (The molecular structures are actually three-dimensional.)

different in embryologic origin from the cells making $T_3$ and $T_4$. The physiology of thyrocalcitonin is discussed later (see Chap. 8).

## IODINE AND THE THYROID GLAND

*Iodine* is the crucial element and the key to the thyroid hormones. It was unknowingly (in the form of seaweed or burnt sponge) used in the treatment of goiter for perhaps several thousand years and has consciously been used for this purpose for over 150 years. Since there is relatively little iodine in the body or in the usual diet, in the course of evolution the thyroid gland developed into a structure for both concentrating iodine and making thyroid hormone.

Iodine in the diet is generally converted to iodide, which is completely absorbed by the gut. The average diet has 100 to 200 μg, but amounts vary a great deal from place to place. Eggs and milk are important sources. The actual requirement is not too well known, but a human can remain in balance on an intake of about 70 μg. Total body iodine is about 20 to 50 mg, with 8 to 15 mg in the thyroid, 0.5 to 2.0 mg in blood, and the remainder mostly in muscle. A small amount of the iodine circulating in the blood is in the form of iodide anion (about 0.2 to 0.3 μg/100 ml); during the course of a day some of the circulating iodide is lost in the urine and some is taken up by the thyroid.

The thyroid gland selectively and actively *takes up iodide*. Not only does it maintain a chemical gradient for iodide ($I^-$) against the serum of 25 to 1 (the so-called thyroid/serum or T/S ratio) but it also continues to take up iodide against both the chemical gradient and an electrical gradient of 50 to 90 mv, the cell interior being electrically negative to the surrounding interstitium. The initial step in the uptake of iodide may be a complexing of iodide with phospholipids in the cell membrane. The mechanism is called the *iodide pump* and is located at the outer, nonfollicular border of the thyroid cell. The function of this pump is dependent on intact cells, and it is energy dependent, requiring oxygen. An ATPase in the cell membrane may be involved somehow in supplying energy for the process. Apparently, the active functioning at the same time of a thyroid sodium pump, with a requirement for potassium, is also necessary, although why is not clear. Other factors important to optimal iodide uptake are the size and the single negative charge of the iodide ion and perhaps phospholipid synthesis in the thyroid cell membrane.

The term iodide "trap" is often used to describe this concentrating mechanism, but this is a bit misleading since a *trap* implies a one-way process. In reality it is a two-way process with the equilibrium in favor of the thyroid. The follicular structure of the thyroid is not required for iodide uptake because the isolated cell can do it, but the follicular structure does seem to enhance it. The iodide pump under special circumstances can concentrate up to a T/S of 500.

The thyroid must take up between 75 and 150 µg of iodide per day to replace what is lost, but it need not all come from the diet for, as we shall see, much is derived from iodide recirculated within the body.

## SYNTHESIS OF THYROID HORMONES

Once in the gland, the iodide is bound to organic compounds within seconds, and some is *synthesized to thyroxine in minutes*. The steps include (1) oxidation of iodide, (2) formation of monoiodotyrosine (MIT), (3) formation of diiodotyrosine (DIT), and (4) coupling of the iodotyrosines to form $T_3$ and $T_4$.

1. The iodide must first be oxidized; only then can it attach to a TYR residue *in the thyroglobulin molecule* to form *monoiodotyrosine*. Hydrogen peroxide, formed in mitochondria from molecular oxygen, is the oxidant. In the thyroid microsomes a *peroxidase* containing a hematin-like coenzyme catalyzes the conversion of iodide to oxidized iodide. Several hemoprotein peroxidase preparations have been made with molecular weights of the enzyme varying from 64,000 to 104,000. The oxidized form of iodide is not really known but may be a protein-bound sulfenyl iodide (Fig. 33).

2. The next step is the iodination of tyrosine. Most of the tyrosine that is iodinated is actually a tyrosyl residue in the intact thyroglobulin molecule, which has a molecular weight of 650,000. Possibly tyrosine or iodine in some kind of free radical form is involved here. No one is quite sure whether this step is really a different reaction with a different enzyme (the postulated "tyrosine iodinase") or whether both steps 1 and 2 are part of a single overall reaction. The latter is becoming a more likely possibility since the isolated hemoprotein peroxidases in vitro can catalyze the oxidation of iodide *and* the formation of MIT from either tyrosine or thyroglobulin. Either the enzyme preparation is im-

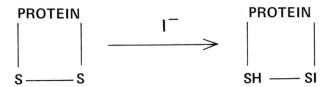

FIG. 33.   One possible form of oxidized iodide in the thyroid gland.

pure or a tyrosine iodinase is unnecessary. The iodine is now considered to be *organic iodine*, as opposed to the inorganic anion. Some of the MIT is in a free form, but most is formed from tyrosine already bound in thyroglobulin.

Tyrosine may itself contribute to $H_2O_2$ formation, by first being decarboxylated to tyramine, which is then oxidized, yielding $H_2O_2$. Furthermore, MIT may also undergo decarboxylation, forming iodotyramine; in this instance, iodotyramine is an inhibitor of the amine oxidase that converts tyramine to $H_2O_2$. The whole system may act as an internal control mechanism for regulating the synthesis of thyroid hormones (Fig. 34). Tyrosine and its reactions may therefore be as important as those of iodine since tyrosine not only is a precursor of MIT but may assist in the oxidation of the iodide.

3. The third step is the formation of 3,5-diiodotyrosine (DIT) by the rapid addition of an iodine at the 5 position, probably by the same mechanism as that forming MIT. Again, a small amount of DIT is free, but most is in the thyroglobulin. The hemoprotein peroxidase in vitro can catalyze the synthesis of DIT as well as MIT and do it almost as quickly; the substrate may be either thyroglobulin or MIT.

4. The last step is the coupling of the iodotyrosines to form $T_3$ and $T_4$. $T_4$ is formed from two molecules of DIT and $T_3$ from one molecule of DIT and one of MIT. $T_3$ is *not* formed by removing an atom of iodine from $T_4$. These hormones are made much more slowly than MIT and DIT. While the coupling process is generally thought to be catalyzed by an enzyme different from the peroxidase, several experiments have suggested that the isolated peroxidase discussed above can in fact catalyze the complete synthesis of $T_4$ or even that coupling is not enzymatic at all but simply depends on the proper oxidizing conditions.

Coupling occurs in the thyroglobulin molecule just as does iodina-

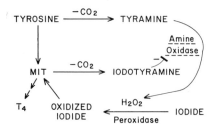

Fig. 34. A possible thyroid system for controlling the synthesis of MIT and therefore thyroid hormones. A bar and − indicate inhibition.

tion. The process is rather mysterious since it is hard to imagine the contortions of the thyroglobulin molecule required to get the iodinated tyrosines into the right position and then, still within the thyroglobulin molecule, have an enzymatic formation of an ether linkage with the removal of an alanine side chain. This nevertheless may be just what happens. Some possible explanations:

1. One of the iodinated tyrosines might become an intermediate free radical, enhancing the reactivity of the molecule.
2. Some of the small amount of free DIT may be oxidatively deaminated to 4-hydroxy-3,5-diiodophenylpyruvic acid, better known as DIHPPA. DIHPPA would then be oxidized to *3-OOH-DIHPPA*, which combines with a bound DIT to form $T_4$ or with a bound MIT to form $T_3$. Recent work does not support the idea of free substances playing a significant role in $T_3$ or $T_4$ synthesis, and it is hard to show the presence of DIHPPA in the thyroid gland. Still, a small amount of DIHPPA can be found in the thyroid (rat) and, if it turned over rapidly, could be important.
3. If $T_3$ and $T_4$ are formed from iodotyrosines within the thyroglobulin molecule without the aid of free forms or free radicals, perhaps the juxtaposition of iodotyrosines in different protein chains of thyroglobulin enhances the reaction.

In addition to all the things going on in thyroglobulin, it has been shown lately that a very small amount of $T_4$ can be made from iodide without going through thyroglobulin. Perhaps this derives from the free iodotyrosines present or from a different iodoprotein that turns over more rapidly.

*Thyroglobulin* (TGB) (650,000 mol. wt.) is a 19S-globulin and a glycoprotein. It has four protein chains and contains 10% carbohydrate by weight. It is synthesized in the thyroid cell and is relatively slowly released into the colloid in the center of the thyroid follicle. The peptide chain is synthesized first at one site in the cell, then the carbohydrate is added, and finally the tetramer is formed. Iodination probably occurs before the molecule is completely put together but at a different cellular site from that of the protein synthesis. While synthesis of the large molecule and of thyroid hormone generally occur in parallel, though the former is slower, thyroid hormone can still be formed even when protein synthesis—including that of thyroglobulin —is completely blocked. So the synthesis of $T_4$ and $T_3$—or the iodination process—is not dependent on the synthesis of TGB or of protein.

$T_3$ and $T_4$ are *stored* in the thyroglobulin of the follicular colloid; in the normal thyroid there is enough hormone to last several months even if no more is made. The large molecular size of TGB makes it a good storage form since it is too large to get out of the thyroid follicle unhydrolyzed.

Quantitatively, TGB makes up about one-third of the entire weight of the thyroid gland; there are about $8 \times 10^{18}$ molecules of TGB in the gland. Estimates of its iodine content vary from 0.2% to 0.9% with somewhere between 6% and 17% of the 115 tyrosyl residues in each molecule being iodinated. There are enough technical problems so that the values are only approximate averages of the available data, but in each TGB molecule there are about:

> 6.0 molecules of MIT
> 5.0 molecules of DIT
> 0.3 molecule of $T_3$
> 1.0 molecule of $T_4$

Note that iodination is not peculiar to TGB. Many proteins can be iodinated and show thyroid hormone activity; farmers have often used iodinated casein as a cheap substitute for thyroid extract. TGB is iodinated in part because it is located in a peculiar place, the thyroid gland, and because its molecular structure is adapted to easy iodination.

To sum up, then, the tyrosines are by and large iodinated and coupled to form the thyroid hormones while they are in peptide bonds in the thyroglobulin molecule (Fig. 35).

### Cellular Site of $T_4$ Synthesis

The fact that these reactions take place in the thyroglobulin molecule does not mean that they take place in the follicular lumen despite the

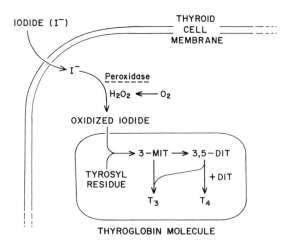

FIG. 35. Overall synthesis of thyroid hormones. For abbreviations, see text or Appendix II.

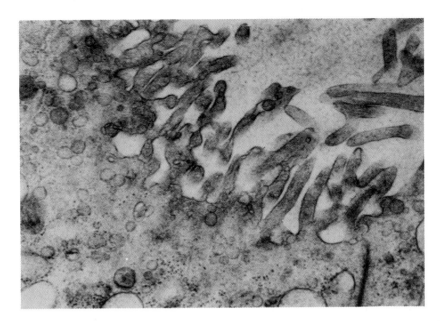

FIG. 36.   The border between the thyroid follicular cell and the colloid in the center of the follicle. Note the many microvilli. In this case TSH is probably stimulating the gland. (From S. L. Wissig, in R. Pitt-Rivers and W. R. Trotter, Eds., *The Thyroid Gland*, Vol. 1. London: Butterworths, 1964.)

fact that most of the thyroglobulin is there. For example, some animals make $T_4$ and have no follicles; and $T_4$ can be made by isolated thyroid cells in the absence of follicles. Nevertheless, it does seem that the follicular structure enhances $T_4$ formation. The most likely site for the iodination of thyroglobulin and $T_4$ formation is at the *border of the follicular cell and lumen*. Electron microscopic work has shown that this border is not a simple membrane; it is a highly infolded structure with many microvilli (Fig. 36).

## SECRETION OF THYROID HORMONES

To release $T_3$ and $T_4$ to the blood, TGB must be broken down. The TGB most recently synthesized is broken down first. Probably some kind of *protease* is involved, and the whole process is enhanced by TSH. MIT and DIT must be released as well, yet not much of either of these compounds is normally found in the thyroid vein. Why not? Because there is a *deiodinase* in the thyroid which rapidly removes the iodine from MIT and DIT but does not affect $T_3$ and $T_4$. This intrathyroid iodide can then be resynthesized into TGB. As much as one-third of the thyroid iodine may turn over each day in this way. The deiodinase reaction serves to prevent iodine loss from the body because if MIT and DIT were secreted they would be lost in the urine. The reaction is stimulated by TSH; this is probably the reason TSH causes the release of a certain amount of iodide ($I^-$) from the thyroid gland into the blood, some of the iodide spilling out instead of being re-utilized.

Thus one may have two iodide "pools" within the thyroid gland, one derived from outside the gland via the iodide pump and the other from within the gland via the deiodinase reaction. There is some experimental evidence that these "pools" exist and they may be of significance, since the iodide derived from deiodination seems to be more easily reutilized into TGB. However, the "two-pool" concept, implying that all iodide in the gland is not freely exchangeable, is not universally accepted.

The two-pool idea has also been applied to the organic iodine in the gland in an attempt to explain certain experimental findings. The smaller pool, about 5% of the organic iodine, is the one mainly involved in the deiodination reaction, and the bigger pool, containing the large bulk of thyroid iodine, is the origin of the $T_4$ and $T_3$ secreted by the gland. Remember, though, that "pools" are concepts designed to fit experimental findings; a new experiment may change everything.

Each day $T_4$, $T_3$, some iodide, a small amount of thyroglobulin, and perhaps a bit of MIT and DIT are secreted by the thyroid gland. Estimates of total organic iodine secretion range from 50 to 120 μg per day. Most of it is $T_4$, and about 60 to 150 μg of $T_4$ are secreted each day (note that $T_4$ is two-thirds iodine by weight; thus 67 μg of $T_4$-

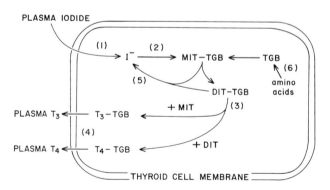

FIG. 37.   Conversion of plasma iodide to plasma thyroid hormones by the thyroid gland. Sites of possible metabolic defects in the overall process are numbered. For abbreviations see text or Appendix II.

iodine equals 100 μg of T$_4$). T$_3$ was thought to account for only about 5% of the daily thyroid secretion of iodine, but recent work suggests that the amount is larger. While most publications on the subject make the tacit assumption that T$_4$ is the main thyroid hormone, if certain reasonable assumptions are true there may be 25 to 50 μg of T$_3$ (representing 12 to 25 μg of iodine) secreted each day. As we have said, T$_3$ is three to five times more active than T$_4$. Under normal conditions, then, T$_3$ is probably as important metabolically as T$_4$.

The whole process by which plasma iodide is converted into plasma thyroxine can be represented as in Figure 37. This sequence of events is of direct clinical importance, since metabolic blocks or abnormalities can occur at any of the numbered points 1 to 6. It is easily seen that thyroxine deficiency could result from any of these blocks.

## THYROID HORMONE METABOLISM

### Plasma Binding and Turnover

In the blood, T$_4$ and T$_3$ are largely *bound to protein*. The known binding proteins are:

1. Thyroxine-binding globulin (TBG). Described in 1952, human TBG is a specific globulin migrating between the α$_1$ and α$_2$ peaks of globulin on electrophoresis; hence the name, *inter-α-globulin*. Its molecular weight lies somewhere between 50,000 and 80,000; different workers report different results. It is present in small amounts but binds T$_4$ very strongly (the $K_A$ is on the order of $10^9$ to $10^{10}$) and accounts for perhaps 45% to 60% of the bound T$_4$ in plasma. T$_3$ is bound only one-third as strongly as T$_4$ to TBG; about 75% of plasma T$_3$ is bound to TBG.
2. Thyroxine-binding prealbumin (TBPA). Described in 1958, this protein is so named because it migrates ahead of the albumin on electrophoresis. It has a weaker affinity for T$_4$ than TBG (the $K_A$ is $2$–$3 \times 10^8$), but there is more of it; thus it binds somewhere around 15% to 35% of the plasma T$_4$. T$_3$ does not bind to TBPA at all. TBPA decreases nonspecifically with many illnesses.
3. Albumin. The binding power of albumin is the lowest of the three (the $K_A$ is $2$–$6 \times 10^5$), but there is so much of it that it still accounts for about 15% of the plasma T$_4$. Albumin binds T$_3$ even less strongly, but since TBPA does not bind T$_3$ at all, albumin accounts for about 25% of bound T$_3$. Albumin also binds whatever MIT and DIT are found in plasma.

Plasma T$_4$ has a half-life of seven days, and about 10% turns over each day; plasma T$_3$ has a half-life of 1.5 to 3.0 days and turns over faster, about 30% per day. $T_3$ turns over faster in part because it is bound less tightly to protein.

## Physiologic Activity and Plasma Levels

The important point of all this is that the protein-bound hormone is in all likelihood physiologically inactive. Only the small amount of hormone that is *free* and not bound to protein can readily get out of the blood and act on the tissues of the body. *The free $T_4$ and $T_3$ are the physiologically active hormones.* Of course, the truly active hormone is that which gets into the responsive cells, but it is impractical to measure and in general the levels of free hormone seem to correlate nicely with the physiologic state.

Nevertheless, the total *protein-bound iodine* (PBI) does change with gross changes in physiologic state and is a useful clinical test. The normal value is 6 µg/100 ml (range 4 to 8 µg/100 ml). Almost all of this iodine is $T_4$, and thus the plasma level of $T_4$ is about 9 µg/100 ml or $1.2 \times 10^{-7}$ M. However, 99.94% of this is bound to protein. There is then only 5 mµg/100 ml of free $T_4$ or about $7 \times 10^{-11}$ M. Measurement of free $T_4$ would be even more valuable clinically than that of the PBI but at present it is a rather expensive test.

If most of the PBI is $T_4$, clearly the level of $T_3$ is low. Measurements of total and free $T_3$ were attempted for many years, but the attempts met with limited success until 1967. At that time some elegant work by the Naumans and Werner showed that the total plasma $T_3$ is 0.3 µg/ 100 ml, that 99.5% is protein bound, and that the level of plasma free $T_3$ is 1.5 mµg/100 ml or $2.4 \times 10^{-11}$ M.

## Distribution

The distribution of all the $T_4$ outside the thyroid gland shows that only part of it is in the plasma despite the intense binding by plasma proteins. About 25% is in the plasma and another 25% in the rest of the extracellular fluid, which also has some TBG in it. More interesting is that the liver and other tissues apparently take up $T_4$ and keep it in a form exchangeable with plasma $T_4$; thus the liver contains 15% to 30% of the $T_4$ outside the thyroid and other tissues have the rest. In the liver the $T_4$ is inside the cells but is nevertheless readily exchangeable with the plasma $T_4$ by direct transfer between plasma-binding proteins and hepatic binding sites. As regards pregnancy, little $T_4$ or $T_3$ usually crosses the placenta; the fetus must therefore supply almost all its own thyroid hormone. However, with high doses of $T_3$ to the mother, significant amounts of $T_3$ do get into the fetal circulation.

## Catabolism

Many peripheral tissues not only take up $T_4$ and $T_3$ but deiodinate them as well. Exactly which tissues do so is a matter of controversy at present, but the liver and kidney are important and for the body as a whole this is the main reaction for $T_4$ and $T_3$ degradation. One possible mechanism: $T_4$ binds to tissue, and a single iodine is removed, leaving bound $T_3$. Another iodine is then removed, leaving bound DIT. The DIT is then released and deiodinated by another system.

Much of the iodine, released as iodide, goes back through the blood to the thyroid while some appears in the urine. The latter accounts for 85% to 90% of the daily iodine loss from the human body, amounting to about 60 μg of urinary iodide per day if the person is in balance on an intake of 70 μg per day.

Some of the thyroid hormones, however, are not deiodinated but conjugated. In man, conjugation seems to be a relatively minor metabolic pathway for thyroxine. Conjugation usually occurs at the hydroxyl group with the formation of sulfates or glucuronides. For the most part, the liver does the conjugating, and the conjugates then go into the bile and the gut. Precisely what happens to the conjugated hormones in the human intestine is not at all clear. Some are hydrolyzed back to $T_4$ and $T_3$ and reabsorbed from the small intestine. The reabsorption may be limited by an uncharacterized protein in the lumen of the gut, which may explain why only about one-half to two-thirds of $T_4$ and about 80% of $T_3$ given by mouth is actually absorbed.  There is no doubt that this enterohepatic circulation exists; its importance is another question.

Another part of the conjugated $T_3$ and $T_4$ appearing in the intestinal lumen is not resorbed. These compounds pass through to the colon, where they are hydrolyzed by bacteria. Since the colon apparently does not absorb $T_3$ or $T_4$, the hormones appear as such in the stool. The iodine lost in this way seems to be lost even when there is a deficiency of iodine; it amounts to about 15% of the daily iodine loss or about 10 μg per day when in balance on an intake of 70 μg per day.

## THE ACTIVE FORM OF THYROID HORMONES

It seems most reasonable that the free, unbound, and unconjugated hormones in plasma are the ultimately active forms, but there is no certainty regarding the active form of the hormone in the responding tissues. Although the problem was considered by Kendall in the late 1920's, most of the uncertainty arose because of the discovery of $T_3$. Since it is more potent than $T_4$, some workers have felt that something other than $T_4$ is the actual stimulator of tissues. Some of the ideas are:

1. $T_3$ is the active form. The theory is that $T_4$ is deiodinated by tissue to $T_3$ which is still bound to tissue. Having acted, $T_3$ is then deiodinated, and the remaining biologically inactive material is

further metabolized. $T_3$ itself, of course, is active without further change.

2. Since some tissues can deaminate and decarboxylate $T_3$ to tri-iodothyroacetic acid (TRIAC), and TRIAC is indeed active in some systems, some have thought that TRIAC is the active form, a theory adding to the features of 1.

3. Many tissues can deiodinate $T_4$. If deiodination were necessary for metabolic activity, then $T_3$ might be the active substance, as in 1. Or the released iodine could be the active substance, $T_4$ and $T_3$ simply being an elaborate iodine carrier. It has been recently shown, however, that deiodination does not increase oxygen consumption per se.

The whole problem is not solved. For the moment $T_4$ and $T_3$ *must be regarded as active per se* until better evidence is available.

## ACTIONS OF THYROID HORMONES

Removal of the thyroid in the young mammal has many effects. The major easily observable ones are:

1. Low oxygen consumption or a decreased metabolic rate
2. Poor growth
3. Poor maturation and development in many body systems
4. Poor central nervous system development and function

If thyroid hormone is given before too much damage has occurred, *all these effects will be reversed*. Except that it is more potent and seems to act more quickly, $T_3$ seems to be identical in action to $T_4$.

### Oxygen Consumption, Protein Synthesis, and Increased Metabolism

The effect on oxygen consumption, where $T_4$ increases the use of oxygen, is still not completely understood. This is called the *calorigenic* effect and was first noted and defined by Magnus-Levy in 1895. It is a long-term effect since it takes many hours to reach a peak, although some change may be seen after an hour or two. This is the only readily available measure of the influence of $T_4$ on *tissues* and clinically is still used as a thyroid function test (the basal metabolic rate or BMR).

How does $T_4$ increase oxygen consumption? $T_4$ is known (see below) to speed up a number of metabolic processes, and since the effect on oxygen consumption is a somewhat delayed one, it may be that the increase in oxygen consumption is simply the end result, the primary effect of $T_4$ being whatever it does to increase the affected processes. The converse approach, however, that $T_4$ specifically affects oxygen consumption, with many of the other effects following from this, is the one usually taken.

$T_4$ enhances free fatty acid (FFA) release by increasing the sensitivity of adipose tissue to the effects of catecholamines, an effect mediated by adenyl cyclase and cyclic AMP, and perhaps in some more direct way. $T_4$ sometimes increases circulating epinephrine. Fatty acids and epinephrine are themselves calorigenic and could mediate a similar action of $T_4$. However, even when there is no fatty acid or catecholamine response to $T_4$, $T_4$ still increases oxygen consumption. Thus, the increased oxygen consumption due to $T_4$ may be in part mediated by catecholamine effects and fatty acid oxidation, but something else is going on as well.

A major focus of research has been the mitochondria, the locus of oxidative phosphorylation and the enzymes of the respiratory chain. Large amounts of $T_4$ have been shown to act directly on liver mitochondria to cause a swelling which in turn causes partial uncoupling of oxidative phosphorylation. The uncoupling results in an increased oxygen consumption in order to maintain the energy supply at the normal level. Some sort of structural change in the mitochondria, then, may be the direct cause of the uncoupling and the increased oxygen consumption.

However, although swelling and uncoupling of oxidative phosphorylation occur in liver mitochondria, they are not seen in the mitochondria of skeletal muscle despite the fact that $T_4$ causes an increased oxygen consumption in both. Further, the amounts of $T_4$ needed to cause uncoupling are far above those found naturally in vivo. Swelling of the mitochondria and uncoupling of phosphorylation cannot explain the calorigenic action of $T_4$.

The mitochondria are nevertheless the likely site of the action of $T_4$ on oxygen consumption. With physiologic doses of $T_4$ one can show a definite increase in the $T_4$ content of mitochondria, suggesting a specific localization of $T_4$. At these levels of $T_4$ one can see a rise in phosphorylation along with the increased oxygen consumption. Thus the P/O ratio (oxidative phosphorylation) does not change, and $T_4$ may actually cause an increase in available energy supply.

It has also been shown that the mitochondria of liver use oxygen in at least two ways, described as stage 3 respiration (the oxygen used in the ADP $\rightarrow$ ATP conversion process) and stage 4 or controlled respiration (the oxygen consumed after ATP is formed). $T_4$ added to mitochondria from hypothyroid rats did not change stage 3 respiration but did tend to keep stage 4 respiration at normal levels. Furthermore, the fact that the changes are reversed by removing the $T_4$, provided it is removed early enough, suggests that $T_4$ has a direct effect on the mitochondrial respiration not mediated—at first—through other mechanisms such as increased protein synthesis. It is fair to say that the picture is not yet clear but that $T_4$ acts somehow to affect the mitochondrial membrane with a resulting increase in oxygen use.

Is the effect on oxygen consumption the primary action of $T_4$? Many have suggested it is. A major problem in accepting this idea is the existence of tissues which seem to require $T_4$ for optimum function but which show no increase in oxygen consumption when it is given. These include organs such as the brain, spleen, and testes. The brain of a young and growing animal *does* respond to $T_4$ with an increase in oxygen consumption but the adult brain does not. Yet cerebral function in the adult is patently impaired in thyroid deficiency, so $T_4$ must do something important without raising the amount of oxygen used. Either $T_4$ and $T_3$ have more than one basic action or the effect on oxygen consumption is secondary to a more fundamental action.

A recent candidate for the primary action of $T_4$ is its effect on protein synthesis. Some work has been published showing that actinomycin blocks the oxygen consumption effect of $T_4$, the implication being that $T_4$ acts primarily to increase nuclear and messenger RNA synthesis. An effect closer to the site of protein synthesis has somewhat better experimental backing. For example, many different enzymes, both in the mitochondria and cell sap, are affected by $T_4$. The findings with different enzymes are somewhat contradictory when in vivo work is compared with in vitro changes; nevertheless, these experiments do show widespread effects of $T_4$ on protein synthesis.

Thyroxine increases protein synthesis in muscle, kidney, reticulocytes, and liver. In most tissues, it also increases protein breakdown, including that of collagen, thus increasing protein turnover, and it does so in the very tissues that show no effect on oxygen consumption—the brain, spleen, and testis. The immediate locus of the effect on protein synthesis seems to be the ribosome or the polysome. In the liver $T_4$ acts on the polysome to increase amino acid incorporation into protein, perhaps by increasing the transfer of activated amino acids (bound to sRNA) to the protein-synthesizing site. In reticulocytes $T_4$ may somehow act on the ribosome to increase amino acid incorporation by enhancing elongation of the peptide chain.

Over the short term, at least, in many instances the increased protein synthesis need not be preceded by a higher RNA synthesis—another indication of direct action on protein synthesis. While the effect may be on the ribosome or polysome, as suggested above, $T_4$ could also somehow stabilize existing mRNA and have the same end result. Furthermore, over longer time periods (one to two days) or under different experimental conditions there *is* a rise in RNA synthesis, and the stimulatory effect on several enzyme activities in the cell sap (glycogen synthetase, some enzymes of the glycolytic pathway) can be blocked by actinomycin D.

Can any of this be related back to the mitochondria? The answer is, at least partly, yes. For one thing, the increased transfer of amino acids to protein in liver ribosomes and polysomes seems to be secondary to the release of an unknown factor from the mitochondria. For another, at physiologic levels of $T_4$ or $T_3$ one can see in liver mitochondria an increase in total protein synthesis and in the activity of enzymes such as α-glycerophosphate dehydrogenase. These effects on the mitochondria of liver might be related to an increased synthesis of the enzymes of the respiratory chain; they at least seem to correlate well with the changes in oxygen consumption by the intact liver. However, with appropriate manipulations one can show some increase in mitochondrial oxygen consumption with $T_4$ when there is no increase in either amino acid uptake or synthesis of respiratory chain components.

To sum up: It is entirely possible that thyroid hormones have major effects on both oxygen consumption and protein synthesis which, though generally parallel, are sometimes independent of one another. Under certain conditions one can show an effect on mitochondrial oxygen consumption without affecting protein synthesis. In some tissues there is an increase in protein synthesis and no effect on oxidation. The increased protein synthesis may be secondary to a mitochondrial effect whether or not oxygen consumption changes, or it may be in part mediated through a change in mRNA synthesis, or perhaps both mechanisms play a role. In any case the calorigenic effect is not the only effect of thyroid hormone. Finally, while the effect of a normal amount of $T_4$ is an increase in protein synthesis, excessive $T_4$ causes a large increase in protein breakdown leading to muscle wasting and a negative nitrogen balance.

Many other processes are speeded up. Whether these actions are due to the effect on oxygen consumption or protein synthesis or both is not certain, but the general picture is one of increased metabolism. Thyroid hormones stimulate an *increase* in:

1. *Carbohydrate turnover* with increased gluconeogenesis, increased glycogen breakdown (an effect not related to epinephrine) and increased peripheral utilization of glucose. If there is excess $T_4$ the blood glucose can be elevated.
2. *Fat turnover* with increased fatty acid synthesis, mobilization, and oxidation, particularly when there is a relative lack of carbohydrate.
3. *Cholesterol turnover* with an increase in both synthesis and excretion, so that the net result is a loss of cholesterol from the blood and total body.
4. *Milk production* during lactation. These hormones are sometimes used in dairy cattle to increase their yield.

5. *Calcium mobilization* from bone, which is probably due to a direct effect on bone with a resulting increase in bone turnover and may result in an elevation of serum calcium.
6. *Magnesium turnover* with a tendency to increase exchangeable magnesium and to increase intracellular magnesium concentration when total exchangeable magnesium is constant.
7. *Heart rate* and *contractility*. The main action appears to be an increase in the total force produced. Thyroid hormone may stimulate the heart by increasing the amount of, or sensitivity to, catecholamines, although some work suggests that neither is an appropriate explanation.
8. *Total peripheral resistance*, under some conditions, perhaps by increasing the sensitivity to catecholamines (controversial). The rise in systolic blood pressure occasionally seen with excess thyroid hormone is probably due to the action of $T_4$ on the heart.
9. *Red cell production* by the bone marrow—probably a direct effect; important clinically in explaining in part the anemia of hypothyroidism.
10. *Hydrocortisone secretion*, probably due both to a direct effect on the adrenal and to an increased ACTH output. $T_4$ also increases the catabolism of hydrocortisone to cortisone and the reduced metabolites in the liver. The net result is no change in plasma hydrocortisone levels.
11. *Growth hormone secretion*. There is also an increase in the growth stimulation caused by GH. These effects probably account for a good part of the action of $T_4$ in maintaining skeletal growth.

A number of these effects may in fact be a response to the presence of both the catecholamines and thyroid hormone, particularly the effects on glycogen breakdown, fatty acid mobilization, and possibly heart rate. The amount of catecholamines need not be increased, although $T_4$ may increase the amount found in, for example, the heart. What thyroid hormones may do is *increase the sensitivity* of some tissues to the catecholamines. There is reasonable evidence to support this idea if one considers only β-adrenergic responses; note that the effects just mentioned (on glycogen, fat, and the heart) are all β-adrenergic responses. It might be regarded as another fairly basic, though unexplained, action of thyroxine and $T_3$.

*Growth*

The effect on growth and on the other observed deficiencies, all of which are correctable with $T_4$, does not seem well correlated with the effect on oxygen consumption, but that may be because these other effects occur over a much longer time. Regarding growth, one can show (in some species) growth due to $T_4$ without an increase in oxygen consumption. The growth defect is best seen in the patient who has been hypothyroid since birth and not treated. This is the classic cretinous dwarf, now very rare in this country. The influence of $T_4$ on protein synthesis may be important here, and in addition $T_4$ acts by enhancing growth hormone secretion, action, or both.

### Maturation and Differentiation

Maturation and differentiation too are speeded up by thyroxine, and they appear to be different from the effects on growth. Here, not simply enlargement of tissues is involved but a change in structure and organization. For example, growth hormone will cause bones to get longer, but the epiphyses will not calcify and close. $T_4$ will cause bone growth initially, then later help in closing the epiphyses. Another example: in the frog, $T_4$ is needed to transform the tadpole into the adult frog, a process involving both maturation of the animal and differentiation of certain tissues.

### Nervous System Development and Function

The hypothyroid patient is dull, apathetic, and often not mentally alert. If the patient is young and the brain had not completed its development before hypothyroidism occurred, it may never do so even if treated; this aspect of $T_4$'s action may simply be part of the effect on maturation. $T_4$ has then clear-cut importance in the development and function of the central nervous system. Very little is known, however, of how it acts. One can show an increased uptake of thyroid hormone by the young, maturing brain compared to an older one. Thyroxine increases the maturation of brain tissue both in vivo and in vitro, under some conditions without an increase in oxygen consumption. But to date thyroxine has not been shown to have any consistent biochemical effect on the adult brain, and the problem is still with us.

## CONTROL OF THYROID HORMONE
## SECRETION

The main regulator is *thyrotropin* (TSH). The thyroid gland does have some autoregulatory capacity. Thus if the plasma inorganic iodide is low, or the thyroid iodine content is low, the thyroid gland of itself tends to pick up more iodide from the blood, raising the thyroid/serum (T/S) ratio. Furthermore, there are internal control systems. One has been mentioned: regulation of the synthesis of MIT by iodotyramine. Another is the tendency of the thyroid gland to make more $T_3$ and less $T_4$ when faced with a shortage of iodine; since $T_3$ is more potent, more efficient biologic use of the available iodine is thus possible. Nevertheless, without TSH, the thyroid gland simply does not function well, and these other mechanisms play a small role at best and may even be due to the effects of TSH.

### TSH and the Thyroid Gland

The basic effects are similar to those of ACTH on the adrenal cortex: TSH *stimulates thyroid hormone secretion* relatively quickly, and, over the long term, *stimulates growth of the thyroid gland*. A great deal of work has been done to find an action which is early, and therefore perhaps *primary*, and which would account for both the fundamental effects. This work has resulted in a multitude of findings; a selected synthesis of these observations follows.

TSH binds to the thyroid cell at some superficial site. The binding is rather tight ($K_A = 3 \times 10^8$). Since phospholipase C mimics many of the following effects of TSH on the thyroid gland, it has been suggested that, after binding to the cell, TSH changes the phospholipid membrane in some way, thereby causing all the other effects.

Two of the earliest effects of TSH on the interior of the thyroid cell are: (1) an *increase in glucose uptake* and *oxidation*, largely via the hexose-monophosphate shunt (HMP shunt), and (2) an *increase in colloid droplets* in the thyroid follicular cells, representing resorption of colloid from the follicular lumen.

The effect on *glucose oxidation* is duplicated by TPN (NADP). Since TSH increases the TPN content of the thyroid, it has been suggested that TSH increases DPN (NAD) conversion to TPN, that TPN increases glucose oxidation by the HMP shunt, and that all the other effects of TSH follow from this. While the increased ribose synthesis via the HMP shunt may be related to the increased RNA synthesis seen later, in some species (e.g., the dog) the effect on glucose oxidation does not seem to be any earlier than the effect on thyroxine secretion. That the effect of TSH on TPN and glucose metabolism is its primary effect is an idea that must be viewed with caution.

The *increase in colloid droplets* in the thyroid cells represents resorption of colloid from the follicular lumen. Once inside the thyroid cell, the droplets are attacked by lysosomal enzymes, particularly an acid protease, and a short time later there is an increase in thyroxine secretion. Some have suggested that this is the primary effect of TSH, and that many of the metabolic changes in the gland (including the increased glucose uptake) are secondary to the higher cellular activity induced by TSH.

In fact, while neither of these two early effects of TSH can be said with certainty to be the cause of the other, recent work suggests that *both* may be due to the *stimulation of cAMP synthesis* by TSH. Furthermore, in some species TSH increases phospholipid synthesis in the thyroid, which also is mediated by cAMP. Here, then, TSH probably stimulates adenyl cyclase activity in some thyroid cell membrane with a resulting increase in synthesis and concentration of cAMP. Do not accept this whole idea completely, however; the findings are accurate but cannot be clearly shown in all species examined, so that the issue is somewhat clouded and a conclusive statement cannot be made.

For the moment, then, one can assume that TSH binds to a thyroid cell membrane and stimulates cAMP synthesis by activating an enzyme found in cell membranes, adenyl cyclase. Either directly or via cAMP, TSH induces some change in phospholipids, presumably again in thyroid cell membranes. The result is greater oxidation of glucose and resorption of colloid, plus several other effects now described.

1. *Increased sodium uptake,* an effect which is somehow linked to a later increase in iodine uptake.
2. *Increase in thyroglobulin breakdown and thyroid hormone secretion,* which is related to the colloid resorption noted above. Along with this one sees the expected increase in intrathyroid deiodination of MIT and DIT and an increase in iodide release from the gland. Somewhat unexpected is the finding that some of the iodide discharged does not come from thyroglobulin but is iodide just recently taken up by the gland.
3. *Increased synthesis of thyroid hormones* in all its aspects: more peroxidase activity, more MIT and DIT formation, and more synthesis of $T_3$ and $T_4$. Recent experiments suggest this may be an earlier effect than was formerly thought.

Finally, about two or three hours after TSH has been given to a rat (longer in larger species), there is:

4. *Increase in thyroid cell volume,* perhaps the earliest effect related to actual growth of the gland, and in *purine synthesis.*
5. *Increase in iodide uptake,* which is therefore a later, secondary effect of TSH, not primary as was once thought. Normal sodium-potassium flux across the thyroid cell membrane is necessary, suggesting that the TSH effect on phospholipid synthesis may be important here.

In a more general sense, TSH seems necessary for the *follicular structure* of the gland, of obvious importance in the effective storage of thyroglobulin.

How much of all this could be due to a basic effect on protein synthesis? There is a good deal of evidence that TSH has significant effects on protein synthesis. TSH causes a definite increase in amino acid uptake and incorporation into protein. There is an increased synthesis of the protein part of the thyroglobulin molecule. The effects on protein synthesis may in part be mediated by an increase in mRNA synthesis, suggested, for example, by the localization of TSH in the thyroid cell nuclei. However, a number of other facts indicate that the effect on protein synthesis is not primarily via increased synthesis of mRNA. TSH also localizes on the thyroid cell membrane. The synthesis of thyroglobulin protein can continue despite actinomycin; thus the mRNA involved is relatively stable, and constant synthesis of mRNA is not required. More important, puromycin does not seem to block the TSH stimulation of thyroglobulin iodination, thyroxine synthesis, or thyroxine secretion, showing that protein synthesis is not essential for the action of TSH on many aspects of thyroid hormone formation and secretion. The later effects of TSH, on the other hand, may in fact require synthesis of both mRNA and protein for their appearance.

There is some work showing that the effect of TSH on early protein synthesis, i.e., that not requiring mRNA synthesis, depends on the effect on glucose uptake and oxidation. One can then construct conceptually two pathways of action for TSH after it initially causes changes in the thyroid cell membrane. In one direction, a stimulation of glucose metabolism is connected to enhancement of protein, RNA, and eventually DNA synthesis with growth and multiplication of cells. In the other direction, there is a stimulation of thyroid hormone synthesis and release without any necessary connection with the synthesis of protein or nucleic acid. Clearly links exist between the two pathways—for example, protein synthesis must sooner or later be necessary for thyroglobulin synthesis—but the nature of these links is not clear—another area for interested and curious minds.

### Control of the Secretion of TSH and Thyroid Hormones by Negative Feedback

A clear negative feedback relationship between TSH and thyroid hormone secretion was first described in 1931. Simply stated, more $T_4$ lowers TSH secretion and less $T_4$ raises TSH secretion. The former was demonstrated in animals in 1931 and the latter for the first time in man in 1965. Human plasma TSH rises from a normal value of about 1 mμg/ml to 15 mμg/ml or more in primary hypothyroidism.

As with the adrenal cortex, the mechanism is not as simple as that. The hypothalamus plays a role, and one can make a partial analogy with ACTH and the adrenal cortex.

There is a TSH-stimulating site in the hypothalamus–median eminence which is different from sites stimulating the secretion of the gonadotropins and ACTH. This site seems to act as an integrator for nervous system stimuli from many sources, the most immediate being other hypothalamic areas. For example, there are TSH-stimulating and -inhibiting areas in the upper anterior and posterior hypothalamus, respectively. Extracts of the hypothalamus–median eminence contain a TSH-releasing factor which acts on the pituitary, but this material is not yet well defined. It is abbreviated TRF and is different from CRF and LH-RF. Extracted TRF stimulates TSH secretion from the pituitary in several species including man; energy is needed for this stimulation, and it may be mediated by cAMP.

How much control does the hypothalamus have? $T_4$ implanted in the hypothalamus decreases TSH secretion. On the other hand, $T_4$ implanted in the pituitary also decreases TSH secretion and apparently does so more effectively than the hypothalamic implant. Section of the pituitary stalk, eliminating hypothalamic effects, cuts down but does not eliminate either TSH secretion or the ability of $T_4$ to regulate TSH secretion. The transplanted pituitary seems capable of secreting a small amount of TSH. Finally, even if TRF reaches the pituitary, $T_4$ or $T_3$ can block its action on TSH secretion.

The present feeling on the inhibition of TSH secretion by thyroid hormone is, then, that the pituitary plays a major role. The hypothalamus probably exerts a sustained tonic effect on TSH secretion and has a large but not always determining part in the negative feedback inhibition of TSH secretion by thyroid hormones.

What of the reverse—when decreased $T_4$ stimulates TSH production? The mechanism may be just the opposite of the above, but one cannot assume this. The roles of the pituitary and hypothalamus are less clear here, but hypothalamic mediation is probably more important. In animals, a drop in thyroxine secretion increases the amount of TRF in the hypothalamus, and, with the hypothalamus separated from other neural connections, one can show that most of the effect of low levels of $T_4$ in increasing TSH secretion is mediated by the hypothalamus. Moreover, the area of hypothalamus involved is probably different from the area mediating TSH suppression. It is even possible that a third hypothalamic area is involved: one that is sensitive to decreased $T_4$ which then transmits the information to the area responsible for increasing TSH secretion.

What is the true regulator of the hypothalamus and pituitary? Again, the answer is not clear. It probably is the level of plasma $T_4$ and $T_3$. Presumably, the *unbound free hormone* is the significant substance. However, some have thought that something else acts on the hypothalamus and pituitary; the action may somehow be a function of the BMR or even of deiodination of $T_4$. This particular problem arose because changes in TSH secretion did not correlate well with changes in PBI. With the assays for TSH and free thyroxine in plasma now available, it seems that the inverse correlation of plasma TSH and plasma free thyroxine is good; thus, free thyroxine is probably the determinant of TSH secretion. As with hydrocortisone and ACTH, this thought assumes a correlation between plasma levels and biologic effect. It may be that the immediate regulator is the amount of thyroid hormone in the cells of the hypothalamus or pituitary, which in turn happens to correlate well with the level of free hormone in the plasma.

Note that the negative feedback system works only within a certain range. When $T_4$ is totally absent, all tissues slow down, including the pituitary, and TSH secretion, rather than rising, may actually fall; so *some* thyroid hormone is needed for TSH to be secreted at all.

### Secretion of TSH, Stress, and Other Factors

TSH secretion is affected by stimuli which are not involved in the negative feedback system but act by direct central nervous system stimulation, much as various stresses increase ACTH secretion. The effects are generally less rapid, however.

1. In rats, goats, and humans, *cold* increases TSH secretion, an effect necessary for survival, at least in unclothed animals. Since the response is only partially blocked by hypothalamic implants of $T_4$ into the usual TSH-stimulating area, it may in part be a direct reaction on the pituitary. However, it is more likely that a different TSH-stimulating area is involved or that the implanted $T_4$ is overwhelmed by the effect of cold, for the effect is clearly mediated by the hypothalamus. Large hypothalamic lesions do block the effect, as does section of the pituitary stalk, and the effect can be duplicated by local application of cold directly to the hypothalamus.
2. *Emotional stress* can cause increased TSH secretion that is also not inhibited by $T_4$. However, in the rat, the stress of being picked up seems to decrease TSH secretion, perhaps in some way secondary to the increased ACTH secretion occurring at the same time. Circulating catecholamines are apparently not important in increasing TSH secretion.
3. *Light* may indirectly stimulate TSH secretion in some species.
4. The hypothalamic *areas controlling temperature and hunger* are near the TSH hypothalamic areas in the anterior hypothalamus. These areas may influence TSH secretion; all three may work together to supply fuel and maintain body temperature at a proper level.

Other factors affect $T_4$ secretion, but their relationship to TSH secretion is not clear.:

1. *Hydrocortisone* is necessary for normal thyroid function and for optimal $T_4$ action on oxygen consumption. In excess, hydrocortisone may decrease iodine uptake and $T_4$ secretion, possibly by inhibiting TSH action. Or it may act on peripheral tissues to block deiodination of $T_4$, which might result in the above findings. The overall effect in man is minor, and it is often difficult to show any effect.
2. *Estrogen* and perhaps progesterone increase the plasma thyroxine-

binding globulin, causing a transient decrease in free thyroxine and thus a transient increase in TSH output. Estrogen may also have a minor stimulatory effect directly on the pituitary.

3. *Exercise* lowers the plasma free $T_4$, probably by increasing peripheral utilization of $T_4$.
4. *Fasting* decreases $T_4$ secretion.
5. *Aging* may be associated with a decreased $T_4$ turnover.
6. *Iodide* itself in relatively large amounts can cause decreased $T_4$ release and decreased iodine binding.

There is an exception to everything. As expected, removing the pituitary drops TSH secretion and $T_4$ secretion as well. An occasional patient, however, will have apparently normal thyroid function even after complete hypophysectomy. What controls thyroid function under these peculiar circumstances is not clear.

Summing up: Under normal circumstances, TSH is the main regulator of thyroid function. The exact primary effect of TSH on the thyroid is uncertain, but it may well be on the thyroid cell membrane, and cAMP is probably the mediator of the other effects seen. In any case, thyroid hormone secretion is increased. TSH secretion is regulated in turn by the plasma levels of free thyroxine (acting on both pituitary and hypothalamus) and is also increased in response to cold and perhaps other stimuli, the latter responses being mediated by the central nervous system.

## CLINICAL THYROID DISORDERS

Clinically, a good deal of the physiologic information is useful. It helps in the understanding of the common clinical tests of thyroid function:

1. *Radioiodine uptake,* usually measured at 24 hours, measures more than simply uptake since by the end of a full day most of the iodide has been incorporated into thyroglobulin. A shorter test that measures the radioiodine uptake at 10 minutes or two hours more accurately reflects the function of the iodide pump.
2. *Protein-bound iodine* (PBI) test measures exactly that; the PBI is largely $T_4$.
3. *Red cell* or *resin uptake* assays the saturation of the binding proteins.
4. *Basal metabolic rate* (BMR) was mentioned earlier.

If results of these tests are above normal, the patient is usually *hyperthyroid;* if they are below normal, the patient is usually *hypothyroid.* There are exceptions, of course. For example, the radioiodine uptake may be elevated in a patient who is euthyroid (i.e., normal in thyroid hormone secretion) but who has a goiter; the PBI is elevated in pregnancy because of increased binding proteins although the patient is again euthyroid.

One can see how anything which *decreases thyroid hormone secretion* would increase TSH secretion. If $T_4$ secretion continues to be low (hypothyroidism), the persistently elevated TSH secretion would eventually cause an enlarged thyroid, providing the thyroid gland was capable of responding. Any enlarged thyroid is called a *goiter*. For example, iodine deficiency in the diet can cause goiter although if the diet includes seafood and iodized salt, it would not be a likely cause of goiter. Any of the metabolic blocks noted earlier could also produce goiter. Other causes such as inflammatory disease or tumors have a less obvious relation to TSH, but, surprisingly, many patients, including some with metastatic thyroid cancer, apparently have TSH-dependent lesions and therefore improve when given thyroid hormone.

In some patients the increase in thyroid size compensates for the low secretion of $T_4$ and brings the latter up to normal. The patient has therefore *simple goiter* or *euthyroid goiter*. On the other hand, even though large, the thyroid may not be able to make much $T_4$; the patient then has *goiter and hypothyroidism*. Of course, if the thyroid gland is fibrotic and incapable of responding to TSH, there will be no goiter; the patient then has *hypothyroidism without goiter*. Thyroid hormone is the treatment for hypothyroidism and most patients with goiter.

The opposite, *hyperthyroidism* or excessive $T_4$ secretion, leads to some predictable findings. The patients are usually thin because of fat mobilization and protein catabolism. They are weak, probably because of the latter. They sweat a lot because of the increased sympathetic activity and heat production. They prefer the cold because of the increased $O_2$ consumption and heat production. They also have conditions which are not yet well explained: bulging eyes, or exophthalmos, and, rarely, thick, lumpy skin over the shins, or pretibial myxedema. These mysterious changes may have something to do with the *long-acting thyroid stimulator* or LATS, which is thought by many to be the cause of the excessive secretion of $T_4$ in the first place. LATS is a circulating globulin, but why it is present no one knows, although it may be an unusual type of antibody.

Treatment of hyperthyroidism is the removal of the excess $T_4$. One can remove iodine from the diet, thus limiting the thyroid's ability to make hormone, block the iodide pump with thiocyanate or perchlorate, block organification of iodine and coupling of iodotyrosines with propylthiouracil or methimazole (the antithyroid drugs), block release of thyroxine with large doses of iodides, selectively destroy part of the thyroid gland with radioiodide, or remove part of the gland surgically. In most cases, the preferred initial therapy today is propyl-thiouracil.

## BIBLIOGRAPHY

### Physiology

Bastomsky, C. H., and McKenzie, J. M. Cyclic AMP: A mediator of thyroid stimulation by thyrotropin. *Amer. J. Physiol.* 213:753, 1967.

Coval, M. L., and Taurog, A. Purification and iodinating activity of hog thyroid peroxidase. *J. Biol. Chem.* 242:5510, 1967.

Halasz, B., Florsheim, W. H., Corcorran, N. L., and Gorski, R. A. Thyrotrophic hormone secretion in rats after partial or total interruption of neural afferents to the medial basal hypothalamus. *Endocrinology* 80: 1075, 1967.

Hoch, F. L. Early action of injected L-thyroxine on mitochondrial oxidative phosphorylation. *Proc. Nat. Acad. Sci. U.S.A.* 58:506, 1967.

Ingbar, S. H., and Freinkel, N. Regulation of the peripheral metabolism of the thyroid hormones. *Recent Progr. Hormone Res.* 16:353, 1960.

Krause, R. L., and Sokoloff, L. Effects of thyroxine on initiation and completion of protein chains of hemoglobin in vitro. *J. Biol. Chem.* 242:1431, 1967.

Krishna, G., Hynie, S., and Brodie, B. B. Effects of thyroid hormones on adenyl cyclase in adipose tissue and on free fatty acid mobilization. *Proc. Nat. Acad. Sci. U.S.A.* 59:884, 1968.

Myant, N. B., and Witney, S. The time course of the effect of thyroid hormones upon basal oxygen consumption and plasma concentration of free fatty acid in rats. *J. Physiol.* (London) 190:221, 1967.

Nauman, J. A., Nauman, A., and Werner, S. C. Total and free triiodothyronine in human serum. *J. Clin. Invest.* 46:1346, 1967.

Nicoloff, J. T., and Dowling, J. T. Estimation of thyroxine distribution in man. *J. Clin. Invest.* 47:26, 1968.

Nishinaga, A., Cahnmann, H. J., Kon, H., and Matsuura, T. Model reactions for the biosynthesis of thyroxine: XII. The nature of a thyroxine precursor formed in the synthesis of thyroxine from diiodotyrosine and its keto acid analog. *Biochemistry* (Washington) 7:388, 1968.

Odell, W. D., Wilber, J. F., and Utiger, R. D. Studies of thyrotropin physiology by means of radioimmunoassay. *Recent Progr. Hormone Res.* 23:47, 1967.

Pastan, I., and Macchia, V. Mechanism of thyroid-stimulating hormone action. *J. Biol. Chem.* 242:5757, 1967.

Pitt-Rivers, R., and Trotter, W. R. (Eds.). *The Thyroid Gland* (2 vols.). London: Butterworth, 1964.

Schultz, A. R., and Oliner, L. The possible role of thyroid aromatic amino acid decarboxylase in thyroxine biosynthesis. *Life Sci.* 6:873, 1967.

Seljelid, R. Endocytosis in thyroid follicle cells. *J. Ultrastruct. Res.* 18:1, 1967.

Vought, R. L., and London, W. T. Iodine intake, excretion and thyroidal accumulation in healthy subjects. *J. Clin. Endocr.* 27:913, 1967.

Yip, C. C., and Hadley, L. D.   Involvement of free radicals in the iodination of tyrosine and thyroglobulin by myeloperoxidase and a purified beef thyroid peroxidase. *Arch. Biochem.* 120:533, 1967.

## Clinical

McKenzie, J. M.   The long-acting thyroid stimulator: Its role in Graves' disease. *Recent Progr. Hormone Res.* 23:1, 1967.

Means, J. H., De Groot, L. J., and Stanbury, J. B.   *The Thyroid and Its Diseases* (3rd ed.). New York: McGraw-Hill, 1963.

Stanbury, J. B.   The metabolic errors in certain types of familial goiter. *Recent Progr. Hormone Res.* 19:547, 1963.

World Health Organization. *Endemic Goitre.* Monograph Series No. 44. Geneva: W.H.O., 1960.

# 8. The Hormonal Control of Calcium Metabolism

Can these bones live?
—EZEKIEL 37:3

TETANY, or carpopedal spasm, a spastic twitching of the muscle, is a common clinical finding, though not now as common as it once was. Though many physicians carefully described it in the early and middle nineteenth century, they had no clue to the cause. In 1880 Weiss reported that removing the thyroid gland from patients with various thyroid diseases sometimes resulted in tetany. Thus he at least focused attention on the fact that something in the neck was necessary to prevent tetany.

There was indeed something in the neck. Although never connected with tetany or calcium metabolism, the structures we now call parathyroid glands were described in the mid-nineteenth century, well before Weiss's description, but he unfortunately had not heard of them. The most likely reason for this oversight is that none of the descriptions were in humans and none were in "popular" journals. Owen described them in the Indian rhinoceros—not a common laboratory animal—in 1852, Leydig the same year in the salamander, and Remak in the cat in 1855. The year Weiss made his report, Sandström found and nicely described human parathyroid glands and bestowed upon them their present name. However, few knew of his discovery, which was published in Swedish in a relatively obscure journal and the article was not translated into English, for example, until 1938.

So it was not until 1891 that Gley rediscovered the parathyroid glands (in animals), found Sandström's paper, and showed that, if these glands were removed, tetany would occur. He originally thought that both the thyroid and parathyroid glands had to be removed to cause tetany but finally concluded in 1897 (as had Vassale and Generali in 1896) that removal of the parathyroids alone was sufficient.

By 1909 MacCallum and Voegtlin, after showing that injections of parathyroid material reversed the tetany of a parathyroidectomized dog (1905), had hit upon the remarkable discovery that injections of calcium would do the same thing. A great deal of brilliant work was then done by many workers, and for that matter is still being done today, in the study of parathyroid hormone—what it is and how it works. Assays for calcium had to be improved since the bioassay for the hormone depended on them. Better extracts of the parathyroid gland were needed. The crude extract mentioned above was given to dogs; humans were treated with crude preparations as early as 1907. Much better active extracts were made by Hanson (1923–1925), but perhaps the best for many years were those of Collip (1925). Collip

119

combined his extraction procedure with the best calcium assay of the time, thereby making a major impact on parathyroid research with effects that lasted for several decades. In fact, not until 1959 were better preparations of parathyroid hormone made (Aurbach).

The basic facts, now well established, are that lack of parathyroid hormone causes *hypocalcemia* and, if severe enough, *tetany*, and that *parathyroid hormone* (PTH) restores the serum calcium to normal. We now know that parathyroid hormone also affects phosphate metabolism; that *vitamin D*, a "skin hormone," is necessary to have a normal serum calcium; and that *calcitonin*, now often called *thyrocalcitonin* (TCT), reduces the serum calcium when it rises too high. TCT was at first thought by its discoverer to be a parathyroid hormone (Copp, 1961) but was later shown to be present in the thyroid gland (Munson, 1963); hence the new name.

## Parathyroid Hormone (PTH)

Phylogenetically, the parathyroid glands are a development of terrestrial animals. Fishes, for example, do not have any. One can reasonably speculate that, when the bony structure became solid and heavy enough to support an animal out of water, the bone became a calcium "sink" and not enough calcium was getting to the other tissues of the body. Parathyroid hormone, and the glands secreting it, evolved to correct the problem and get the calcium out of the bone. In man there are usually four glands, each weighing only 25 to 40 mg.

PTH has been purified to a high degree only in the past five to six years. The best preparations are bovine. Bovine PTH is a polypeptide containing 80 amino acids and has a molecular weight of about 8500. There is some uncertainty in these figures since different researchers have come up with slightly different results. Only about one-third of the molecule is actually necessary for biologic activity. In arbitrary bioassay units, activity is 2800 to 3000 units/mg. The human PTH has not been as well characterized but is a peptide of somewhat different composition containing 83 to 85 amino acids.

PTH comes principally from the chief cell of the parathyroid gland. Estimates of the amount secreted per day range from about 100 units in the rat to 3000 units in man and much more in the cow. If the molecule of human PTH is about the same size as the bovine molecule, then man secretes about 1 mg per day, which is a lot considering the small weight of the glands. Since extraction of the glands indicates that PTH makes up less than 0.01% of the gland's weight, it becomes clear that most of the secreted hormone is not stored but must be synthesized only a short time before it is secreted. In this sense, the parathyroid glands are much like the adrenal cortex and not at all like the thyroid gland.

Whether PTH in the blood is bound to anything is not known. The amount in plasma was found by bioassay to be 1 to 12 units/ml. This is too high, since recent work, using a radioimmunoassay method, showed in man a range of 0 to 3 mU/ml or about 0.3 mμg/ml in terms of bovine PTH. The measurement in man in terms of human PTH has not been done because of problems in getting enough pure human PTH. The plasma level is high in hyperparathyroidism, and thus the assay may be clinically useful when it is more widely available.

By bioassay, the plasma half-life of PTH in the dog is about three hours while in the rat it is less than one hour. In fact, PTH probably disappears faster than this since, according to immunoassay, the half-life in the cow is only 18 minutes.

PTH can be found in the urine but only in small amounts, approximately 20 to 30 units per day in man. This level correlates well with the hyperparathyroid or hypoparathyroid state, but the assay is too tedious and complex for routine clinical use.

## VITAMIN D

Rickets, a disease of bone in which the bones are soft and do not calcify, was at one time thought by Londoners to be due to the heavy fog, a proposition that now might be considered laughable. It is, however, correct. The disease was effectively treated with sunshine (1850) and cod liver oil (1872), but no one knew why these maneuvers worked nor did they become widely accepted. Some of the key observations are those of Hess, who showed that cod liver oil contains something that is good for treating rickets (1917), of Huldschinsky, who found that radiating the skin with ultraviolet light is also good for rickets (1919), and of Windhaus, who isolated the active substance found in the body, a sterol now called vitamin $D_3$ (1936) (Fig. 38).

Vitamin D is made in the skin—which might therefore be called an endocrine gland—whenever sunlight or ultraviolet light strikes it. The actinic energy converts 7-dehydrocholesterol to vitamin D. Vitamin D

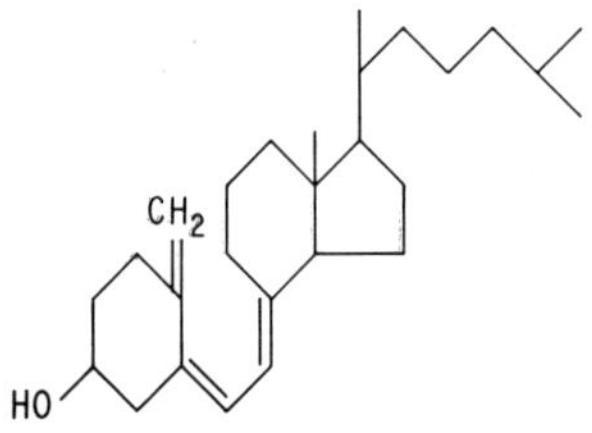

FIG. 38. Vitamin $D_3$.

may also be found in a few oily foods of animal origin. When eaten, vitamin $D_3$ may change to another active compound which, if bile is present, is then absorbed. Whatever the nature of the compound absorbed from the intestine, in the circulating blood vitamin $D_3$ almost certainly must change to 25-hydroxycholecalciferol for complete biologic activity; the hydroxylated sterol seems to be the truly active compound. The normal level in the plasma of an adult human being is about 25 mµg/ml. The plasma half-life of vitamin D is initially about 2 days, but after several days the rate of disappearance slows so that the plasma half-life is then several weeks.

Wherever there is little sun and not enough vitamin D in the diet, vitamin D deficiency can develop. In children, the result is rickets; in adults, osteomalacia. About 400 units of vitamin D in the diet is enough to prevent these diseases even in the absence of sunlight; in the United States, where practically all milk sold contains vitamin D, rickets is uncommon. In general, assuming a fair exposure to the sun, little is actually needed in the diet in an adult who is neither pregnant nor lactating.

## Thyrocalcitonin (TCT)

Experiments were done that unwittingly demonstrated thyrocalcitonin as early as 1958. However, in 1961, Copp, reasoning that there must be something that actively lowers serum calcium when it gets too high, was the first to look for such a hormone, find it, and give it a name, calcitonin. He thought it was another hormone of the parathyroid gland, but all now agree, ever since Munson showed that it could be extracted from the thyroid glands of rats (1963), that it is in fact a secretion of the thyroid gland, at least in mammals. It is now usually called thyrocalcitonin (TCT).

TCT has now been found in the thyroid glands of many mammalian species including the dog, rat, sheep, goat, pig, and man. It is, however, *not* found in the thyroid gland of the chicken, an obscure fact that throws a great deal of light on the true origin of TCT. Birds, including chickens, have a structure called the ultimobranchial gland, separate from the thyroid, that contains much TCT. Embryologically, in mammals a similar gland begins as an outpouching of the posterior pharynx from the fifth pharyngeal pouch but it does not remain a separate gland, instead becoming mixed with the thyroid gland. The only evidence, then, of this "other gland" is histologic; in the thyroid gland, next to the follicles that make $T_4$ and $T_3$, are lighter-staining cells known as *parafollicular*, or *light*, or *C* cells. These cells are the source of TCT.

TCT is a single-chain polypeptide. For a while, its size was not certain since different investigators had different preparations with molecular weights ranging from 3000 to 9000. In 1968, however, four different groups, two in the United States and two in Switzerland, established that porcine TCT contained 32 amino acids in a particular sequence (Fig. 39). Even more impressive, three of these groups have synthesized the molecule and established the validity of the proposed structure. The actual molecular weight is 3604.

Several of these groups have also shown that human TCT has 32 amino acids. Human TCT differs from porcine TCT at 18 of the 32 amino acid positions in the peptide chain. Quite remarkably, these groups have already synthesized human TCT; since species differences may be important, the availability of human TCT is a major advance in human biology. In arbitrary units, when assayed in rats, pure porcine TCT has about 200 units/mg while human TCT has about 120 units/mg. The most potent TCT found to date seems to be salmon TCT, which has 3000 to 5000 units/mg and may therefore be of great clinical use.

The only common assay for TCT to date is a bioassay which is not too sensitive, so it is not yet clear that TCT circulates in normal plasma in all species (see p. 143). However, the weight of evidence now indicates that it does. Detectable levels of about 0.1 mμg/ml have been found in normal rabbit blood using a newly developed radioimmunoassay, and the half-life in rabbit plasma is 5 to 15 minutes. The immunoassay cannot be used yet with human plasma, but the older bioassay has detected high plasma levels of TCT in a few patients with a thyroid tumor probably derived from parafollicular cells, and it has also detected TCT in normal human plasma after the plasma is concentrated.

## Actions of PTH, Vitamin D, and TCT

The discussion so far has centered on calcium. In fact, however, the metabolism of magnesium and phosphate are closely connected in

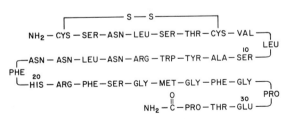

Fig. 39.  Porcine thyrocalcitonin. Every tenth amino acid in the sequence is numbered. Human thyrocalcitonin has a different sequence.

many ways with that of calcium and will be discussed where pertinent. For many years it has been known that *parathyroid hormone* has two major effects: (1) It *maintains the serum calcium* up to its normal level of 10 mg/100 ml and (2) it *increases renal phosphate clearance.* A good deal of controversy went on for a long time over which of these was primary. Different theories were constructed in an attempt to explain how one caused the other, based on the idea of a single action for a single hormone. By 1955, however, it was generally agreed that each was a *separate* action of PTH. In 1961 the pure hormone was finally shown, under appropriate conditions, to cause each action in the absence of the other.

*Vitamin D* also appears to have more than one action. It is required not only for *calcification of new bone* but also for *maintenance of the serum calcium.* It has effects on the kidney, too, of which more later.

At the moment, it seems that the only important action of *thyrocalcitonin* is to *lower the serum calcium* whenever the level rises higher than normal.

The rest of the discussion will try to explain how these three hormones bring about their effects, in large part by seeing what they do to bone. In addition, PTH has effects on magnesium metabolism that are less clear but may be of even more fundamental importance than the actions on calcium.

## Calcium, Magnesium, and Phosphate Metabolism

Some knowledge of calcium, magnesium, and phosphate metabolism is essential to an understanding of the actions of PTH, vitamin D, and TCT, since calcium turns out not to be the only element affected by these hormones.

CALCIUM.   Calcium is required for many functions of the body: for bone and teeth formation, blood coagulation, normal muscle and heart contractility, normal function of the nervous system, and perhaps other things not yet well understood. Its major role in many membrane transport systems accounts for its importance in muscle, heart, and nerve function.

The plasma concentration of calcium is maintained within a narrow range, about 9 to 11 mg/100 ml. More or less than this will upset many of the functions just noted, so keeping the level within this narrow range is very important to the body. Not all the calcium in plasma is important. About 45% to 55% of the plasma calcium is bound or complexed. Only about *5 mg/100 ml* (or 2.5 mEq/liter) is *free ionized calcium* and is *physiologically active.* Most of the rest is bound to albumin; one can therefore have normal physiologic levels with a low total calcium if the plasma albumin is low. A small amount is complexed (about 10% to 15%) with citrate, bicarbonate, and phosphate and is also not physiologically available. The distribution in one study, with a total serum calcium of 10.0 mg/100 ml, was approximately:

$$\text{Bound} \begin{cases} \text{Globulin} & 0.8\,\text{mg/100 ml} \\ \text{Albumin} & 3.7\,\text{mg/100 ml} \end{cases} \text{Nondiffusible: 4.5 mg/100 ml}$$

$$\begin{cases} \text{Complexed} & 1.0\,\text{mg/100 ml} \\ \text{Ionized} & 4.5\,\text{mg/100 ml} \end{cases} \text{Diffusible:} \quad 5.5\,\text{mg/100 ml}$$

The diffusible fraction roughly corresponds to the concentration found in the extravascular extracellular fluid. Note also that "diffusible" and "ionized" are neither synonymous nor equal.

The effects of *hypocalcemia* are well known; *tetany* is caused by an increased excitability of both neurons and motor end-plates. *Hypercalcemia*, seen, for example, in hyperparathyroidism and some cancers, is equally bad and can cause bradycardia, cardiac arrhythmias, decreased renal concentrating ability, abdominal pain, and changes in the psyche as well as depressing neuromuscular excitability.

Figure 40 outlines calcium balance insofar as we know it; many of the values given are approximations. The figure makes clear that many things are involved in the total metabolism of calcium. The serum calcium could be influenced in any of a number of ways, and it is assumed a priori that hormones are only one influence on the circulating calcium level, albeit the major one. The overall net absorption from the gut is about 100 mg per day, and, when in balance, the calcium in the urine and sweat should equal the net absorption from the gut. Bone is, of course, an immense reservoir of calcium that turns over relatively slowly in toto.

MAGNESIUM. The magnesium in the body is, outside the bone, mainly an intracellular ion. The relation with cellular calcium is much the same as the relation between potassium and sodium. There tends to be a constant intracellular $Mg^{++}/Ca^{++}$ ratio as well as $K^+/Na^+$ ratio. In both cases the ratio inside the cell is high, with a higher concentration of magnesium and potassium in cells and a higher concentration of calcium and sodium outside cells. Nevertheless, a great deal of magnesium is in bone—about half to two-thirds of the body content of 25,000 mg (2000 mEq)—although its exact place in the bony crystal structure is not clear.

Magnesium has many important roles, the best known having to do with nucleic acid and protein metabolism. It is needed for DNA synthesis, stabilizes both DNA and RNA, helps bind mRNA to the ribosome, and is important for the formation of amino acid-sRNA complexes and for the function of many enzyme systems.

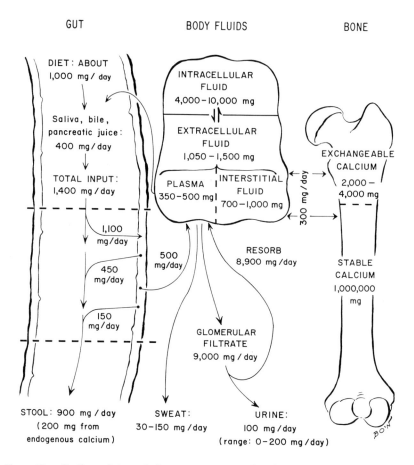

FIG. 40.   Daily calcium balance in man and calcium content of various compartments of the body. Note that the intestinal wall itself takes up and excretes calcium as well as effecting net absorption into the blood. Because of difficulties in analytic techniques, many of the amounts shown are only approximate. Daily rates are indicated in milligrams per day and contents of compartments in milligrams.

It is not surprising, then, that the *plasma level* is fairly constant at about *2.4 mg/100 ml* (or *2.0 mEq/liter*), but little is known about what keeps it so constant. About 55% is free, ionized magnesium. The effects of hypomagnesemia and hypermagnesemia are much like those resulting from similar changes in plasma calcium; the only way to be certain as to the cause of tetany, for example, is to measure both calcium and magnesium in the plasma.

We eat about 25 mEq (300 mg) of magnesium each day, most of

which is found (as one might guess) in chlorophyll. About one-third is absorbed from the gut.

PHOSPHORUS. In the body, phosphorus is ubiquitous, and its role in a host of biochemical reactions is well known. Still, bone contains 80% of the total body phosphorus, most of which is in bone crystals. *Plasma contains 3 to 4.5 mg/100 ml* of inorganic phosphorus, mostly as phosphate. Some is bound to protein and some is complexed or circulates as undissociated phosphate salts; together these fractions make up perhaps a third of the total plasma phosphate. The ionized phosphate circulates in two major forms, $HPO_4^=$ and $H_2PO_4^-$, with a ratio favoring the former by 4/1. Only a very small amount of trivalent phosphate anion ($PO_4^{\equiv}$) circulates as such.

Of the 900 mg or so in the diet, about 70% is absorbed by the gut and the rest appears in the stool. When it is in balance, therefore, one should find 600 to 700 mg per day in the urine.

### Regulation of Plasma Levels of Calcium, Magnesium, and Phosphate

The maintenance of the *plasma* or *serum calcium* at $10 \pm 1$ mg/ 100 ml is the business of PTH and vitamin D, which together keep the level up to 10 mg/100 ml, and of TCT, which keeps it down to 10 mg/ 100 ml. Other factors which are probably important are noted below.

PTH, in many cases, seems to have an effect on *serum magnesium* similar to that on serum calcium; for example, a lack of PTH can cause a low serum magnesium. However, just the opposite can occur, e.g., low PTH causing high serum $Mg^{++}$ and excess PTH resulting in low serum $Mg^{++}$. For the moment PTH can be regarded as keeping the serum $Mg^{++}$ up to 2.4 mg/100 ml, but one should keep an open mind as new information develops. While TCT has no effect on serum $Mg^{++}$, other hormones such as vitamin D, $T_4$, and aldosterone are all capable of lowering it.

Because PTH directly affects its clearance by the kidney, *serum phosphate* is in large part regulated by PTH, the net effect of PTH being to lower serum phosphate. In this instance PTH and TCT work in concert because both decrease serum phosphate, although by different mechanisms.

Finally, the levels of *serum calcium* and *serum phosphate* tend to vary inversely; a higher calcium is associated with a lower phosphate and vice versa. This is in part a physicochemical relationship and in part a hormonally regulated one. The relationship is only a crude one, and there are often exceptions. Nevertheless, it is seen often enough in various diseases to be of both physiologic and clinical importance.

The actual levels of calcium, magnesium, and phosphate in blood, though closely regulated by hormones, are in reality the result of the actions of these hormones on several tissues: the gut, the kidney, and the bone. The remainder of this section discusses these effects and concludes with some remarks on the influences of these hormones on other tissues of the body.

### Factors Affecting Absorption from the Gut

CALCIUM. Dietary calcium, mostly derived from milk and milk products, is not the only calcium to enter the intestine. Bile, saliva, and pancreatic juice contribute about 400 mg per day. Furthermore, the lower small intestine secretes calcium into its lumen (150 mg per day). While we know a fair amount about the regulation of calcium absorption, there is not much information on the regulation of endogenous calcium input to the intestine except that calcium secretion by the gut wall is *not* affected by PTH.

What we see as a net absorption of 100 to 200 mg per day, or about 15% of dietary intake, does not reflect the true daily absorption of calcium by the upper small intestine, which actually absorbs 30% to 50% of the calcium presented to it. The net absorption of 15% can also be greatly increased whenever there is a shortage or a higher need for calcium. Under some circumstances, such as active body growth or lactation, the need for calcium is higher. As much as 2000 to 3000 mg may be required in the diet and as much as 60% may be absorbed. If a patient has a large, healing fracture or is recovering from rickets, absorption of calcium may be almost 100%.

The two principal factors known to *increase calcium absorption* are vitamin D and PTH.

*Vitamin D* is probably essential to the process and appears the more important of the two. A metabolite of vitamin D acts even faster to increase calcium absorption; its nature is not completely clear but it is probably 25-hydroxycholecalciferol. We do know that $Mg^{++}$ is needed for optimal activity of vitamin D.

How does vitamin D work? There is evidence that the vitamin localizes in the intestinal mucosa and seems to bind specifically to the nuclear membrane of the mucosal cells. Experiments suggest too that vitamin D increases the permeability of the cell to calcium, that it increases a calcium-binding protein in the cell, and that it increases the release of calcium from the mucosal cells into the blood stream. Finally, vitamin D seems to increase the permeability of the nuclear membrane of the mucosal cell to calcium. When all this is put together, a reasonable mechanism can be proposed: Vitamin D selectively binds to the intestinal cell and then to its nuclear membrane, increasing the entry of a critical substance (calcium?) into the nucleus. The nucleus now sets machinery in motion to increase the synthesis of enzymes required by the calcium transport system, which ultimately results in more calcium coming into and going through the mucosal cell.

The effect of *PTH* is still mildly controversial, but most workers now agree that it increases calcium absorption. It will do so, however, only if adequate vitamin D is present.

Other factors that may increase calcium absorption are:

1. Growth hormone.
2. Thyroxine (may inhibit absorption or increase secretion into gut at high doses).
3. Previous low calcium diet (secondary to PTH?).
4. Low intestinal pH.
5. Lactose in the diet.
6. Bile salts, probably by increasing the solubility of calcium in lipids.

There is no certainty regarding the importance of any of these under normal circumstances.

*Decreased calcium absorption* is hard to demonstrate but may be seen with the opposite of some of the above (e.g., deficient growth hormone or thyroxine), when the diet is high in *fat, oxalate, phosphate,* or *magnesium,* or when there is *renal failure.* Fat, oxalate, and phosphate tend to bind calcium and thus decrease absorption although the usual amount of dietary phosphate has no significant effect. Magnesium may compete with calcium for the absorptive pathway, resulting in less calcium absorption, but this is not at all clear since some work suggests just the opposite. *Glucocorticoids, thyroxine* in excess, and *thyrocalcitonin* can all lower calcium absorption, but these effects either are not yet confirmed or occur only under nonphysiologic conditions.

MAGNESIUM.    Studies attempting to analyze what affects magnesium absorption are confusing, except that they support the generally reciprocal relation between calcium and magnesium just mentioned. High calcium in the diet decreases magnesium absorption and vice versa. Vitamin D may or may not increase absorption, PTH has a probable effect on increasing resorption, and TCT may decrease it. Aldosterone surprisingly has an effect; it decreases net absorption, probably by increasing secretion into the gut. No specific transport system has been defined in the intestinal mucosa.

PHOSPHATE.    Again, there is no known specific mechanism for absorbing phosphate, although absorption is enhanced by several things that enhance calcium absorption: low intestinal pH, previous low-calcium diet, and perhaps PTH and vitamin D.

*Factors Affecting Resorption and Excretion by the Kidney*

CALCIUM.    Urinary calcium, normally less than 200 mg per day, may be increased by a number of hormones, including growth hormone, thyroxine, cortisol, PTH, and vitamin D. PTH of itself increases renal resorption of calcium somewhat, but, because it raises the serum calcium, the net effect is an increased urine calcium. $T_4$ and cortisol may do essentially the same thing, but vitamin D and possibly growth hormone (in humans) seem to act directly on the kidney to decrease calcium resorption. At the same time, however, vitamin D is necessary for PTH to exert its resorptive effect on filtered calcium. The effect of vitamin D may thus be dose dependent, the overall effect being generally to increase calcium excretion.

On the other hand, TCT injected into an animal reduces the urinary calcium, perhaps directly although the effect may be secondary to a lower serum calcium.

MAGNESIUM.   Here again, though investigation has not been so intensive, PTH raises daily urinary excretion, despite the fact that PTH can directly act on the kidney to increase resorption of $Mg^{++}$. It does so probably because of an increased filtered load of $Mg^{++}$ due to bone resorption. This is perhaps a bit surprising, since some work suggests that $Ca^{++}$ and $Mg^{++}$ compete for the same resorptive sites in the kidney; if PTH directly increases renal resorption of calcium, one would expect decreased resorption of $Mg^{++}$. It is possible that the competitive resorptive sites are different from the locus of action of PTH. Aldosterone, $T_4$, and perhaps vitamin D also increase urinary $Mg^{++}$ excretion, thereby accounting in large measure for the drop in serum $Mg^{++}$ caused by these three hormones.

TCT, as with urinary calcium, decreases urinary magnesium.

PHOSPHATE.   About two-thirds of the phosphate lost by the body each day appears in the urine. Thus the kidney would seem to be the main regulator of the serum phosphate level. Phosphate is resorbed in the proximal tubule and (in some species at least) secreted back into the lumen of the distal tubule.

*Parathyroid hormone* causes an *increase in phosphate clearance* by the kidney, probably due to an inhibition of resorption in the proximal tubule. There is suggestive evidence that PTH will increase secretion as well. This is a rapid action of PTH, occurring in less than one hour, whereas in man a rise in serum calcium takes four to six hours. Further it is a *direct* renal effect since it can be demonstrated with direct renal artery infusion of PTH.

Unlike the rise in serum calcium induced by PTH, the increased phosphate clearance ($C_p$) is not blocked by actinomycin; thus mRNA synthesis is not essential. Nor is vitamin D needed for this action although it may be necessary for optimal phosphate clearance. PTH does, however, cause an increase in adenyl cyclase activity in the renal cortex and in urinary cyclic AMP excretion *before* the increase in $C_p$.

Furthermore, protein synthesis may be required. Since a high serum calcium alone can increase $C_p$, part of the action of PTH on $C_p$ may be indirect, but at best this indirect effect plays only a minor role since the rise in serum calcium does not occur until later. The mechanism is still under investigation, but now one may speculate: PTH directly stimulates renal cortical adenyl cyclase activity, and the resulting increase in cAMP increases the activity of essential proteins (enzymes?) involved in the rejection of phosphate.

The physiologic significance of this action of PTH is not clear at present. One might conjecture that a phosphate diuresis would help the body get rid of the phosphate mobilized during bone resorption and by lowering serum phosphate enhance the hypercalcemic action of PTH since any lowering of serum phosphate tends to raise serum $Ca^{++}$. Whatever it means, it is useful clinically to speak of tubular resorption of phosphate or phosphate clearance because these can be measured in patients and may help in the diagnosis of hyperparathyroidism.

TCT, in some species at least, acts much like PTH on urinary phosphate, causing an increase in phosphate excretion. However, the effect may not be a direct one but may be secondary to the TCT-induced hypocalcemia. (How is this explained?)

Vitamin D probably has an opposite action and causes a slight rise in phosphate resorption, although this seems to be minor. Growth hormone does the same thing by direct renal action. On the other hand, dihydrotachysterol, a vitamin D analogue, decreases phosphate resorption just as PTH does.

## Hormones and Bone

The *major effect of PTH on calcium metabolism* is due to its *action on bone*, in which it promotes the mobilization of calcium into the blood. As we shall see, PTH also plays a role in the remodeling of bone structure. Whether these actions are different or simply represent different results of the same action is not yet clear.

BONE STRUCTURE AND CONTENT.   Bone is about two-thirds mineral and one-third organic material. The *mineral* is thought to be predominantly a complex calcium phosphate salt called *hydroxyapatite* [$3\ Ca_3 (PO_4)_2 \cdot Ca(OH)_2$]. However, bone also contains a great deal of sodium (1500 mEq or one-third the body's content), carbonate, citrate, and magnesium (1000 mEq or one-half the body's content). Many of these ions can substitute for calcium and phosphate in the crystal structure; in any case, the mineral is by no means a perfect hydroxyapatite crystal. In addition, recent work shows that a fair fraction of bone mineral is not crystalline at all but that as much as 30% is amorphous calcium phosphate [$Ca_3(PO_4)_2$]. The *organic matrix* is mostly *collagen*—90% to 95% in mature bone. Collagen contains a large amount of hydroxyproline, an amino acid found only in collagen. The remainder of the organic matrix consists of *ground substance* (mostly mucopolysaccharides) and *cells.*

One can divide the calcium in bone into two types, which are actually concepts rather than physical loci (Fig. 40). *"Exchangeable" calcium* is that calcium which exchanges relatively quickly with serum calcium, i.e., within a few hours or days, depending on the definition, and involves little or no change in the haversian systems. A small amount of the exchangeable calcium is not actually in bone but is in tissues such as cartilage and fibrous tissue. The definition of just how much calcium is exchangeable is difficult; its calculation depends on a number of assumptions, such as the straightness of a nonlinear curve and whether or not resorption of stable bone occurs during the period of exchange. By far the greater part of bone calcium is the *stable bone calcium,* which does not readily exchange with serum calcium. When changes occur in stable calcium there is probably remodeling of haversian systems, and the changes involve the formation of new bone and the resorption of old bone. A certain fraction of stable bone calcium does exchange slowly with serum calcium without the formation or resorption of bone mineral. This process of *long-term exchange* is slow and in humans does not involve more than 1% to 2% of the total bone calcium in an entire year.

Bone is a reasonably active tissue on the whole. It gets between 3% and 10% of the cardiac output. The crystalline mineral is separated from the blood by the capillary endothelium and also by a thin layer of bone cells. The cell types of bone are the *osteoblast,* the *osteocyte,* and the *osteoclast.* Originally, the osteoblast was thought to be responsible for bone formation and the osteoclast for resorption, but the matter is more complex than that. The osteocyte, for example, may be a relatively inactive osteoblast yet be concerned principally with calcium mobilization. Furthermore, all three types may simply be different forms of the same basic cell.

BONE FORMATION.    As one might expect, bone formation is faster in younger than in older people. The osteoblast makes "osteoid," a mixture of mucopolysaccharide ground substance and collagen. The collagen is not laid down in its final structural form until it is outside the cell, where actual calcification occurs. The structure of bone collagen seems to be at least partially specific since some other forms of collagen, in vitro, do not act as a support for bone crystal.

The next step is calcification of the collagen. What initiates calcification? The answer is not really known but there is enough information to allow a reasonable theory. In order to have precipitation of bone salt, there must be a nucleus or "seed" to start things off and enough of the right ions in the surrounding fluid. The collagen fibril is the "seed." The surrounding fluid, if it is similar in unbound ion concentration to plasma, contains $Ca^{++}$, $HPO_4^=$, and $PO_4^\equiv$ in amounts close to the solubility products of $Ca_3(PO_4)_2$ and $CaHPO_4$. $Ca_3(PO_4)_2$ precipitates when the ion product is about $1 \times 10^{-25}$ and the plasma ion product is $1 \times 10^{-23}$; $CaHPO_4$ precipitates somewhere between $1 \times 10^{-6}$ and $3 \times 10^{-7}$, while the plasma ion product is about $0.8 \times 10^{-6}$. (Why plasma remains supersaturated with respect to $Ca_3(PO_4)_2$ is unknown.) Thus the nucleus and ions are present.

Collagen also acts as a template, directing the shape of the bone spicule. Since metabolic activity seems necessary for bone formation, local enzymes may well be involved. We also know that added phosphate stimulates the formation of bone mineral. So perhaps a phosphoprotein or phospholipid, made by the osteoblast, is broken down by local enzymes and releases its phosphate very near the collagen fibril. Here the phosphate might combine with calcium from the serum and start the whole process going. In addition, it is possible that some unknown local factor or the bone cells themselves increase the local concentration of calcium. Whether amorphous calcium phosphate or an actual crystal is made first is not certain; recent work suggests that in the main the amorphous salt is made first and acts as a precursor for bone crystal, more of the amorphous salt becoming crystalline as time passes. The amorphous salt is more soluble than the crystal; the change to the latter may account for the decreased solubility of older bone, and the ratio of amorphous salt to crystal may determine how much "exchangeable calcium" there is.

Between certain areas of bone is an electric gradient; for example, the bone marrow is electrically negative (10 to 15 mv) with respect to an adjacent joint cavity, and bone is probably electrically negative to the adjacent periosteum. These differences, which may be due to streaming potentials or the effects of bone acting as a semiconductor, might also play a role in the deposition of calcium. The electric potential seems to be of definite importance in the formation of new bone under the stress of bending or after a fracture. The stress of bending, for example, causes the appearance of an electric current, with the bone acting as a special type of semiconductor. The concave surface of the bent bone becomes electrically negative to the convex surface. New bone forms on the concave surface to "fill in the space" and better resist the bending; one sees an increase in collagen deposition, cellular activity, and apatite formation. Not yet clear is the precise relation between these electrical events and the chemical and cellular phenomena just noted.

In any case, even in vitro small crystals can be seen forming on the collagen matrix, with the displacement of water. Most of the calcium in newly formed bone—about two-thirds to three-fourths—is laid down rather quickly in a few hours, very possibly because the predominant ions of plasma relevant to calcification are $Ca^{++}$ and $HPO_4^=$; when $CaHPO_4$ forms, it is not too stable and tends to change into tricalcium phosphate or hydroxyapatite. In this form it has much less solubility, and consequently there tends to be rapid precipitation of more surrounding $Ca^{++}$ and $HPO_4^=$ ions.

So much for initiating calcification. What stops it and prevents bone from becoming a piece of solid limestone? Once again, not much is really known and all that can be offered is reasonable speculation. It is possible that bone formation is inhibited, when enough bone salt and crystals have formed, by a "crystal poison" on the surface of recently made bone mineral. Further crystallization can occur, perhaps, only when the "poison" is removed. The "poison" may be a complexed phosphate or, more probably, pyrophosphate. Removal of pyrophosphate may permit both new crystallization and resorption; that is, removal of pyrophosphate makes the bone salt more reactive and allows bone crystals to act as nucleators for more crystal formation. The enzyme that breaks down pyrophosphate, pyrophosphatase, is a type of alkaline phosphatase, and we know that bone alkaline phosphatase activity is increased during periods of bone formation. It is reasonable to suggest that a rise in the activity of pyrophosphatase correlates with the formation of new bone mineral and that it may also be associated with increased bone resorption (see below).

As more and more bone is formed, the osteoblast becomes surrounded by bone mineral and "trapped" in the midst of haversian systems. The cell now is relatively quiescent, and is called an osteocyte.

BONE RESORPTION.   Which brings us to the other half of the story. Bone is not only formed continuously but also resorbed at varying rates. The osteocyte probably accounts for a good portion of rapidly resorbed calcium. The osteoclast, a larger multinucleated cell, seems to be associated with the bone resorption that leads to structural remodeling of bone. It may not, however, be essential for bone resorption since some species of amphibians appear to have few osteoclasts.

Bone is constantly being remodeled in response to the stress of weight bearing or gravity. The remodeling process includes, of course, formation of new bone as well as resorption of old bone. Osteoclasts appear to resorb actively both bone mineral and the collagen matrix. In bone undergoing active resorption, osteoclasts can be seen close to the resorbing site, and small crystals of bone have actually been seen inside osteoclasts.

BONE TURNOVER.   One can, then, form a mental image of the haversian systems as structures made of a calcium salt–collagen complex with blood circulating through them at a slow but reasonable rate. The blood does not flow directly over bone crystal, of course, since the endothelium of the capillaries and probably the cells of bone lie between blood and crystal. The exchangeable calcium is presumably at the surface of the calcium-collagen complex and most readily available to the bone interstitial fluid and thus to the blood. The more crystallized, stable calcium is "deeper" and less accessible. When the need arises, the osteoblasts make new bone and the osteoclasts break down old bone, thus remodeling bone in response to various stresses. If the need is for more calcium in the blood, the osteocyte works a bit harder and dissolves some of the bone salt.

The overall process of formation and resorption, exclusive of simple exchange, is called *bone turnover* and often involves *bone remodeling*. Quantitation of turnover in man is difficult because it is so slow; all measurements involve certain untested assumptions, and thus all results must be viewed with caution. Present measurements indicate that the total daily turnover in man involves about 600 mg of calcium per day, 300 mg going into new bone and 300 mg being resorbed from old bone. However, *bone turnover* implies that all bone is the same, when it clearly is not. Some bone, e.g., thin trabeculae, may turn over completely in a few months while other parts of the skeleton, e.g., thick cortical bone, may turn over only once in 50 years.

EFFECT OF HORMONES ON BONE. Bone alone in the absence of PTH shows some remodeling (i.e., bone formation and resorption) and maintains the serum calcium at the low but steady level of 5 to 6 mg/100 ml. Some of the latter is probably a physicochemical effect, i.e., a result of dissolution of bone salt to maintain the solubility product ($[Ca^{++}]^3 \times [PO_4^{\equiv}]^2$) at a given level. However, it seems that bone must be metabolically active even to maintain the serum calcium at 5 to 6 mg/100 ml. More than the physical chemistry of calcium phosphate must be involved. The exchangeable calcium is the main source of the blood calcium under these circumstances.

Bone alone is not enough. Parathyroid hormone is required to maintain the serum calcium at the normal level of 10 mg/100 ml and does so by resorbing bone calcium. Furthermore, the classic experiment of Barnicot (1948) showed that a parathyroid graft causes resorption of bone from the adjacent area of a nearby bone graft and at the same time the formation of new bone just beyond the area of resorption. Thus PTH is needed for optimal bone remodeling as well as for optimal mobilization of calcium. With both these effects of PTH, part of the action seems to be on exchangeable bone calcium but most of it appears to be on the stable bone calcium since the release of hydroxyproline parallels the release of calcium.

How does PTH do all this? Although they may not be truly independent actions, it is conceptually convenient to think of *calcium mo-*

*bilization* and *bone remodeling* separately, particularly because the former occurs quickly and the latter takes several hours to days to become apparent. Vitamin D and TCT also have significant roles to play, as noted below.

*Calcium Mobilization.*    Although there is a report that PTH mobilizes calcium from dead bone, most workers agree that oxygen consumption, i.e., metabolic activity, is necessary for PTH to act. Calcium mobilization by PTH from bone into the blood probably has to be viewed as a two-component system. There apparently is an early phase and a later phase, the one occurring in minutes and the other in several hours.

The *early phase*, the mobilizing of a small amount of calcium, is not inhibited by actinomycin, so mRNA synthesis is probably not necessary. The already matured osteocytes may be the responsible cells since, after PTH is given to an animal, bone resorption seems to occur around them. Protein synthesis may be required although mRNA synthesis is not; the osteocyte shows an increased proline uptake after PTH, another indication that it is the responsible cell.

The *later phase*, accounting for most of the calcium mobilized by PTH, probably does involve mRNA as well as protein synthesis. This gradual, slower release of relatively large amounts of calcium *is* inhibited by actinomycin. It seems to be dependent on the formation or differentiation of new bone-resorbing cells.

What does PTH do to the osteocyte? At present a definite picture is hard to draw, but there are several proposed mechanisms, any or all of which may be operative, and all of which have at least some experimental backing.

1. PTH increases adenyl cyclase and then cAMP concentration, which then mediates the hypercalcemic response.

2. PTH stimulates an increase in bone and plasma citrate concentration. The calcium can then be chelated with the citrate and removed. Against this idea: One can, under certain conditions, show a rise in serum calcium after PTH without an increased serum citrate; further, the total organic acid made by bone is not enough to complex the calcium released.

3. PTH stimulates an increase in organic acid production by bone, including lactate, thus reducing the local pH. The lower pH, simply by physicochemical means, can then cause bone dissolution. In vitro, bone powder releases enough calcium to the surrounding medium to maintain a calcium concentration in the solution equal to that of the ionized calcium in plasma *if* the pH of the medium is between 6.7 and 7.0. Unfortunately, no one really knows what the pH of bone is, PTH action is not enhanced by a low pH, which one would expect if this idea is valid, and there is a poor correlation between the amount of

acid produced and the calcium mobilized. Nevertheless, if the bone pH is in fact relatively low, it would explain in part why plasma appears supersaturated with respect to $Ca^{++}$ and $PO_4^{\equiv}$, since the solubility product is higher at the lower pH.

4. PTH increases appropriate enzyme activities which lead to calcium release. Several enzymes do show increased activity, but generally by the time they do, the serum calcium has already gone up. Nevertheless, adenyl cyclase is probably an exception (see above). Furthermore, this kind of action, though not explaining the early rise in calcium release, may well be pertinent to the later rise that accounts for most of PTH's action.

One may construct a theory involving enhanced enzyme activity based on analogies with certain experiments on the effect of PTH on renal mitochondria (Rasmussen): (a) PTH stimulates increased magnesium entry into the bone cell (osteocyte); (b) PTH enhances the affinity of $Mg^{++}$ and the enzyme pyrophosphatase; (c) $Mg^{++}$ activates pyrophosphatase; (d) pyrophosphatase breaks down pyrophosphate, which coats the bone mineral and inhibits resorption; (e) with less pyrophosphate, bone mineral dissolves much more readily, perhaps enhanced by one of the mechanisms listed above.

In this proposed mechanism the primary effect of PTH is not on calcium at all, but on magnesium. It is really not a direct effect on enzyme activity but on ion transport by membranes.

5. PTH may increase the "pumping" of calcium from the bone cell to the extracellular fluid, another postulated membrane effect based on experiments with renal mitochondria.

Regarding the last two (4 and 5), as with any work using isolated mitochondria, one never knows whether the in vitro conditions are in any way similar to those in vivo. Nevertheless, some sort of membrane effect may be operating in the action of PTH, viz., the effect on adenyl cyclase, generally an enzyme associated with cellular membranes.

So we are once again left with speculation—fascinating, interesting, and pointing the way to more experiments, but nevertheless speculation. We *can* say that both living bone cells and some change in the solubility of bone mineral are involved in the calcium mobilization induced by PTH.

*Vitamin D* is a necessary requirement if PTH is to mobilize calcium from bone; it localizes in bone cells just as it does in the cells of the intestinal mucosa. Its major influence is probably on the later phase of calcium release, implying perhaps an effect on cell growth or differentiation. This synergistic action of PTH and vitamin D requires magnesium; perhaps mechanism 4, just above, has something to do with it. Without vitamin D, PTH will not work and the serum calcium stays the same (in rats, dogs, and humans). The reason may be that vitamin D makes calcium available to the site of action of PTH, and without vitamin D no calcium is available. Vitamin D alone, without PTH, is equally ineffective unless taken in very high doses. Small doses of each, ineffective if given alone to a parathyroidectomized animal, when given together raise the serum calcium to normal, nicely pointing out the interrelation between the two hormones.

*Thyrocalcitonin* drops the serum calcium. In humans, the effect is probably best seen with human TCT, but porcine TCT works almost as well. TCT acts principally on bone, where it decreases calcium resorption and may increase calcium incorporation, although the latter point is not settled. The former suggests an anti-PTH effect, but the latter indicates that the action of TCT must be more than simply to antagonize PTH. This has in fact been shown since in vitro TCT acts on bone in the absence of PTH and in vivo TCT lowers serum calcium even when the parathyroid glands are removed. TCT's action is opposite to that of PTH but it does not act by inhibiting the secretion or action of PTH itself.

Just what TCT does to bone cells is not clear. Some work suggests it antagonizes the early phase of calcium release (see above) because its action is not inhibited by actinomycin; other work indicates an action on the later phase. The presence of vitamin D neither adds nor detracts from the action of TCT.

PTH also increases mobilization of *magnesium* from bone, and so does vitamin D. The effects of PTH and vitamin D are similar, then, to their effects on calcium; practically nothing more is known about them (a fertile field for future research).

*Bone Remodeling.* It is likely that the primary effect of PTH in this regard is to *increase bone resorption.* The early effect on bone formation is a bit uncertain but probably adds up to an initial decreased bone formation; later, probably as a secondary reaction to the higher resorption, there is an increase in bone formation as well. At this stage the net effect of increased resorption and formation amounts to an increased turnover, and, given the appropriate stress, one finds an appropriate remodeling of bone.

*After PTH* has been given, there is a very early rise in the uptake of amino acids and in collagen synthesis by bone cells, but shortly thereafter the predominant early effect of *decreased bone formation* is manifest. One sees in bone decreases in (1) oxygen consumption, (2) amino acid uptake by osteoblasts, (3) osteoblast activity, (4) incorporation of glycine into bone matrix, and (5) conversion of proline into the hydroxyproline of bone collagen. Some of the confusion may be due to the problem of adequately separating the several types of bone cells.

In addition, one sees *increased bone resorption,* which is partly due to increased osteoclast activity. PTH has been observed to increase the number of osteoclasts in bone even when the bone is incubated in vitro, correlating with the finding of increased RNA and DNA synthesis after several hours and with the fact that actinomycin blocks the osteoclast response. The extra osteoclasts are probably derived from mesenchymal cells; PTH stimulates the differentiation.

The osteoclast effect is not the whole answer, however, to the question of the action of PTH on bone resorption. One can, under appropriate experimental conditions, show normal calcium mobilization and bone resorption with no change or even a decrease in the number of osteoclasts. The osteoclast response is perhaps an indirect one secondary to some other action. The osteocyte may also play a role, involved as it is in calcium mobilization.

Whether or not the osteoclasts are the direct mediator of increased bone resorption, PTH does cause lysis of the bone matrix by acting on some bone cell(s). Activation of hydrolytic enzymes found in lysosomes of the cells is a possibility. One can show an increase in collagenase, an enzyme that destroys collagen, and in the breakdown of collagen. With the supporting structure of bone gone, calcium is released. Since this phase of bone resorption rather resembles the later phase of calcium mobilization, many of the mechanisms proposed for the latter may apply here as well.

For a while the early decrease in bone formation no doubt enhances the effect of PTH on net bone resorption. However, when observations are continued long enough after PTH has been given, one sees a *secondary increase in bone formation*. Experiments show an increase in oxygen consumption, in uptake of uridine by bone cells, in RNA and DNA synthesis (at least in certain areas of bone), in incorporation of proline into the hydroxyproline of bone collagen, and in the synthesis of bone mucopolysaccharide. There is also more incorporation of inorganic phosphate into bone and, of course, more gross new bone formation as in the classic experiment of Barnicot noted previously.

There is then *increased bone turnover* with PTH, reflected ultimately in a higher turnover of both components of bone matrix, polysaccharide and collagen, and in an increased metabolic activity of bone. Some have suggested that the late rise in bone formation is simply a reaction to greater bone resorption, but PTH may in fact have a more direct action on this process (see below re vitamin D).

A major problem in untangling and putting together these many effects of PTH is that the doses given to experimental animals are often far in excess of anything likely to be encountered in the body. Although the broad outlines are clear, a cautious, skeptical approach is best when considering detailed mechanisms.

*Vitamin D* is an integral part of the process of bone remodeling. Like PTH, it increases both the resorption and the formation of bone and therefore increases bone turnover. Its main action, however, is on bone formation rather than on bone resorption and thus it differs from and complements PTH. Vitamin D is, for example, necessary for the initial calcification of bone matrix, or osteoid, and therefore one might postulate a prime action on the osteoblast. Nevertheless, it is equally essential for mobilization of calcium from bone, as noted above. Possibly both these actions are related; the vitamin may increase the resorption of older bone and thus enhance the calcification of osteoid simply by supplying more calcium.

PTH and vitamin D again act synergistically. Although it has not been conclusively demonstrated, osteoid seems not to calcify well without PTH even in the presence of vitamin D. Overall, then, vitamin D and PTH act together to enhance bone formation, bone resorption, and calcium mobilization and so help to regulate bone remodeling and the serum calcium.

*Thyrocalcitonin,* as expected, "dumps" calcium into bone, which action tends to decrease bone resorption, perhaps to increase bone formation, and, overall, to decrease bone turnover. TCT also decreases the number of osteoclasts. However, as in its action on serum calcium, TCT does not act simply by antagonizing PTH. It actually increases the mass of bone, which probably would not happen simply in the absence of PTH; TCT, for example, increases the amount of calcium deposited at the site of a healing fracture. Furthermore, while TCT reverses the demineralization caused by PTH, it does not seem to block the increased collagen resorption of the latter. All of which suggests an action on both osteoclasts and osteoblasts different in quality from that of PTH, though not enough work has been done with this newly discovered hormone to be sure. TCT may thus be very important to the process of bone remodeling in addition to its importance in regulating serum calcium.

So far, it must seem that all that is needed for bone to be happy are PTH, vitamin D, and TCT. Not so. Other hormones are required. Growth hormone, for example, is obviously needed for normal bone growth; without it the patient is short. In vitro, growth hormone increases the growth of cartilage, increases amino acid uptake by bone, and is perhaps the pituitary factor necessary for new bone formation. Thyroxine seems necessary for normal bone formation, and so are the gonadal hormones.

### Effects of Parathyroid Hormone, Vitamin D, and TCT on Other Tissues

While the above effects are the more readily observed ones, only in recent years have tissues other than bone, kidney, and gut been investigated with any great interest. The fact that the parathyroid-deficient patient with a low serum calcium has *increased* calcium deposition in several nonbony tissues, such as the lens of the eye and the basal ganglia of the brain, prompted workers to examine the effect of PTH on the body as a whole.

In general, PTH increases calcium and phosphate flux across cell membranes. It also helps maintain the normal sodium/potassium ratio across the cell membrane, which tends to be reversed by the accompanying higher serum calcium. The tendency, then, is for PTH to cause an increased calcium inside muscle cells (though apparently not in nervous tissue, where it may actively keep calcium out) with a decrease in intracellular phosphate and sodium. Here again vitamin D plays a similar but not identical role; it tends to increase intracellular calcium but has no effect on sodium or phosphate. Vitamin D is probably not needed for these actions of PTH, a situation similar to that in the kidney and clearly different from that in the bone.

Such effects would seem to be of some importance, but not enough is known about them to say more. Further, the abnormal deposits of calcium in the PTH-deficient patient are still not explained.

Practically nothing is known about the action of TCT on these tissues nor is anything certain about the effects of the three hormones on the magnesium in the tissues. Relative to $Mg^{++}$, we do know that thyroxine is needed for optimal transport of $Mg^{++}$ in and out of cells. In view of the possible importance of PTH on magnesium metabolism, and of the widespread interest in TCT, the next few years should show marked improvement in our understanding of these problems.

## CONTROL OF THE SECRETION OF PTH, VITAMIN D, AND TCT

### PTH

Here a classic feedback system operates. A drop in serum calcium stimulates more secretion of PTH, and a rise in serum calcium turns it off (Fig. 41). A drop in serum calcium of only 0.3 mg/100 ml is enough to increase PTH secretion within a matter of minutes, providing the drop is below a critical level of approximately 9 mg/100 ml. A rise in serum phosphate also increases PTH secretion, but this is an indirect effect and is due to the moderate drop in serum calcium that occurs with an elevated serum phosphate. Most of the secreted hormone is newly synthesized because little seems to be stored by the gland. Hypocalcemia increases the uptake of many amino acids by the parathyroid gland in vitro. It is entirely possible, then, that a low serum calcium stimulates increased amino acid uptake, with the increase in PTH synthesis and secretion a secondary effect. It is not completely clear yet, but DNA and RNA synthesis may not be obligatory; one would think protein synthesis necessary since the hormone

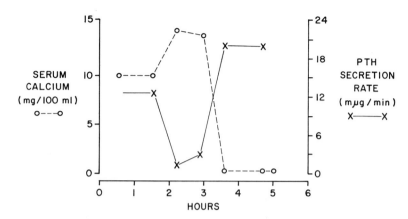

FIG. 41.   Changes in secretion of PTH from a goat's parathyroid gland resulting from changes in the concentration of calcium in the perfusing blood. (From A. D. Care, L. M. Sherwood, J. T. Potts, Jr., and G. D. Aurbach, *Nature* [London] 209:55, 1966.)

is a fairly large peptide, but perhaps synthesis of all cell proteins is not required. A drop in serum magnesium also increases PTH secretion, but not much is known of the relative importance of this effect.

The opposite, a higher serum calcium, shuts off PTH secretion and, as one would predict from the above, is associated with decreased amino acid uptake by the gland; once again, the effect is more likely to be mainly on PTH synthesis than on secretion alone. A rise in serum magnesium does the same thing, though nothing is known of the mechanism.

### Vitamin D

As we have said, one may consider vitamin D a "hormone" of the skin, and we have several times called it a hormone, but in fact there is no evidence to suggest that the amount made by the skin or absorbed by the intestine is in any way determined by changes in calcium metabolism. As far as we know, the skin makes more vitamin D whenever exposed to sunlight. The amount of pigmentation, however, may act as a crude regulator; thicker, darker skin cuts down vitamin D synthesis, and thinner, lighter skin does the opposite. So tanning of the skin or genetically darker skin may protect against vitamin D toxicity in very sunny areas of the world.

### TCT

There is no question that a rise in serum calcium stimulates the secretion of TCT, perhaps mediated by cAMP. The reverse is also likely—a fall in serum calcium tending to inhibit or shutting off completely the secretion of TCT. As with PTH, a negative feedback system probably operates, but it differs in its effect on and response to the serum calcium. At present the bioassay for thyrocalcitonin is relatively insensitive and does not easily detect TCT in normal (i.e., normocalcemic) plasma (see p. 123). It is difficult, then, to state definitely that TCT is secreted all the time in greater or lesser degree; perhaps it is secreted *only* when the serum calcium is high. Since rats did not seem to have any TCT in their blood unless the serum calcium was elevated, the latter idea found early favor. However, more recent work with rats indicates that TCT is present in normocalcemic rat blood; TCT is also present in blood containing normal amounts of calcium in pigs, rabbits, and humans. The rabbit, for example, has about 0.1 mμg/ml and shows a sharp rise within 15 minutes after calcium is injected into the blood stream.

Some workers in this field feel that TCT may be more important in bone remodeling than in the regulation of serum calcium because (1) it may be needed only when the serum calcium is high and (2) it may have little value even here since patients without a thyroid gland seem to have no trouble keeping their serum calcium down to normal. No firm conclusions on this topic are yet possible, for (1) may not be true and another study examining (2) indicates that patients with poorly functioning thyroids do indeed have a problem in lowering the serum calcium. Further work with the radioimmunoassay will probably supply the answers to this question. For the moment, the overall impression is that TCT is important for both bone remodeling and the control of serum calcium, and that in controlling the serum calcium the secretion of TCT can be stimulated or suppressed by a rise or fall in serum calcium.

In sum, parathyroid hormone and vitamin D are responsible for maintaining the serum calcium up to 10 mg/100 ml from the basal level of 5 mg/100 ml, while TCT keeps it close to the normal level by damping any tendency to go over 10 mg/100 ml. The two hormones, PTH and TCT, thus exert a particularly tight control over the serum calcium since the serum calcium is affected by a double negative feedback control system.

### Other Factors Involved in Control of Serum Calcium

We have noted the importance of thyroxine in bone formation; it tends to increase serum calcium (ionized and total) when too much is given, and may play some role in maintaining a normal serum calcium under normal circumstances. *Growth hormone* may have a similar action. In addition, some pituitary extracts have a hypocalcemic action. The *central nervous system* may also play a role, at least in maintaining calcium intake. Rats that have had their parathyroids removed will specifically select a diet with a higher calcium content. Purely *phys-*

*icochemical* effects via the maintenance of a constant ion product of calcium and phosphate are likewise of some importance, but there are instances when both calcium and phosphorus change in the same direction. The maintenance of a constant ion product has a subsidiary part at best in regulating serum calcium.

## CLINICAL DISORDERS OF CALCIUM METABOLISM: A BRIEF SKETCH

### PTH

*PTH deficiency*, or hypoparathyroidism, leads to hypocalcemia and tetany. It may occur spontaneously or after operations on the neck, particularly on the thyroid gland. Logically, one should treat with PTH, but since this is scarce and must be injected, calcium and vitamin D are usually used, given in large doses and by mouth. One peculiar form of hypocalcemia, pseudohypoparathyroidism, looks like PTH deficiency but in fact the patient has normal or elevated PTH secretion. The defect lies in the tissues, which are incapable of responding to the hormone. In this instance calcium and vitamin D are the only treatment since PTH does not work.

*Excessive PTH*, or hyperparathyroidism, perhaps first described in 1923, causes hypercalcemia and kidney stones. The net effect of too much PTH on the bone is resorptive; many parts of the skeleton may become thin, and in severe cases cystic areas appear in the bone. The best test for the disease, though many have been proposed, is still the measurement of serum calcium, but it must be done carefully and if necessary repeatedly. It would probably be better to measure just the ionized portion of the serum calcium but this is at the moment technically difficult; it may on occasion be of great help. Assay of plasma PTH might be the best test, but the technique is not widely available, and, more important, many patients with hyperparathyroidism seem to have PTH values in the normal range. Note that many things other than excessive PTH cause hypercalcemia: excess $T_4$ and diseases such as sarcoid or some cancers. Certain cancers, however, seem to secrete something similar to PTH, perhaps PTH itself; the resulting hypercalcemia is then a form of hyperparathyroidism but is not due to disease of the parathyroid glands.

Treatment is surgical. One removes the abnormal parathyroid tissue (usually a single adenoma, occasionally several hyperplastic glands) or attempts to remove a PTH-secreting tumor. If there is an urgent need to lower serum calcium rapidly, one might give TCT; since it is not generally available, oral or intravenous phosphate solutions are an effective emergency treatment. Occasionally surgery is not possible and the elevated calcium must be controlled chronically. Oral phosphate solutions or, if available, injections of a long-acting preparation of TCT seem to be the best choice.

## Vitamin D

*Deficiency of vitamin D* causes rickets or osteomalacia, or "soft bone" disease. The serum calcium tends to be low, and extra PTH is secreted in an attempt to make up the deficit. It usually doesn't work, however, although much phosphate appears in the urine since the phosphaturic effect of PTH does not require vitamin D. An unusual form of rickets is called "vitamin D–resistant rickets" because the usually very effective therapy, vitamin D, does not work except in high doses. This form of rickets may be due to poor metabolism of vitamin D to its active metabolite (25-hydroxycholecalciferol).

*Vitamin D toxicity* results from eating too much vitamin D or, in some instances, from an increased sensitivity to the usual amounts of the vitamin. The principal finding is hypercalcemia. Treatment is avoidance of vitamin D and sunlight.

## TCT

Ever since TCT was discovered, physicians have been looking for patients who might reveal syndromes of abnormal secretion of TCT. The search for *deficiency of TCT* has not really been successful although some of the patients mentioned above lacking thyroid tissue might well be deficient in TCT. *Excessive TCT secretion* has been found and confirmed by discovering excessive TCT in the plasma of a few patients with an unusual thyroid tumor, medullary carcinoma of the thyroid, which probably derives from the parafollicular cells of the thyroid. Excess TCT is possibly the cause of the very dense bone (osteopetrosis) seen in some patients with no other apparent disease.

## Osteoporosis

None of these disorders involving PTH, vitamin D, or TCT, however, are particularly common. Far more often seen in patients is the general thinning of bone called *osteoporosis*. In this condition the serum calcium is normal. There is a loss of bone mass, both organic and mineral. For many years one of the dominant theories of the cause of osteoporosis was that bone formation was decreased in the face of a continuing normal bone resorption rate. Recent work has shown normal bone formation and sometimes increased bone resorption in some patients with osteoporosis. A better way of looking at it, proposed by Heaney, is to consider that osteoporosis is due to many factors all of which impinge on the mechanisms responsible for calcium homeostasis. Implicitly, then, what we call osteoporosis is probably due to several different diseases, all acting in some way to increase the rate of bone resorption.

If, for example, *estrogen or androgen deficiency* caused bone to become hyperresponsive to PTH, one would see increased bone resorption followed by a transient rise of serum calcium. This would cause, along with damping by TCT, a lowering of the PTH secretion rate in order to maintain serum calcium at the normal level. However, a lower PTH level would cause the intestine and kidney to lose more calcium, thus throwing the organism as a whole into negative calcium balance and eventually causing osteoporosis. Clinical support for this idea is seen in the fact that postmenopausal women, who are estrogen-deficient, commonly get osteoporosis, yet some work suggests that it may be prevented simply by taking extra calcium by mouth. Simple *deficiency of calcium in the diet* may cause, or aggravate, osteoporosis, although this is controversial. In such cases, as before, the presence of PTH is probably necessary for osteoporosis to appear. The *immobilization* required for treating a major fracture (and for flying in a space capsule) may result in osteoporosis. Here, bone for some unknown reason becomes more sensitive to thyroxine and PTH, and net resorption increases. Perhaps *too much meat in the diet* can cause osteoporosis by subjecting the body to an excessive load of acid which requires alkaline bone salt for buffering. Since chronic metabolic acidosis (seen in certain patients with severe renal disease) does cause loss of bone mineral, this idea is not completely far-fetched, but there is little evidence to support it at present.

Treatment of osteoporosis is often unsatisfactory. One may usually reverse immobilization easily enough, and feed the patient more calcium. One may replace missing estrogens—no doubt a good idea when indicated. Fluoride (which increases bone density), phosphate (which may increase bone formation), and TCT have been proposed as therapies. All probably have some value, but none have been used long enough to prove that they are effective and, in any case, until a specific cause is found in the patient at hand, effective treatment will be difficult.

## BIBLIOGRAPHY

*Parathyroid Hormone*

Aurbach, G. D.   Isolation of parathyroid hormone after extraction with phenol. *J. Biol. Chem.* 234:3179, 1959.

Barnicot, N. A.   The local action of the parathyroid and other tissues on bone in intracerebral grafts. *J. Anat.* 82:233, 1948.

Berson, S. A., Yalow, R. S., Aurbach, G. D., and Potts, J. T., Jr.   Immunoassay of bovine and human parathyroid hormone. *Proc. Nat. Acad. Sci. U.S.A.* 49:613, 1963.

Chase, L. R., and Aurbach, G. D.   Parathyroid function and the renal excretion of 3'5'-adenylic acid. *Proc. Nat. Acad. Sci. U.S.A.* 58:518, 1967.

Potts, J. T., Jr., Aurbach, G. D., and Sherwood, L. M.   Parathyroid hormone: Chemical properties and structural requirements for biological and immunological activity. *Recent Progr. Hormone Res.* 22:101, 1966.

Rasmussen, H., Shirasu, H., Ogata, E., and Hawker, C.   Parathyroid hormone and mitochondrial metabolism. *J. Biol. Chem.* 242:4669, 1967.

Wells, H., and Lloyd, W.   Effects of theophylline on the serum calcium of rats after parathyroidectomy and administration of parathyroid hormone. *Endocrinology* 81:139, 1967.

### Thyrocalcitonin

Copp, D. H.   Parathyroids, calcitonin, and control of plasma calcium. *Recent Progr. Hormone Res.* 20:59, 1964.

Munson, P. L., and Hirsch, P. F.   Discovery and pharmacologic evaluation of thyrocalcitonin. *Amer. J. Med.* 43:678, 1967.

Potts, J. T., Jr., Niall, H. D., Keutmann, H. T., Brewer, H. B., Jr., and Deftos, L. J.   The amino acid sequence of porcine thyrocalcitonin. *Proc. Nat. Acad. Sci. U.S.A.* 59:1321, 1968.

Raisz, L. G., Au, W. Y. W., Friedman, J., and Niemann, I.   Thyrocalcitonin and bone resorption. *Amer. J. Med.* 43:684, 1967.

Sherwood, L. M.   Relative importance of parathyroid hormone and thyrocalcitonin in calcium homeostasis. *New Eng. J. Med.* 278:663, 1968.

Tashjian, A. H., Jr., and Melvin, K. E. W.   Medullary carcinoma of the thyroid gland. Studies of thyrocalcitonin in plasma and tumor extracts. *New Eng. J. Med.* 279:279, 1968.

Tauber, S. D.   The ultimobranchial origin of thyrocalcitonin. *Proc. Nat. Acad. Sci. U.S.A.* 58:1684, 1967.

Tenenhouse, A., Rasmussen, H., Hawker, C. D., and Arnaud, C. D.   Thyrocalcitonin. *Ann. Rev. Pharmacol.* 8:319, 1968.

### Vitamin D

Arnaud, C., Rasmussen, H., and Anast, C.   Further studies on the interrelationship between parathyroid hormone and vitamin D. *J. Clin. Invest.* 45:1955, 1966.

Loomis, W. F.   Skin-pigment regulation of vitamin-D biosynthesis in man. *Science* 157:501, 1967.

Stohs, S. J., and DeLuca, H. F.   Subcellular location of vitamin D and its metabolites in intestinal mucosa after a 10-IU dose. *Biochemistry* (Washington) 6:3338, 1967.

### Bone and Mineral

Belanger, L. F., Belanger, C., and Semba, T.   Technical approaches leading to the concept of osteocytic osteolysis. *Clin. Orthop.* No. 54:187, 1967.

Bell, N. H.   Dynamics of bone metabolism. *Ann. Rev. Med.* 18:299, 1967.

Fleisch, H., Russell, R. G. G., and Straumann, F.   Effect of pyrophosphate on hydroxyapatite and its implications in calcium homeostasis. *Nature* (London) 212:901, 1966.

Harris, W. H., and Heaney, R. P.   Skeletal renewal and metabolic bone disease. *New Eng. J. Med.* 280:193, 253, 303, 1969.

Simkiss, K.   Phosphates as crystal poisons of calcification. *Biol. Rev.* 39:487, 1964.

Termine, J. D., and Posner, A. S.   Amorphous/crystalline interrelationships in bone mineral. *Calc. Tiss. Res.* 1:8, 1967.

Walser, M.   Magnesium metabolism. *Ergebn. Physiol.* 59:185, 1967.

*Clinical*

Jackson, W. P. U.   *Calcium Metabolism and Bone Disease.* London: Arnold, 1967.

# 9. The Endocrinology of Reproduction

> The omnipresent process of sex, as it is woven into the whole texture of our man's or woman's body, is the pattern of all the process of our life.
> —HAVELOCK ELLIS,
> *The New Spirit*

THE endocrine secretions involved in reproduction can be viewed as essential for the survival of the species whereas those discussed so far are principally concerned with the functioning of the individual. The glands to be considered here are the *ovary* and *testis*. In addition, the *pituitary* and, in pregnancy, the *placenta* play an essential role.

Just as there is a negative feedback control of the endocrine secretion of a gland, so too there seems to be a similar control over the reproductive ability of a species. When the species' population becomes too great, the ability of the individuals in that population to bear young is cut down. This is true for animals ranging from the mouse to the elephant. Man, however, seems at present to be an exception; overcrowding has not, apparently, diminished fertility. Consequently we now must spend a great deal of time and effort in expanding contraceptive programs.

## SECRETIONS OF THE FETAL GONAD

For the individual, although reproduction cannot occur until after puberty, the endocrinology of reproduction begins long before—in utero, in fact. While a second X chromosome is needed for a normal ovary to develop from the cortex of the undifferentiated gonad and a Y chromosome for a normal testis to develop from the medulla, the chromosome constitution alone is not the whole story. Successful reproduction depends not only on normal gonads but also on the proper growth and development of the central nervous system and of the internal and external genitalia.

### Central Nervous System

The central nervous system (CNS) is important because both the sexual behavior and gonadotropin secretion that occur later at puberty are dependent on it and are in part "built into" the brain during fetal life. Whether or not the fetus is exposed to testosterone makes a great deal of difference later on. In animals such as the rat, if the fetus makes (or is given) testosterone, one will see male sexual behavior and a non-

149

cyclic LH secretion after puberty. If there is no testosterone, the adult will behave like a female and secrete LH cyclically. Even in humans, extra androgen in utero may result in generally normal feminine behavior in adulthood, but the woman is clearly more masculine than is normal.

In adulthood, human sexual behavior depends also on the gonadal hormones secreted and their effect on the CNS. Once the behavior pattern is established, its maintenance apparently depends on the CNS; libido beyond puberty is in large part psychologically determined. Still, normal adult sexual behavior probably requires proper conditioning of the CNS, preferably in utero.

### Genitalia

The genitalia, internal and external, are of obvious importance in reproduction. While most of their growth takes place at puberty, the development and initial growth that occur in utero must first be normal for the pubertal changes to occur.

One may recall that the chromosome-dependent gonadal differentiation into ovary or testis is followed by a *ductal* differentiation into male or female internal genitalia. The müllerian duct system in women develops into the fallopian tube, the uterus, and the upper one-third of the vagina, and the wolffian duct system atrophies. This same pattern would occur in the male except for the presence of the fetal testis. The testis makes a substance, the *testis inducer,* the presence of which depends on the Y chromosome and which causes the müllerian system to atrophy and the wolffian duct to differentiate into the epididymis, the vas deferens, and the seminal vesicles. The inducer does not seem to be solely an androgen since, while androgens will stimulate wolffian development, they will not cause atrophy of the müllerian system. It is not clear what this inducer is, nor is it necessarily secreted (it may act after simple local diffusion), but it is clearly of hormonal quality.

The testis of the male fetus is also responsible for the proper development of the male external genitalia. In this instance the androgen *testosterone* is the agent involved, and there seems little question that the development of the penis, the fusion at the median raphe (ensuring proper location of the urethra), and the development and median fusion of the scrotum are all dependent on the secretion of the fetal testis. The gonadotropin stimulating the testosterone secretion is probably of maternal rather than fetal origin, coming either from the mother's pituitary or the placenta, more likely the latter. In the absence of the testis, no testosterone will be made, and the corresponding female external genitalia will form: the clitoris, labia minora, and labia majora.

After birth there appears to be relatively little gonadal activity until puberty, but the stage has been set.

## PUBERTY

Adolescence: a stage be-
tween infancy and adultery.
—ANONYMOUS

"Puberty" literally has to do with the appearance of hair in particular areas of the body. It has come to mean, however, the time of life when sexual maturity occurs and reproduction becomes possible. In this sense, of course, much more than the appearance of pubic hair is involved.

At about 11 years of age in girls (a little later in boys), *pubic hair* appears and begins to grow. This is probably an *adrenal* as well as a *gonadal* function. Presumably an adrenal androgen (testosterone?) in girls, and perhaps in boys, is secreted at about the same time that the ovaries or testes begin to increase their function.

Shortly thereafter *girls* show an increased secretion of *estrogen* which soon becomes cyclic and which stimulates the development of the breasts and genitalia. One can now easily detect, even with the relatively crude assays available, *urinary gonadotropin.* Sometime later, about the age of 13 and two years after pubic hair growth started, *axillary hair* begins to grow and the *onset of menstruation* (the *menarche*) takes place. The *ovulation* which precedes menstruation is at first erratic and only occasional, but after a variable period regular *cyclic ovulation* begins. For unknown reasons, perhaps nutritional, the age at menarche has been decreasing over the last 100 years; in Norway, for example, menarche appeared at age 17 in 1840 and at age 13.5 in 1950. Even in the last 50 years in the United States the age has dropped from 14.2 to 12.9 years.

In *boys*, hair growth appears at about the same time in the sequence, and the pattern is similar except that the processes involved are *testosterone secretion, development of facial hair and genitalia,* and *seminal emission* with the production of *spermatozoa* instead of *ova.*

At puberty, the growth rate increases noticeably in both boys and girls; this is the *pubertal growth spurt.* It is probably due to the gonadal hormones, testosterone and estrogen, which stimulate growth directly and which also increase the secretion of growth hormone (see Chap. 11).

### Cause of Puberty

Why does puberty occur when it does? An entire book devoted to this problem was published in 1965 without a definite answer, but clearly the central nervous system and hypothalamus are important. A girl who is blind, for example, has an earlier puberty than other girls.

Many bits of evidence are available and provide clues. Small amounts of gonadotropins are present before puberty. The difference is that they are present in lesser amounts than after puberty. For example, in the normal adult, average values in the urine are 5.6 units/liter for follicle-stimulating hormone (FSH) and 4.7 units/liter for luteinizing hormone (LH); in children the values are 2.2 and 0.4, respectively. The gonadotropins are in fact necessary to the prepubertal child for the development and maintenance of the gonads during this relatively quiescent phase. The gonads before puberty secrete a small amount of estrogen or androgen, depending on the sex. Furthermore, the ovaries have a normal response to gonadotropin given by injection.

If the pituitary and gonads are thus capable of functioning, the prepubertal individual must lack a proper stimulus to gonadotropin release. Most of the evidence to date supports the thesis that FSH and LH are completely dependent on hypothalamic stimulation for their secretion, as opposed to the lesser degree of dependence of adreno-corticotropic hormone (ACTH) and thyroid-stimulating hormone (TSH).

The next step was to see whether the gonadotropin-releasing factors were present or absent in the prepubertal hypothalamus. When looked for, both FSH-RF and LH-RF were found in the prepubertal hypothalamus. Presumably, *brain centers* higher yet than the median eminence are responsible for the pubertal stimulation of gonadotropin release.

The "trigger" to the release of gonadotropin is not known. One mechanism involved, although not explaining the basic problem, may be as follows:

1. Before puberty, gonadotropin release is inhibited by the small amount of estrogen or androgen made by the prepubertal gonad.
2. In some way as yet unknown, at the time of puberty the central nervous system, perhaps the anterior hypothalamus, becomes less repressed by the small amount of gonadal hormone. (In the female, the ovary may make a little progesterone, which could cause less suppression of the CNS.)
3. With the CNS centers now less suppressible—which means in functional terms that they are less sensitive to given amounts of sex hormone—larger amounts of the hypothalamic releasing factors flow to the pituitary and more gonadotropins (FSH and LH) are released. In the rat, an increase in LH-RF secretion has been shown at the time of sexual maturation. In humans, the increase in LH secretion is greater than the increase in FSH secretion; puberty is associated then with a drop in the FSH/LH ratio.
4. All this increases the estrogen or androgen production. At a higher circulating estrogen level, the CNS centers will again respond by inhibiting gonadotropin secretion, and a new equilibrium is established. The difference is that now the estrogen or

androgen level is high enough to cause the biologic effects recognized as puberty.

Whether the decreased inactivation of estrogen by the liver seen at this time has anything to do with it is not known. Equally uncertain is the place of a gonadotropin inhibitor found in the urine of children under 6 years of age.

What seems certain is that the *stimulus for puberty* comes from within the *central nervous system* and that *gonadotropin secretion precedes ovarian or testicular development and secretion.*

## The Ovary and Reproduction in the Female

The secretions of the normally functioning ovary are cyclic and are predominantly *estrogens* in the earlier *follicular* stage of the cycle with the addition of *progestins* in the later *luteal* stage. One may almost regard the ovary as two separate endocrine glands depending on which stage is considered, the *follicle* and surrounding tissue being the secreting gland in the first stage and the *corpus luteum* ("yellow body") in the second. Besides the estrogens and progestins, a tiny amount of testosterone is also secreted and can be found in the ovarian vein. It is not clear yet whether the testosterone is secreted by the same cells that secrete estrogen and progestin; possibly it comes from different cells, e.g., the ovarian interstitial tissue.

### Estrogens

Many substances may be estrogenic. The word literally means "causing estrus." Estrus or "heat" is the sexually active state found in most mammalian females and occurs about the time of ovulation. It is derived from a Greek word meaning "gadfly," an insect which makes cattle nervous and irritable, a state resembling that of sexual activity. No such state can be demonstrated, however, in the human female, and for practical purposes an estrogen is usually defined in terms of other actions and not according to its ability to cause estrus.

The main *active estrogen* secreted by the ovary is *17β-estradiol.* Estrogenic activity was first shown in ovarian extracts in 1923 by Allen and Doisy, and the first estrogen to be isolated was estrone in 1929 (Doisy, Butenandt). There are many *synthetic* estrogens other than estradiol; in fact, a great deal of the estrogen used clinically is synthetic. One of the more potent ones (*stilbestrol*) is not a steroid at all, and was discovered as a by-product of investigations concerning carcinogenesis.

BIOSYNTHESIS.   17β-Estradiol is synthesized along pathways similar to those of the adrenal cortex. The difference lies in the lack of 21- or 11-hydroxylation in the ovary and in the predominance of the pathway from Δ⁴-androstenedione through testosterone to estradiol (see Figs. 20 and 42).

Estradiol may also be made without testosterone as an intermediate via direct 19-hydroxylation of Δ⁴-androstenedione and subsequent aromatization, which means the formation of the "benzene" A ring, and reduction. Recent work suggests that the $C_{19}$ may not be hydroxylated at all. One possibility is that the $C_{19}$ methyl group is first removed from Δ⁴-androstenedione, which is then aromatized to estrone and then reduced to estradiol. Another possibility is that the oxidative attack takes place on the 1β-hydrogen and not on the $C_{19}$ methyl group; at the same time, the $C_{19}$ is lost and the double bond ($\Delta^{10 \to 1}$) formed.

The overall yield of the reaction progesterone ⟶ estradiol has been estimated to be about 5%. In the follicular phase, estradiol is made by the follicle and its surrounding cells. The ovarian thecal cells, a layer of cells surrounding the inner layer of granulosa cells, are probably responsible for cleaving off the 2-carbon side chain of progesterone (the $C_{20}$ and $C_{21}$), thus making a $C_{19}$ steroid, Δ⁴-androstenedione. The granulosa cells then convert Δ⁴-androstenedione to testosterone, and both thecal and granulosa cells take part in the final conversion of testosterone to 17β-estradiol. Estradiol is also made by the corpus luteum in the luteal phase and hence is not just a follicular-phase hormone. Hydrocortisone plays a permissive role in estradiol secretion.

There might be a metabolic block in the pathway from testosterone

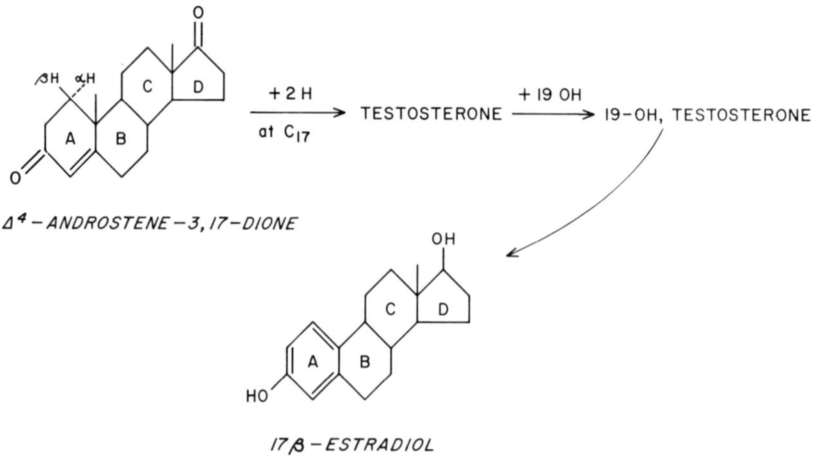

FIG. 42.   The likely final steps in the biosynthesis of 17β-estradiol.

to estradiol in some patients' ovaries, which could cause an increase in testosterone secretion and thus masculinizing of the female. In fact this occurs: In the normal ovary, only 0.2% to 0.3% of progesterone winds up as testosterone; in the abnormal ovary of such patients the amount is demonstrably increased to 0.4% to 2.0%.

The ovary converts a small amount of estradiol to estrone, a less potent estrogen. This reaction involves the reduction of the 17-OH group to a 17-keto group (see Fig. 43).

SECRETION AND BLOOD LEVELS.    Estrogen secretion is *stimulated by LH*, although there is some evidence that FSH may cause a slight amount of secretion. The cellular site of LH action is not known. How does LH act? Probably by stimulating the later steps in estrogen synthesis. For example, in the ovary, LH stimulates the conversion of (refer to Fig. 20 for some of these reactions) (1) cholesterol to 20α-OH-cholesterol, (2) Δ⁵-pregnenolone to Δ⁴-androstenedione, (3) progesterone to Δ⁴-androstenedione, (4) Δ⁵-pregnenolone to estradiol, and (5) testosterone to estradiol. Exactly which step (or steps) is directly stimulated by LH or which step is limiting is also a mystery at this time. Furthermore, despite this biochemical information, there is some recent evidence showing that LH can inhibit rather than stimulate the secretion of estradiol under certain conditions. More work is needed.

Since FSH increases amino acid uptake by the ovary, it is possible that a basic effect on protein synthesis plays a supportive role in the changes in steroid metabolism caused by LH. Not much is known about this, nor is it known whether cyclic AMP is involved—another area for further work. It does seem that $T_4$ enhances the action of LH on estrogen secretion.

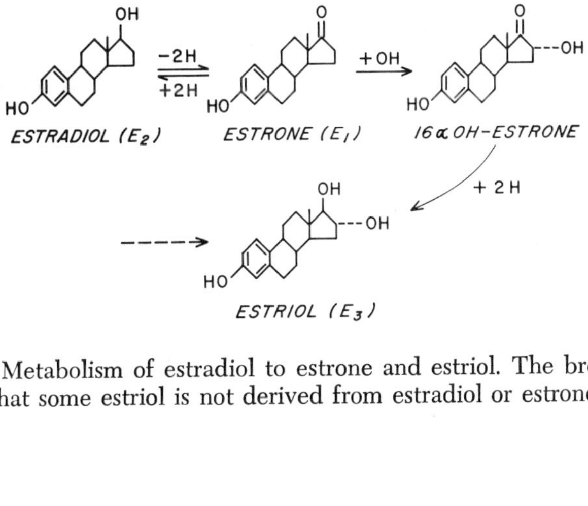

FIG. 43.    Metabolism of estradiol to estrone and estriol. The broken arrow indicates that some estriol is not derived from estradiol or estrone.

The daily *secretion rate* of estradiol in humans is difficult to measure. It is impractical to put a cannula in the ovarian vein, so indirect methods are used. The result is then more properly termed a "production rate" than a secretion rate because estradiol may be formed from estrone outside the ovary, for example, in addition to being secreted by the ovary. Estimates of estradiol secretion in adult women are 90 to 150 µg per day in the follicular stage and 200 to 250 µg per day in the luteal phase. Adult men, for comparison, make about 40 µg per day. Note that there is a *peak at ovulation* and that more is secreted during the luteal phase than the follicular.

In the *blood* of adult women estradiol circulates bound in part to a β-globulin ($K_{41} = 3 \times 10^{10}$). The concentration of estradiol rises from a level of 6 to 8 mµg/100 ml in the follicular phase to a peak at the time of ovulation of 30 mµg/100 ml, then probably drops somewhat to about 20 mµg/100 ml in the midluteal period. The equivalent value in men is only 2 mµg/100 ml.

METABOLISM. Many tissues can convert estradiol to estrone. Since the reaction is often reversible, and estrone is an active but less potent estrogen than estradiol, one can see how this might be a mechanism for regulating estrogen activity at the tissue level. For the body as a whole, the equilibrium is toward estrone.

A major conversion product of estradiol (and the form in which much of it is excreted) is 16α-OH-estriol, or *estriol*, a rather impotent estrogen. Most is made in the liver, from which it may return to the blood. Estriol is not formed simply by the addition of a 16α-OH to estradiol, as one might expect, but is formed via the reaction shown in Figure 43. Based on the number of hydroxyl groups, estrone, estradiol, and estriol are conveniently abbreviated $E_1$, $E_2$, and $E_3$, respectively. Other metabolites of estradiol include 16β-OH-estriol (or epiestriol), 2-OH-estrone—further converted to 2-methoxyestrone (which accounts for about 10% of secreted estradiol)—and a number of 6α-OH, 6β-OH, and possibly 11β-OH compounds. Much of the estriol found, however, is probably not derived from estradiol, as indicated by the broken arrow in Figure 43.

Thyroxine in sufficient amounts causes the catabolism of estradiol to shift more toward 2-methoxyestrone and away from estriol. If both these end products were simply waste and of no physiologic importance, the effect of $T_4$ would be of little moment. Some recent work, however, suggests that the action of estradiol on its chief end-organ, the uterus, is inhibited when more estriol is present. More of this later.

All these compounds have some estrogen activity (in certain cases very little), but just how much of a role they have in vivo is not known. Estrone, because of its relatively high circulating level, may well play a major part along with estradiol.

These hormones and their metabolites are usually conjugated, principally in the liver. The kidney, gastrointestinal tract, and lung have a relatively minor role and account for 20% to 30% of estradiol and estrone metabolism. Glucuronides and sulfates are the main conjugated forms. Glucuronide is conjugated mainly at the 16-OH or 17-OH groups, while sulfate is conjugated principally at the 3-OH group. The conjugates in part are secreted into the bile and thence to the gut, where a certain amount may be resorbed (of estradiol and estrone, at least), and are also secreted back into the blood from the liver, where they circulate about 50% bound to protein. Roughly 75% of $E_1$ given intravenously appears in the bile initially, but ultimately only 7% winds up in the stool and 90% appears in the urine, emphasizing the magnitude of the enterohepatic circulation. What is not known is whether any of the material resorbed from the gut has biologic activity. Another topic for investigation.

Most of the estradiol metabolites are excreted into the *urine*, in both free and conjugated form. To date, almost all measurements have been of the so-called classic estrogens: estradiol, estrone, and estriol. Although they are usually measured as "total" amounts, rather than as the free or conjugated forms, it has been shown that much of the estradiol is not conjugated (is "free") while most of the estrone and estriol is conjugated. The total amount of these in the urine accounts, however, for only a third, at most, of the total estradiol produced. The remainder is probably present as other metabolites, as indicated above, but is not usually included as "total estrogens."

Estimates of urinary estrogens show the sort of changes one might expect from what we have said about secretion, with a peak around the time of ovulation, a second somewhat lower peak in the middle of the luteal phase, low levels in the postmenopausal woman, and similarly low levels in the normal adult man (the accompanying table shows urine values in micrograms per day).

| Estrogens | Ovulation | Mid-luteal | Post-menopausal | Adult Man |
|---|---|---|---|---|
| Estradiol | 9 | 7 | 1 | 1–2 |
| Estrone | 20 | 14 | 3 | 4–6 |
| Estriol | 27 | 22 | 3 | 4–6 |
| "Total estrogens" | 56 | 43 | 7 | 14 |

ACTIONS OF ESTROGEN.  At almost every step of the way estrogen is important for normal female reproductive capacity. While most is known about the rat and mouse, in all likelihood the information is largely applicable, in at least a gross sense, to man. Although $E_1$ (estrone) has estrogenic effects, most biologic estrogen effect in humans is probably due to $E_2$ (estradiol), since plasma estrone levels are the same in men and women.

*Female Reproductive Tract.*   Estrogen acts on the *ovary* to increase the sensitivity of the granulosa cell to FSH; it also increases the mitotic activity of the germinal epithelium. These actions are probably dependent on the dose of estrogen; if it is too large, the resulting decrease in gonadotropin would tend to decrease ovarian activity. Estrogen, in addition, stimulates the motility of the *fallopian tube.*

Most of the work on the actions of estrogen has, however, been concentrated on the *uterus*, principally the uterine epithelium or endometrium of the rat, where many things happen:

1.  Within 15 seconds, *estradiol binds* to a cytoplasmic "receptor protein" in a sterically specific manner. $E_2$ is not concentrated by the uterus but is converted only slowly to other compounds such as estrone. Thus a small amount bound—in the rat a total of 0.01 to 0.1 ng—remains effective for a relatively long time. Estriol binds to this receptor protein as well and may limit the action of estradiol by occupying many of the available binding sites. The estriol/estradiol ratio ($E_3/E_2$) may be important then, a high value indicating less estrogen effect for a given amount of estradiol.

2.  The $E_2$-protein complex may then transfer the $E_2$ to the uterine cell nuclei, to which $E_2$ also binds specifically.

3.  Within the same 15 seconds that $E_2$ binds to its receptor, $E_2$ also *increases cAMP* in the uterus. cAMP in turn stimulates synthesis of both RNA and protein in the uterus; logically then cAMP might reasonably play a major role in what follows. The relation of cAMP to $E_2$ binding, however, has not yet been investigated.

4.  By the time a few minutes have passed, one sees an increase in the uptake of RNA and protein precursors by the uterus, an increase in nuclear RNA synthesis (both ribosomal and messenger RNA), and an increase in nuclear RNA polymerase activity. It seems that an increase in synthesis of a specific (though unknown) protein may be necessary for the increase in nuclear RNA synthesis, and the RNA polymerase might be that protein. Nevertheless, some work indicates that enhanced nuclear RNA synthesis occurs before any increase in the activity of two different RNA polymerases. Suffice it to say that at the moment there is controversy as to whether protein or RNA synthesis is effected first. The increased RNA polymerase activity is, however, necessary for a continued estrogen effect. It is also not yet clear whether the increased RNA synthesis is completely DNA dependent.

5.  A bit later, perhaps at 30 minutes, comes a definite rise in DNA-dependent RNA synthesis; estrogen apparently stimulates this by

increasing transcription at specific sites of the DNA. One can, for example, take uterine chromatin extracted from an estrogen-treated rat, put it into the uterus of an untreated animal, and show an increase in RNA synthesis similar to that of the treated rat. At this time there is also increased blood flow to the uterus and increased permeability to water.

6. By three hours, there is an increase in the number and activity of ribosomes, along with a major increase in total protein synthesis. Most of this is probably directly due to the effect on RNA synthesis noted just above.

7. At six hours, the uterus has grown considerably in weight, almost all of which is due to *water imbibition* and not to an increase in dry weight. Some think that this effect is histamine-mediated. While protein synthesis seems to be required for this effect, RNA synthesis may not be. The effect on water content may also be related to the change in blood flow just noted. At the same time one sees a higher glucose uptake and a higher phosphofructo-kinase activity, both dependent on mRNA synthesis.

8. Over the next 18 to 24 hours, there is a rise in total protein and RNA content and in DNA content and the number of mitoses, and one sees actual *growth of the uterus*, in both muscle and epithelial lining.

As we suggested, there is some argument over whether RNA synthesis is required for many or all of these effects, or whether estrogen can increase protein synthesis, both specific and total, by some direct mechanism. If the latter were the case, the effects on RNA synthesis would have to be viewed as secondary to the synthesis of some specific protein. The answers are not all in yet, but it seems reasonable to attribute at least the major part of the later effect on uterine growth to increased RNA synthesis. The best evidence for this, as noted above, is that if one extracts the RNA from an estrogen-stimulated uterus and injects it into another uterus never exposed to estrogen, the RNA will cause a perfectly good estrogen effect.

Other changes occurring in the endometrium, particularly histologic changes, are discussed later (see The Menstrual Cycle, below).

In the *vagina* both estradiol and estrone are taken up and bound, in contrast to the uterus, which binds only estradiol. The main observable effect on the vagina is increased mitotic activity and *increased keratinization* (or cornification) of the vaginal epithelium, which is associated with development and growth of the vagina. The effect on cornification is useful clinically in making a gross estimate of estrogen activity in patients.

*Secondary Sex Characteristics.*    The primary sex characteristics in females may be considered the second X chromosome or the production of the ovum. The other differences that distinguish female from male are called secondary sex characteristics. In the female, most of these are estrogen induced. They include the proper growth and development of the *reproductive tract* (external and internal genitalia) and of the *breasts, menstruation, feminine fat distribution,* and *feminine hair distribution.* Note that the hair development, e.g., axillary hair, is also influenced by some androgenic stimulus, though whether the adrenal or the ovary is more important is not clear.

*Central Nervous System.* Estrogens have been shown to lower the seizure threshold of the brain. This kind of effect, combined with some progesterone, may be what causes the irritability and sexual receptiveness known in most mammals as estrus. While estrus as such is not apparent in humans, estrogens may well play a role in what we crudely call feminine behavior.

This is probably a primarily hypothalamic effect, since estradiol binds to the hypothalamus and hypothalamic implants of estradiol cause estrus behavior even after the ovaries are removed. Note that this feminine response is "built in" in earlier life (see Secretions of the Fetal Gonad, above), for estrous behavior occurs in an adult female (rat) whether the hypothalamic implant is testosterone or estradiol.

*Other Effects.* Estrogens have a number of other, less apparent effects, many of which are apparent only at high levels of estrogen:

1. There is some effect on the *thyroid* since the thyroid enlarges during adolescence and pregnancy. The goiter may be secondary to an increased renal iodide clearance and thus to relative iodine deficiency.

2. A number of specific *plasma-binding proteins* are increased. Thyroxine-binding globulin, transcortin, ceruloplasmin, and testosterone-binding protein are all increased. Pregnant women or women taking oral contraceptives, for example, have a high PBI yet are not hyperthyroid and have a high plasma cortisol yet do not have Cushing's syndrome. The extra hormone is physiologically inactive because it is mostly bound to the binding protein. The changes in binding proteins are not found in all species; for transcortin, for example, only rodents and primates (among the mammals) show this response to estrogen. The changes in binding proteins and therefore in PBI and plasma cortisol are of obvious clinical importance in testing women who have increased estrogen levels.

3. *Adrenal* corticoid inactivation by the liver and corticoid output by the adrenal may be reduced. Adrenal size may be increased, possibly secondarily to increased ACTH output. Conclusive proof for these actions on corticoid metabolism is lacking.

4. *Lipogenesis* in adipose tissue is increased, perhaps accounting for the different fat distribution seen in women as compared to men.
5. Estrogens may be important in maintaining the structure of *bone,* but evidence is indirect (see Chap. 8, under Osteoporosis).
6. *Salt and water* retention is increased, at least at pharmacologic doses. Estrogens may do the opposite at physiologic levels, i.e., increase sodium excretion, thus secondarily raising the secretion of aldosterone.
7. Water content and mitoses in *skin,* particularly of the vulva, are increased. Used in cosmetics for this action, estrogens remove wrinkles temporarily.
8. *Red blood cell* production may be inhibited.
9. There is some suggestion that estrogens will increase resistance to *infection.*

Once again, it is tempting to speculate that these seemingly minor effects of a hormone may actually be more important than we now suspect.

## Progestins

As with the estrogens, many substances may be progestins. A progestin is defined as a substance which aids in maintaining pregnancy. There are several other actions, and only rarely are substances assayed for maintenance of pregnancy; the usual assay involves one of these other actions or is a physicochemical assay.

The principal progestin in man is *progesterone* (Fig. 44). Progestin activity was suspected in 1903 but not demonstrated in ovarian extracts until 1929. Progesterone itself was isolated in 1934 by several groups.

SYNTHESIS AND SECRETION. The synthetic pathway to progesterone is already well known to the reader (see Fig. 20). The corpus luteum is the major producer of progesterone, but some is secreted by the follicle in the late follicular stage, presumably by the granulosa cells.

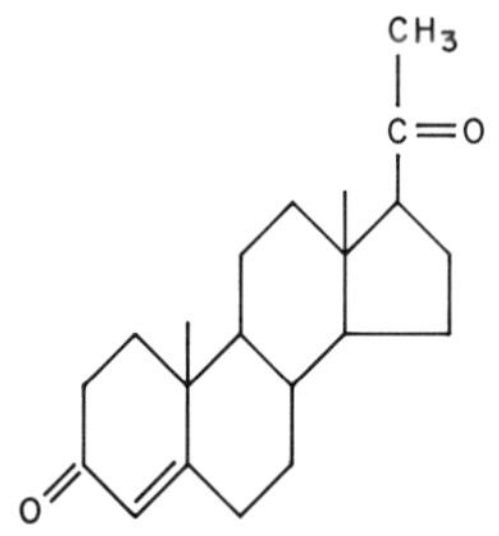

FIG. 44. Progesterone.

Within the corpus luteum it is likely that the luteal cells (which are luteinized granulosa cells) produce the progesterone, possibly with the support of scattered "K" cells. The luteal cells have a decreased capacity for further metabolism of progesterone to other steroids since they have a relative deficiency of 17α-hydroxylase. More progesterone is therefore secreted. Note that estrogen is still made and that the deficiency of 17-hydroxylase is only partial. In the midfollicular stage about 3 to 6 mg per day of progesterone are secreted, increasing to 20 to 40 mg per day in the midluteal stage. The normal male secretes only about 0.75 mg per day, presumably from the adrenals and perhaps from the testes.

STIMULATION OF SYNTHESIS AND SECRETION. The classic teaching, based on work done in the rat, is that progesterone secretion is stimulated by the pituitary gonadotropin, *luteotropin* (LTH). In the rat, luteotropin is identical to prolactin, and the natural tendency has been to identify the two in all other species. However, a luteotropin is defined in a functional sense as anything which either stimulates progesterone secretion in vivo or maintains the integrity of the corpus luteum or both. Confusion will arise if something other than prolactin is luteotropic, or if the two responses defined as luteotropic are controlled by two different hormones, or if the corpus luteum functions well by itself and needs no luteotropin at all. Each of these points should be established for each species to be certain. Caution is the watchword in transferring findings in the rat to humans, although we may often have to do so in the absence of better information. In man, the problem is further complicated by the difficulty in separating prolactin from growth hormone in human pituitary extracts. The two may actually be one hormone; at least they are similar.

In the rat, the mouse, and probably the ferret, there is good evidence showing the identity of luteotropin with prolactin and indicating that prolactin acts as a luteotropin in both senses of the word; i.e., it stimulates progesterone secretion and maintains the corpus luteum in vivo. On the other hand, prolactin is not the luteotropin in some other species. In the pig, the cow, and the sheep, LH is probably the luteotropin; in the rabbit, estrogen itself seems to be luteotropic; and in the guinea pig, no one is sure about anything except that the luteotropin is not prolactin. In humans, there is equal uncertainty and doubt; since prolactin-like material appears in the urine of women during the luteal phase, perhaps prolactin is, after all, the luteotropin in humans.

A possible solution to part of this problem may be at hand because of some recent experiments. Even in rats the story is more complex than the simple statement: "Luteotropin-prolactin stimulates progesterone secretion." The corpus luteum of the rat, incubated in vitro, makes more progesterone if LH is added but does not do so if prolactin is used. This effect of LH in vitro has been amply confirmed in the rat and also has been found in other species such as the cow, the sheep, and the pig, and in the corpora lutea of women. Furthermore, the in vitro findings are probably not artifacts of incubation; under certain circumstances LH given to the rat increases plasma progesterone in vivo. Such experiments attack only one of the two aspects of luteotropin action, that on progesterone secretion. It is beginning to look as though the two luteotropic actions—secretion of progesterone and maintenance of the corpus luteum—may not be both directly due to a single luteotropin. A reasonable idea is that luteotropin-prolactin maintains the structure of the corpus luteum so that LH can then stimulate progesterone secretion. Luteotropin (in those species in which it is not LH) would thus be necessary for both actions to occur but would not be the direct stimulant of progesterone. There is some confirmation of this postulate in work done with perfused bovine corpora lutea. In this preparation LH increases progesterone secretion for a while, but the effect is not lasting; prolactin may allow LH to act for a longer time; both LH and prolactin may be said, then, to be luteotropic. The affair is by no means settled, even in the rat.

A final note on this point: Remember that, while prolactin may not be the luteotropin in some species, it is still necessary for proper lactation.

How does LH act to increase progesterone synthesis and secretion? One suggestion is based on the fact that LH increases glucose uptake, phosphorylase activity, and glucose oxidation by the corpus luteum. There might then be increased TPNH generation secondary to glucose oxidation in the hexose monophosphate (HMP) pathway, and the greater TPNH would in turn increase progesterone synthesis. (Note the analogy to the Haynes hypothesis [see Chap. 5, p. 68] of ACTH action on the adrenal cortex.) Recent evidence, however, suggests that not much of the glucose goes through the HMP pathway and that, although TPNH increases progesterone synthesis, it does so by another mechanism than LH. The increased metabolism of glycogen and glucose may simply be a source of energy for the activated luteal cells.

Another possibility is that LH acts by increasing the synthesis of RNA or some specific enzyme, which would in turn enhance progesterone synthesis. Since both actinomycin and puromycin block the response, RNA and protein synthesis do indeed seem to be important, but exactly what protein or proteins (enzyme?) are needed is unknown.

In any case, LH causes a definite increase in cAMP in the corpus luteum which precedes the increased progesterone synthesis and which is not blocked with puromycin. Furthermore, the ultimate result of LH is a rise in the overall conversion of cholesterol to progesterone, with the critical reaction probably being the hydroxylation of cholesterol to $20\alpha$-OH-cholesterol. Since the cholesterol used in progesterone synthesis comes from both esterified cholesterol in the corpus luteum and plasma cholesterol, it is also possible that the supply of unesterified cholesterol is the limiting factor in this reaction; LH may act to increase the transport of cholesterol across cellular membranes.

Putting all this together, we can suggest that LH stimulates cAMP synthesis by a pathway not involving protein synthesis. cAMP may act at an unknown site, perhaps on the cell nucleus, to increase the synthesis of a critical enzyme (cholesterol hydroxylase? side-chain cleavage enzyme?) or it may act by getting more cholesterol to the reactive site. The result is an increased synthesis and secretion of progesterone. There may be some internal regulation of progesterone synthesis by end-product inhibition; in the corpus luteum in vitro, pregnenolone can apparently decrease acetate's conversion to cholesterol, but whether the same thing occurs in the animal is not certain.

BLOOD LEVELS.  Progesterone circulates largely bound to *albumin* ($K_A = 6 \times 10^4$) and to a fairly specific *globulin* ($K_A = 1 \times 10^7$). The binding globulin may be transcortin or something much like it. Since levels of transcortin are high during pregnancy, they may account in part for the high plasma levels of progesterone at that time. Progesterone has a plasma half-life of approximately five minutes and is therefore rapidly cleared from the blood.

It is difficult to measure actual blood levels, especially in the nonpregnant woman, for technical reasons. Estimations by various methods have led to widely divergent results. Recently, however, newer techniques have given more reliable results. Probably the best estimates in women are about:

| Phase | Plasma Progesterone (µg/100 ml) |
|---|---|
| Preovulatory follicular phase | 0.1–0.3 |
| After ovulation: luteal phase | 1.5 (peak value) |
| Shortly before menses | 0.2–0.4 |
| Pregnancy | 14 (peak value) |

The normal male has only about 0.03 µg/100 ml.

METABOLISM.  Within one hour much of the secreted progesterone is converted to *pregnanediol-3α, 20α*, which is not active as a progestin. Some of it, however, is reversibly converted to 20α-OH- or 20β-OH-$\Delta^4$-pregnenolone (which are progesterone with a 20-OH). These compounds may have some progestin activity, though much less than progesterone. The reversibility may occur in vivo; if so, like estradiol ⇌ estrone, the process would allow a certain amount of local tissue control over progestin activity. In addition, some progesterone seems to be stored in fat (temporarily, at least), in which it is soluble.

The pregnanediol is probably formed mostly in the *liver*, where it is also conjugated. Somewhere between 10% and 30% is then secreted into the bile and thence to the feces.

In addition, there are other catabolic pathways for progesterone and its metabolites, as yet not clearly defined. In any event, only about 20% of the secreted progesterone is found in the urine as pregnanediol, often amounting to less than 2 mg per day, although in the luteal phase urinary pregnanediol may amount to 5 to 10 mg per day. Pregnanediol is what is usually measured to estimate progesterone secretion since blood measurements are difficult. Up to 50% of secreted progesterone is found in the urine in some form; other metabolites account for the 30% that is not pregnanediol.

ACTIONS OF PROGESTERONE.    As with the estrogens, the principal effects of progesterone are on the *female reproductive tract:*

In the *oviduct* (fallopian tube), progesterone decreases motility (opposite of the effect of estrogen).

In the *uterus*, progesterone (1) decreases uterine contractility, which may be related to an increase in intracellular $Na^+$ and $K^+$ and/or to a decrease in sensitivity to oxytocin; (2) enhances estrogen stimulation of overall uterine growth, including the endometrium; (3) causes differentiation of the endometrium so that it is ready for implantation of the blastocyst—the "secretory endometrium"; the proliferative endometrium becomes laden with glycogen, and the endometrial glands become tortuous; (4) is necessary in some undefined way for the further maintenance of pregnancy, perhaps by maintaining the endometrium as in (3).

In the *central nervous system,* progesterone (1) seems to act in general as a CNS depressant but in combination with appropriate amounts of estrogen causes estrus behavior; (2) ordinarily inhibits ovulation, via decreased LH secretion (see below under Control of Gonadotropin and Gonadal Hormone Secretion in the Female); (3) may cause the appearance of maternal behavior in some species.

## The Menstrual Cycle

In normal women, vaginal bleeding, the result of endometrial sloughing, occurs about once a month. Hence the name *menses.* It is an evolutionary invention of primates and is not found in other species. It might be viewed as a monthly failure, since if the pregnancy occurs for which the endometrium was prepared no bleeding takes place.

Although menses occurs about once a month, the actual length of the cycle is highly variable, particularly in younger and older women. The average is indeed once a month, but the deviation in completely normal women is large: mean ± 2 S.D. = 29.1 ± 14.9 days. The length is, however, reasonably constant in the same individual, which, when you think about it, is remarkable.

The observed cyclic bleeding in fact reflects not only a uterine but also an ovarian cycle, under the control of the various gonadotropins. The ovarian *follicular* stage corresponds to the uterine *proliferative* phase with a thickened endometrium and longer endometrial glands, and, after ovulation, the *luteal* stage of the ovary is associated with the *secretory* endometrium with its glycogen-laden cells and tortuous endometrial glands.

THE OVUM AND THE FOLLICLE. The cycling of ovarian hormone secretion is intimately connected with the *periodic release* of the egg or *ovum,* first observed in humans in 1827. While estrus occurs in most mammals about the time of ovulation, the *menstrual flow* appears a half-cycle, or 14 days, after ovulation.

Most mammals, particularly the smaller ones, release several ova at a time. In women, on the other hand, only one follicle develops fully each month and so only one egg is ovulated. Why only one? No one really knows, but the process may be related to the amount of circulating gonadotropin since giving extra gonadotropin to women does cause multiple ovulation. Even though only one follicle normally ovulates, many other follicles develop partially and are in some way needed for the full development of the follicle that does ovulate. Perhaps these smaller follicles make some estrogen which is important for ovulation (see p. 167).

The developing follicle can get as far as the early antral stage without any help from the pituitary; beyond this stage, gonadotropins are needed. Note that the growth and development of the ovum itself are *not* affected by gonadotropins; only the surrounding follicle is stimulated.

HORMONES, THE OVARY, AND THE UTERUS DURING THE MENSTRUAL CYCLE. In the following, human data have been used wherever possible. In the many instances in which they do not exist, however, reasonable extrapolations from animal work have been used.

During the follicular stage there is an increase in the secretion and plasma levels of FSH. FSH alone leads to growth of the follicle. It increases follicular RNA synthesis, amino acid uptake, and amino acid conversion to protein, which no doubt account for the effect on follicular growth. Some LH is also present and appears to augment the growth effect of FSH. LH has also, of itself, been shown to increase RNA and protein synthesis in both the follicle and surrounding interstitial tissue.

The LH is responsible for the gradually increasing *estrogen* secretion that accompanies follicular growth. Estrogen itself seems to act as a stimulus for further follicular growth. The estrogen in turn stimulates *endometrial* protein synthesis and overall growth, with thickening of the endometrium and elongation of the endometrial glands (the *proliferative stage*).

Near the end of follicular development some, but not very much, *progesterone* (and perhaps 20α-OH-progesterone) is secreted from either the follicle or surrounding tissue. Possibly this depends on LH. While usually considered a suppressor of ovulation, which it is in high enough doses, progesterone secretion just before ovulation may be needed for optimum follicular development and at this point in the cycle seems to *facilitate ovulation*. Progesterone may in fact enhance the LH secretion needed for ovulation rather than inhibit it. Perhaps there is a kind of temporary positive feedback system wherein LH increases progesterone secretion which in turn enhances the ovulatory surge of LH. It should be noted here that the evidence that progesterone enhances secretion of LH is best in the rat; in man the point is controversial.

At about the middle of the menstrual cycle there is also a *peak in estrogen secretion*. In all probability the estrogen peak is necessary for ovulation: It *stimulates* or enhances the *sudden release of LH*. The estrogen may be acting on the hypothalamus or pituitary; the latter seems more likely at present.

Both estrogen and progesterone, at this point, combine to bring about estrous behavior (in animals) and perhaps to enhance LH secretion. In addition, in the rat, since estrogen increases plasma prolactin and since plasma prolactin is elevated just before estrus, it is possible that prolactin-luteotropin plays a role in ovulation.

Whatever the stimuli, in the middle of the menstrual cycle occurs a striking, sudden, but transient *increase in LH secretion*—the "ovulatory surge"—which causes ovulation. The high plasma LH is necessary for ovulation. There is a sharp, transient *rise in plasma FSH* as well, which may play some as yet undetermined role in ovulation. In the mouse, FSH does not rise as much as LH so the LH/FSH ratio is relatively high. For the mouse, at least, this high ratio is needed for normal ovulation, which is best at an LH/FSH ratio of about 4/1. In women, as in mice, there is a sharp peak in both plasma FSH and plasma LH; although the rise in LH may occur sooner, it is hard to show much difference between the time of the FSH peak and that of the LH peak. Plasma FSH in women at the time of ovulation rises from a basal level of 10 to 20 mU/ml to about 20 to 50 mU/ml, while plasma LH rises from a basal level of 15 to 30 mU/ml (2 to 4 mμg/ml) to 75 to 150 mU/ml (10 to 20 mμg/ml)—all units in this case being in terms of the newer reference standard (Fig. 45).

LH seems to have a direct action on the follicle, causing it to open and the egg to be released. The wall of the follicle actually becomes

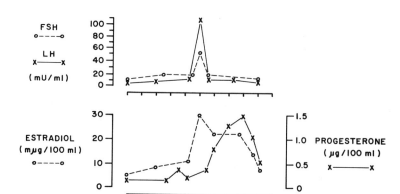

FIG. 45.   Changes observed in plasma levels of FSH, LH, estradiol, progesterone, and basal body temperature during the human menstrual cycle. Although the values shown are approximately correct, the curves are only representational since they are a composite of somewhat differing published data.

thinner (Fig. 46), the cells separate, and collagen fibrils disappear just before rupture occurs. Although the egg is released very close to the opening of the fallopian tube, it is in fact released into the peritoneal cavity and then finds its way into the tube. The fimbriæ of the tube probably have an active role in getting the egg into the tube. We will leave it there and follow it further under the discussion of pregnancy.

The sympathetic nervous system, via catecholamine release—both known to be present in the ovary—may also regulate ovulation by inhibiting it when sympathetic activity is high (at the moment, a speculation).

After ovulation a rapid change takes place in the empty follicle. It is transformed into the *corpus luteum* (first described in 1672 by de Graaf). The principal cell is the luteal cell, which is probably derived from the follicular granulosa cell. The "new" gland then secretes *both estrogen and progesterone* (Fig. 45). Actually, more total estrogen is secreted during the luteal phase than in the previous proliferative phase. Whether the estrogen comes from the new luteal cells or from the older thecal cells is not clear.

Accompanying the increasing progesterone secretion after ovulation

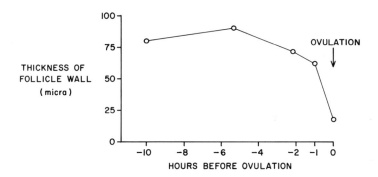

Fig. 46.    Changes in the thickness of the ovarian follicular wall just prior to ovulation in the rabbit. (From L. L. Espey, *Endocrinology* 81:267, 1967.)

there is a rise, in women, in basal body temperature (the morning resting temperature). The higher temperature persists throughout the luteal phase and is a useful clinical indicator of both ovulation and progesterone secretion.

LH is required for the formation of the corpus luteum; hence its name: luteinizing hormone. Whether this is a separate action from ovulation or whether luteinization would spontaneously occur after ovulation is an unanswered question. Some think that LH may simply increase the blood flow to the granulosa cells, thus causing them to luteinize. Once formed, LH stimulates estrogen secretion from the corpus luteum just as it does from the follicle.

Whatever the role of estrogen in causing the ovulatory surge of LH, estrogen plays an important part in the next stage of ovarian and endometrial development. Estrogen seems necessary for the increased *luteotropin* secretion, whatever the luteotropin happens to be (see p. 162), needed for the maintenance of the corpus luteum and its progesterone secretion (the *luteal phase*). We have noted that the rise in estrogen just before ovulation may account for the increased plasma prolactin that occurs about the time of ovulation (in rats, at least). The prolactin may then get the corpus luteum through the early part of its transient life. However, the corpus luteum lasts for two weeks in women and continues to secrete progesterone, and there is prolactin-like material in women's urine right through the luteal phase. Presumably, luteotropin secretion continues, and the estrogen secreted by the corpus luteum during the luteal phase may well be responsible for it. At the same time, estrogen appears to be essential, as a kind of priming agent, for the secretory stage of the endometrium and therefore for the implantation of the fertilized ovum.

The *large amount of progesterone and estrogen* now made causes the endometrial glands to become more tortuous and to produce a more mucous secretion with a high glycogen content. In the endometrial stroma it causes enlargement of cells and a high glycogen content. Glandular growth per se is largely due to the estrogen, while progesterone seems mainly responsible for the stromal changes and for the increase in glycogen and glycoprotein in the glandular epithelium. A proper ratio of progesterone to estrogen is important for optimal change; in the monkey, 1 to 2 mg of progesterone per day and 20 to 40 µg of estradiol per day are about right. The overall endometrial process is called the decidual reaction. This is the *secretory phase.* These changes are at their peak approximately seven to eight days after ovulation, which is about the time of the maximal progesterone and estrogen secretion in this stage.

If implantation of a fertilized blastocyst does not occur, the *corpus luteum* begins to *decrease in function,* and one sees a measurable drop in both progesterone and estrogen secretion. There is an increase in the ovarian enzyme that converts progesterone to $20\alpha$-OH-progesterone which may partly account for the drop in progesterone secretion. What causes the drop? This is another unanswered question. (1) Some have postulated that the corpus luteum has an intrinsically limited life-span; this is probably not true. (2) In some animals a luteolytic or corpus luteum–destroying substance may exist. One of the prostaglandins, $PGF_{2\alpha}$, is a possible candidate. In the rabbit, LH itself may be luteolytic, while in other animals the uterus may contain some luteolytic substance. Luteotropin itself may be luteolytic in the rat. There is no good evidence for such a luteolytic substance in humans. (3) Another possibility is that the corpus luteum disintegrates because of a decrease in luteotropin secretion since one of the functions of luteotropin is to maintain the corpus luteum. Again, good supporting evidence is lacking. Better assays, undoubtedly available soon, will help answer the question.

With the fall in progesterone and estrogen, the secretory endometrium can no longer be maintained. It sloughs, and bleeding occurs: *menstruation.* Apparently, either a drop in progesterone and estrogen or a drop in estrogen alone leads to menstruation, since in anovulatory cycles there is little progesterone production yet menstruation still occurs at about the same time.

The actual bleeding process is thought to be due to the contraction of the spiral arteries, thereby causing ischemia, necrosis, and finally sloughing. However, at least one primate (a monkey) has no spiral arteries and menstruation still occurs. Perhaps some stromal change is responsible. The average blood loss during the menses in women is about 50 ml (range 10 to 200 ml).

## Pregnancy

> The building up of the placenta by the mother and the due performance of function of that wonderful organ require certain favouring conditions . . .
>
> —ENCYCLOPAEDIA BRITANNICA
> (1884)

Let us return to the egg we left in the fallopian tube. For pregnancy to occur, there must be fertilization with a healthy, active, mature spermatozoon (see Spermatogenesis, below). In turn, for this to happen, there must be successful copulation (coitus).

COITUS.   In mammals, including humans, normal mating behavior is essential for normal coitus. Mating behavior is hormonally determined and results from the effects of the gonadal hormones on the central nervous system. Without the CNS effects of the estrogens, progestins, and androgens, no reproduction would occur. In women, sexual desire, or libido, is probably determined by some androgen (testosterone from adrenal or ovary?); estrogen and progesterone are both important as well, if work on rats and monkeys is applicable. While most mammalian females are sexually receptive to the male only at estrus—hence the importance of estrogen—it is certainly not the case for women at the corresponding time: ovulation. Work with other primates suggests that it is true at least in that sexual receptivity seems increased at ovulation relative to other points in the menstrual cycle. In men, libido is clearly related to testosterone secretion, as is sexual activity. Further, the estrogen secretion of the female partner (in monkeys) actually seems related to the sexual activity of the male.

Although not endocrine-mediated except in the broadest sense, the physiology of copulation is of obvious importance; a long and detailed description has been published (*Human Sexual Response* by W. H. Masters and V. E. Johnson).

FERTILIZATION.   Fertilization occurs in the fallopian tube, not the uterus. The spermatozoa must get through the cervical mucus, apparently easier to negotiate at the time of ovulation, and all the way through the uterus. They may be speeded along by prostaglandin made in the seminal vesicles and found in the seminal fluid; prostaglandin seems to stimulate uterine contraction at small dose levels. Oxytocin secreted by the female may also help in the process.

Once in the fallopian tube, how does the spermatozoon locate the

egg? It could be by chance—since there are so many spermatozoa—
or, in some species, by some specific means of recognition. When the
spermatozoon contacts the egg, the egg changes somehow so that
spermatozoa stick to it (agglutinating mechanism). Only one spermatozoon, however, actually penetrates the covering of the ovum, the
zona pellucida, since the egg becomes impermeable to other spermatozoa after the first one has entered. Fertilization is therefore not just
the meeting of spermatozoon and ovum, nor has it occurred when a
spermatozoon gets into the zona pellucida. It is complete only when a
spermatozoon is actually present in the cytoplasm of the egg, and to be
certain, one probably ought to see resumption of cell division. It is not
easy to tell how soon after coitus fertilization can be complete, but in
pigs the whole process can be finished in three hours.

The spermatozoa as they are found in the semen are, in many species,
*not* capable of fertilizing the egg; they must first spend some time in
the female reproductive tract and only then can they stick to and
penetrate the zona pellucida. Exactly why is unclear; the process
depends on some species-specific material in the female reproductive
tract and is called *capacitation*. It may not, however, be necessary for
human fertilization.

Spermatozoa generally live only a relatively short time in the mammalian female, a few days at most, although in dogs they may last 7
to 10 days. In humans, spermatozoa live for only about 24 hours in the
uterus and fallopian tubes.

IMPLANTATION AND THE MAINTENANCE OF PREGNANCY.   Implantation
occurs during the ovarian luteal phase and the endometrial secretory
phase. Both estrogen and progesterone are being secreted.

Cell division begins in the fallopian tube, soon forming the *blastocyst*. For the first seven to eight days after ovulation the blastocyst is
"free-floating" in the tube and uterus, during which time it feeds on
"uterine milk," a secretion of the secretory endometrium. Even though
not attached, the blastocyst still needs the uterus.

If there is too much estrogen, the fallopian tube will contract more
than it should, the blastocyst will arrive in the uterus before the uterus
is ready, and it will not implant. If there is too much progesterone, the
blastocyst is delayed in the fallopian tube, gets to the uterus too late
or is expelled too quickly, and again will not implant. If, however,
there is the proper amount of estradiol and progesterone, the blastocyst arrives at the right place at the right time and, about a week after
ovulation, implants into the endometrium. The implantation site is
near a small blood vessel, which is better for the invasion of the tropho-
blastic cells and ensures adequate nutrition.

There is some evidence that the blastocyst itself requires both estrogen and progesterone to implant, and the endometrium, of course, must be in the secretory phase, which requires both estrogen and progesterone. Thus, estrogen and progesterone are needed for the proper coordination and development of the blastocyst, fallopian tube, and uterus if successful implantation is to occur. Note that the time of implantation corresponds to the time of maximum endometrial development and to about the time of maximal progesterone and estrogen secretion.

Relaxin (see Birth, below) and thyroxine may also play a role in successful implantation. Immunologically, the whole process is fascinating because there is no good explanation of why the blastocyst, a genetically different individual, is not rejected by the host, the mother, as foreign material. An answer to this question might shed much light on the rejection phenomenon in general, a problem of clear importance to those performing transplants of various organs.

Following implantation, the placenta forms with all its vascular supply, absorbing nutrients from the uterine circulation of the mother.

If implantation occurs, menstruation does not. The *corpus luteum* is responsible; the human corpus luteum *continues to function* and secrete progesterone beyond the usual two weeks. The pregnant rat, for example, secretes about 10 µg of progesterone per hour into the ovarian vein. For a while at least the corpus luteum is absolutely essential for the maintenance of pregnancy (except possibly in the elephant).

Why does the corpus luteum continue to function? By definition, we must search for a continued secretion of luteotropin or a decrease in some luteolytic substance.

1. Possibly the *pituitary* continues to secrete a luteotropin. In the hamster, for example, FSH from the pituitary is luteotropic and is required throughout pregnancy. In many other species, including man, the pituitary grossly enlarges during pregnancy, and more acidophil cells appear histologically, suggesting secretion of prolactin. While FSH and LH secretion may be suppressed in most mammals (though FSH is not in women) because of high estrogen and progesterone levels, *prolactin secretion* may be *increased* and it may well be acting as a luteotropin. On the other hand, while helpful, pituitary prolactin-luteotropin secretion is perhaps not essential for prolonging corpus luteum function since women without a pituitary may bear children when given injections containing only FSH and LH. Assays in the two species in which normal levels of plasma prolactin can be detected are contradictory; the pregnant rat has higher than normal plasma prolactin but the pregnant sheep has none at all.

2. The *placenta* is clearly a likely source of a luteotropin. The human

placenta makes two gonadotropins, either of which, or perhaps both, may play a role in maintaining the corpus luteum. These are *human chorionic gonadotropin* (HCG) and *human placental lactogen* (HPL).

*Human Chorionic Gonadotropin.* For many years HCG was the only known placental gonadotropin in man. It was in fact the first gonadotropin detected in body fluids, and its assay has long been the basis of numerous pregnancy tests, including both biologic and the newer immunologic types. The molecular weight of this glycoprotein, which is about one-third carbohydrate, is probably about 55,000 to 60,000. It may be composed of two glycoprotein chains, each with a molecular weight of 25,000 to 30,000. This would account for several reports indicating the molecular weight of HCG to be about 30,000. At present, the most active preparation contains 135,000 U/mg, although most reasonably pure preparations have 12,000 to 20,000 U/mg. It is probably produced by the syncytial cells of the placenta, although older work had suggested that the Langhans' cells were the source.

Although it is a placental hormone, it cross-reacts immunologically with LH from the pituitary and thus must have at least a partially similar structure to that of LH. This phenomenon of cross-reactivity is now used in an immunoassay for LH. HCG itself has predominantly LH-like actions, but under appropriate conditions some FSH-like and luteotropic activity can be demonstrated. When it was the only placental gonadotropin known, it was perforce offered as the placental luteotropin, and it has been shown to prolong human corpus luteum function for a few days.

In pregnancy, with the usual bioassay it is first found in detectable amounts about 35 days after the last menstrual period or at about three weeks of pregnancy. With the more sensitive immunologic method noted above, it can be detected at 10 days of pregnancy. Maximal amounts are in the blood and urine at 60 to 90 days of pregnancy, dropping off to lower levels thereafter. It has a plasma half-life of about 8 hours.

*Human Placental Lactogen.* With the recent discovery of another placental protein, different from HCG, that has luteotropic activity toward the corpus luteum and lactogenic activity toward the breast, we have a better candidate for the placental luteotropin. This discovery did not come as a total surprise; a somewhat analogous substance had been described in the rat almost 30 years before (Astwood). Although it is luteotropic in the rat, firm proof that this human placental lactogen (HPL) maintains human corpora lutea is not available yet; the discovery is too new. It is possible that both HCG and HPL are involved in keeping the corpus luteum functioning, much as both LH and luteotropin probably are in the nonpregnant woman.

HPL appears to be a protein (molecular weight estimated variously at 19,000 or 30,000) made by the syncytial cells. The placenta makes a large amount of it per day (0.3 to 1.0 g). This is reflected in the plasma levels, which rise from barely detectable levels during the fifth week of pregnancy to 1000 to 20,000 mµg/ml just before birth. HPL turns over fairly quickly (plasma half-life of 20 to 30 minutes or less) so that within a day or two after birth none is detectable.

The HPL does not cross-react with LH, as does HCG, but partially cross-reacts immunologically with human growth hormone, a rather remarkable finding. It does not, however, seem to have much, if any, growth activity despite this cross-reaction. Monkey placental lactogen, on the other hand, has a fairly potent growth hormone activity.

HPL appears to inhibit the action of insulin on glucose utilization, much as does growth hormone. It is probably responsible for the mild insulin resistance and glucose intolerance seen in pregnancy.

3. Besides increased luteotropin, there may be a decrease in a *luteolytic* agent. In many animals (though not yet in man), it seems clear that the *uterus* is luteolytic. Implantation of the blastocyst into the uterus somehow blocks or removes this uterine action, thus allowing the corpus luteum to persist. The antiuterine substance is not, however, in the fetus itself.

Whatever the factor or factors responsible, the *placenta*, and perhaps the *pituitary, maintains the corpus luteum* and *progesterone secretion* through the early part of pregnancy, thus maintaining an intact endometrium and allowing pregnancy to continue.

After about two months of pregnancy the human corpus luteum is no longer needed, although it does persist for about six months and ovarian progesterone secretion may persist in small amounts to the end of pregnancy. At the two-month mark, the *placenta* takes over the function of the corpus luteum. It makes increasing amounts of estrogen and progesterone as pregnancy progresses, with peak levels found just before birth. Much of this is de novo synthesis from cholesterol or DHEA in the mother's blood, but a good deal of the estrogen made by the placenta is made from DHEA (or DHEA-sulfate) secreted by the *fetal* adrenal. The fetus and the placenta may be viewed, in part, as an integral endocrine unit. It is possible that the placental gonadotropins noted above stimulate the placenta itself to make these steroids, but this is speculation at the moment. In some animals the placenta is not enough and the corpus luteum is required throughout pregnancy (rabbit).

The placenta also makes corticoids and substances acting like ACTH and TSH, but their function, if any, is not clear.

The maximum amounts of estrogen and progesterone found during pregnancy are roughly as follows (note the different order of magnitude; urine values are in milligrams per day, while in nonpregnant women the corresponding values [see p. 157] are in micrograms per day):

|  | *Urine*<br>(mg/day) | *Blood*<br>(µg/100 ml) |
|---|---|---|
| Estradiol | 2 | 0.4–1.5 |
| Estrone | 2 | 1–5 |
| Estriol | 16 | 1–8 |
| Progesterone | — | 11–14 |
| Pregnanediol | 80 | 50 |

Most of the estradiol in the urine seems to be free and most of the estrone and estriol conjugated. The high progesterone levels in plasma are the result of an increase in progesterone secretion to between 200 and 500 mg per day and a rise in the plasma binding protein.

*Progesterone's major role* in pregnancy may be to prevent excessive uterine contractions and expulsion of the fetus. In truth, exactly what estrogen and progesterone do during pregnancy is not well known, but without them, pregnancy fails.

Thyroxine and hydrocortisone are also required for the successful completion of pregnancy. In this indirect sense, if the patient is otherwise untreated, the pituitary is required in all species including man, since the placenta does not make thyroxine and it is not certain that it secretes hydrocortisone.

### Birth

Man alone, at the very moment of his birth cast naked upon the naked earth, does she abandon to cries and lamentations.

—PLINY THE ELDER,
*Natural History*

Birth does not occur at a given number of days after ovulation any more than the menstrual cycle takes a given number of days. Nevertheless, within any species the length of gestation is surprisingly constant. In man, about 270 days after conception is the usual length.

What causes birth? The precise trigger mechanism is not known. A number of factors probably play a part but much is sheer speculation. Possibilities include:

1. A drop in plasma progesterone which causes increased uterine contractility (there is evidence against this in man).
2. A decrease in the ability of progesterone to suppress uterine motility.
3. An increased plasma level of oxytocin.
4. An increased sensitivity of the uterus to oxytocin.
5. An increased plasma level of prostaglandins.

6. A drop in relaxin, which may then cause increased uterine contractility.

There is not much human evidence available to suggest either accepting or rejecting the last five possibilities. It may even be that something in the hypothalamus/pituitary of the *fetus* is needed to initiate birth.

*Relaxin* has not been discussed yet. In 1926 Hisaw isolated a substance from the ovaries of pregnant pigs (probably from the corpora lutea) which relaxed the interpubic ligament of guinea pigs and was thus thought to aid delivery of the fetuses. Called relaxin because of this action, it is now known to be a peptide (9000 mol. wt.) and has been found in the ovaries (corpora lutea) of pregnant mice and pregnant women as well as the pig. Material similar in biologic activity can be isolated from the uterus and placenta of several animals, including man, but whether it is identical in all is not known. It is another hormone that is defined essentially by its actions, and its physiologic role might be clarified by more work in this area. We can demonstrate several actions of the extracted material:

1. It may *stimulate* the growth of *endometrial blood vessels,* perhaps enhancing nidation (see Implantation and the Maintenance of Pregnancy, above).
2. It *relaxes the interpubic ligament* in some species, which may require the additional presence of growth hormone. This action occurs in guinea pigs, mice, and rats and probably helps birth by allowing easier egress of the fetuses. There is little relaxation of this ligament in the pregnant woman.
3. It can cause *softening of the uterine cervix.*
4. Under some conditions it can stimulate *uterine growth.*
5. It has a *uterine-relaxing* effect.

If the second and third actions have any significance in humans, then a rise rather than a drop in relaxin would aid birth. If the last two mean anything, it is possible that a drop in relaxin secretion might induce the onset of labor. In any case, there is no firm evidence for either a rise or a fall in relaxin at the time of birth, nor does anyone know whether relaxin is secreted in the nonpregnant female.

As to changes in oxytocin level or oxytocin sensitivity, there is also nothing to confirm either of these as the initiator of uterine contraction at term. However, once labor has started, a demonstrable rise in plasma oxytocin (in the cow and goat) does take place, which would help in the later expulsion of the fetus from the uterus. Finally, there is a rise in plasma levels of prostaglandins (perhaps PGE or PGF or both) during labor, but it is not clear whether this rise is a cause or result of the birth process.

After the birth of the fetus, the placenta follows and, as expected, there is a sharp drop in progesterone, estrogen, HCG, and HPL secretion.

## Lactation

> There is no finer investment
> for any community than putting milk into babies.
> —WINSTON CHURCHILL

The ability to secrete milk from the breast is the reason mammals are called mammals. With the exception of man, who has learned to use other animals' milk, it is as essential for survival of mammalian species as reproduction. An analogous process—crop sac secretion—is essential for propagation of pigeons and doves, and curiously, like lactation it requires prolactin.

Three processes, more or less distinguishable, are involved in lactation: (1) breast development, (2) milk secretion, and (3) milk release from the breast.

BREAST DEVELOPMENT.   An obvious point, but one sometimes forgotten, is that breast development for lactation takes place in pregnancy. So it is the hormonal state of the *pregnant* mammal that must be considered.

In women, the initial development of the breasts at puberty is due to estrogens. During pregnancy the development of the *ductal* portion of the glandular tissue of the breast is predominantly influenced by *estrogen,* which binds to breast tissue much as it does to the uterus; that of the more distal *alveoli* and *lobules* is affected mainly by *progesterone.* This is strictly a matter of emphasis; both steroids are present all through pregnancy. They alone, however, are not sufficient for optimal breast development.

Much of the study of breast development has been done in rats and mice, and the experiments are usually carried out by injecting various hormones rather than measuring them in the blood. Perhaps the following results apply to women, perhaps not; they do allow reasonable thoughts on the subject.

Thyroxine must be present for anything to happen. Then, in addition to estrogen and progestin, full differentiation of the breast epithelium requires insulin, hydrocortisone, and prolactin and/or growth hormone. The insulin somehow enhances DNA synthesis by increasing the activity of DNA polymerase and, together with hydrocortisone, is needed for epithelial cell division. Final differentiation of the cell then occurs with prolactin/growth hormone. For 30 years there have been persistent suggestions that a mammogen separate from prolactin was needed for breast development. It seems that this is not the case and that prolactin is the mammogen. Prolactin/growth hormone probably acts synergistically with estrogen and progesterone and not simply in an additive way. It would be reasonable to say that optimal breast development needs *estrogen, progesterone, thyroxine, hydrocortisone, insulin,* and *growth hormone/prolactin,* or substances of similar activity.

One might guess (though it is not proved) that *placental lactogen* (HPL) is a major factor in breast development in women during pregnancy and that in the above scheme of required hormones HPL takes the place of growth hormone/prolactin. Certainly women have high levels of this lactogen in blood during pregnancy which continue to be high right up to the time of birth.

It might be postulated, then, that estrogen and progesterone, with the support and direct stimulation of the placental lactogen, in the presence of adequate insulin, hydrocortisone, and thyroxine, cause breast development in pregnant women. Note that many of these hormones are made by the placenta. $T_4$ may have an indirect as well as a general supportive action, as it may increase pituitary prolactin output, although we are not sure it does so in pregnancy.

MILK SECRETION.   Why is there no secretion of milk in pregnancy if all the hormones noted above are at work? This is a particularly good question in view of the high levels of HPL found. Once again, the answer is not really known. The high levels of estrogen and progesterone may inhibit the action of pituitary prolactin or placental lactogen in this respect. It may be that the placental lactogen does not cause milk secretion in the human but stimulates only breast development. This would be teleologically sensible since the placenta is gone when milk secretion starts. Perhaps the secretion of pituitary prolactin is suppressed, and without it, no matter how much HPL there is, milk production is impossible.

After birth, the pituitary is essential for both initiation and maintenance of lactation. *Prolactin* is the key for both, although in some animals growth hormone is a good substitute. Prolactin activity can be demonstrated in the blood and urine during lactation, while it cannot be shown after lactation stops.

How is lactation initiated? The following is perhaps the most reasonable explanation: When estrogen and progesterone secretion drops precipitously after the passage of the placenta, prolactin secretion rises. In sheep, plasma prolactin goes from zero to 300 m$\mu$g/ml (Fig. 47). Hydrocortisone secretion also rises somewhat at this time and is probably important in the initiation of lactation. A small amount of estrogen has to be secreted by the ovary to stimulate prolactin secretion; suckling by the newborn also helps in this respect. The prolactin may be the cause of the epithelial proliferation that occurs one to three days postpartum.

Once lactation is started, its maintenance requires a number of

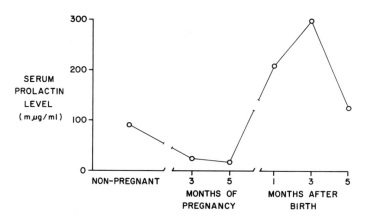

FIG. 47.   Changes in serum prolactin during pregnancy and lactation in the ewe. (From Y. Arai and T. H. Lee, *Endocrinology* 81:1041, 1967.)

hormones. In general they are the same as the ones needed for breast development: prolactin, a small amount of estrogen (perhaps to maintain prolactin secretion), and normal amounts of thyroxine and hydrocortisone and therefore TSH and ACTH. Some animals require insulin and growth hormone as well (goat). There also seems to be a need for normal parathyroid hormone secretion; if PTH is deficient, the resulting hypocalcemia leads to little or no milk production.

Perhaps as important as any of these hormones is *good nutrition* and a *proper mental state*, since a poor diet or severe emotional upset can inhibit milk secretion.

What exactly does prolactin do to the breast? There is scant information on this point, but we do know that prolactin increases DNA synthesis and cell proliferation, and that it stimulates the synthesis of several components of milk: fatty acids, lactose, and casein. The secretion process itself is not well understood. It is not analogous to what goes on in the sebaceous glands, as many have thought, where the glandular cells contribute to the secretion. The sweat gland offers a better analogy, since no part of the cell seems to be destroyed in the process.

THE RELEASE OF MILK FROM THE BREAST.   The removal of milk from the breast is not a simple, passive, mechanical process. Suckling the infant, or milking a cow, actively stimulates the ejection of milk from the breast. Suckling sets off sensory impulses which find their way to the hypothalamus, where oxytocin secretion is stimulated. Once the oxytocin is released to the blood stream, it causes contraction of the myoepithelial elements in the walls of the breast alveoli. Thus, we see a rapid release of milk or "let-down." Note that milk secretion is not increased directly, only the rate of removal from the breast.

As we have said, *suckling* or nursing seems to enhance the secretion of *prolactin* as well as *oxytocin*. It was once thought that the effect of suckling on prolactin secretion was indirect and that the increased oxytocin was the final stimulus to prolactin. Recent work has shown this idea to be wrong. Suckling does increase prolactin secretion, but the effect is separate from that on oxytocin. As with oxytocin, the nervous stimuli of suckling are received in the hypothalamus, where there is probably a *decrease in prolactin-inhibiting factor* (PIF) (of which more later), thus allowing an *increase in prolactin secretion*. There is also a rise in growth hormone and ACTH secretion (in some animals), both of which would help lactation. Nature's own contraceptive seems to result from the same mechanism. Mothers often continue nursing the child longer than necessary to avoid having another child immediately. Along with the decrease in prolactin-inhibiting factor in the hypothalamus that follows suckling, there is a parallel decrease in LH-releasing factor. This, of course, tends to diminish LH secretion and therefore ovulation. Although fairly effective, suckling is not really a reliable contraceptive.

Another interesting sidelight: The hypothalamic area that controls the prolactin-inhibiting factor is about the same area concerned with appetite suppression. Thus, stimuli which block PIF secretion also cause increased eating. This makes good sense teleologically since more food is needed by the mother during lactation.

Clearly, then, both the anterior pituitary gland and the neurohypophysis are needed for good lactation.

If the milk is not removed, there is of course no "let-down." If enough time passes (several days) without removing the milk, milk secretion will stop despite a normal pituitary. Just why is not too clear, but the process is probably related to the absence of suckling and a local pressure effect: The milk-swollen alveoli directly inhibit further milk secretion by these alveoli, and without suckling, the secretion of prolactin and oxytocin stops.

Clinically, to inhibit milk secretion in mothers not wishing to nurse their child, estrogens and testosterone are often used. The assumption is that large doses of either will inhibit prolactin secretion. It is not certain that using these hormones is any better than doing nothing.

### Control of Gonadotropin and Gonadal Hormone Secretion in the Female

So far, the discussion has centered around end-organ response to gonadotropins. Yet the periodicity or cycling of the menstrual period is dependent on the cyclic release of gonadotropins. Their release in turn is dependent on the hypothalamus.

That the central nervous system was involved in the secretion of gonadotropins was first suspected in 1932 (Hohlweg and Junkmann). In 1936 the hypothalamus was proposed as the crucial brain locus, but this was finally proved only in 1957, when estrogen implants into the hypothalamus were shown to decrease gonadotropin release. Work since then, using implantation, electric stimulation, and animals with hypothalamic lesions, has given firm foundation to this concept.

As we have seen, the initial pubertal stimulus to the hypothalamic-pituitary-gonadotropin system is unknown. But once begun, it continues cyclically until the menopause, at which time the ovary fails for unknown reasons. The reason for cycling is also a mystery. One can only suggest the existence of some central nervous system integration which responds to changes in circulating hormones and to various other nervous stimuli so as to maintain a more or less regular rhythm in gonadotropin secretion.

The importance of nervous influences is particularly well shown in the functional amenorrhea (lack of menstruation) that often occurs in young women shifted to a new environment or subjected to unusual emotion strain, e.g., going to college. The condition usually reverts to normal, but while it is present there is deficient gonadotropin secretion.

The analysis of the *negative feedback control* of gonadotropin secretion is obviously complicated, since we must deal not only with the hypothalamus, pituitary, and ovary but also with three different gonadotropins and two ovarian steroids. In addition, the cycling of these secretions should be explained, although no present theory does so.

One problem is that many of the possible interrelationships among all the above have not been examined enough times or in enough species. Technical difficulties in measuring the hormones are a major hindrance but one which is yielding to new advances. Another problem is that of extrapolating to man from animal work, a necessity because many of the required studies (brain operations, etc.) can never be done in man.

Nevertheless, a general scheme can be formulated, keeping these qualifications in mind. Once again, we shall roughly follow the sequence of the menstrual cycle but with the emphasis on the hypothalamus and pituitary and control mechanisms therein. Luteotropin is considered a discrete hormone, ignoring the problem of its identity in man.

A number of *external stimuli* can affect gonadotropin release; whether stimulation or inhibition results depends on the stimulus and the species. For example, extra light increases egg production in hens (i.e., ovulation) and this finding is put to practical use by chicken farmers. In the rabbit and cat, coitus is the stimulus for LH release and therefore ovulation. The smell of a strange male can inhibit luteotropin release in mice—and thus inhibit implantation. And, as we have noted, emotion or psychologic change can inhibit gonadotropin release in women.

Other glands are needed—e.g., the *thyroid,* to produce thyroxine for its general metabolic effect, and perhaps the *pineal,* which has a completely clouded role at present. In some animals, at least, increased pineal activity seems to inhibit gonadotropin secretion.

Let us now consider the gonadotropins one at a time. Keep in mind that in vivo all are present at the same time in greater or lesser amount.

FSH. A small amount of estrogen, probably in combination with a small amount of progesterone, enhances FSH release and probably accounts for the small rise in plasma FSH that occurs in the follicular phase. So we have a kind of indirect positive feedback. A further increase in estrogen or a great increase in progesterone (e.g., during pregnancy) seems to partly inhibit FSH release—the expected negative feedback phenomenon. Estradiol can specifically bind to both the hypothalamus and the pituitary; while some of the inhibitory effect may be due to a direct action on the pituitary, most seems to be mediated through the hypothalamus. There are several hypothalamic areas known to be inhibitory to FSH secretion: anterior hypothalamus, arcuate nuclei, paraventricular nuclei, and posterior median eminence. The median eminence again seems to act as a final common pathway for FSH stimulation and inhibition; it contains an FSH-releasing factor (FSH-RF) which may be about the same molecular size as vasopressin. FSH-RF specifically stimulates FSH secretion by the pituitary, probably by a process involving synthesis of protein.

Note that although FSH does not seem to stimulate estrogen secretion to any great degree except indirectly through follicular growth, its secretion is most sensitive to the level of estrogen. Thus, this is not a direct negative feedback system.

FSH may be involved in a direct negative feedback system of a different sort. There is some evidence suggesting that FSH itself can directly inhibit the secretion of FSH-RF by the hypothalamus—the so-called short-circuit feedback loop.

FSH AND LH. A small amount of estrogen and progesterone (i.e., the follicular stage) is actually a stimulus to LH release as it is to FSH secretion. This combination may be responsible for the "ovulatory surge" of LH secretion necessary for ovulation and for the rise in FSH secretion that accompanies it. With still higher levels of these steroids, but perhaps still within the physiologic range, the release of FSH and LH is somewhat inhibited. The combination of estrogen and progesterone seems to be more effective in the inhibition of FSH and LH secretion than progesterone alone.

LH AND THE HYPOTHALAMUS. Again, the effects on FSH and LH are in general mediated through the hypothalamus and are not due directly to the pituitary. There is controversy, however, regarding estrogen and the stimulation of the ovulatory surge of LH. Estrogen does indeed localize in the pituitary, and some work suggests that it directly stimulates LH release from the pituitary. Most workers feel that this is mediated by the hypothalamus, and certainly in those animals ovulating only after coitus the hypothalamus is the determining area for LH secretion.

Be that as it may, the *shutting off* of the ovulatory surge of LH is probably due to a combination of (1) estrogen and progesterone acting on the hypothalamus and (2), at least in animals ovulating with coitus, cessation of stimuli to the hypothalamus.

In the hypothalamus, one can demonstrate an LH inhibitory area in the anterior hypothalamus and at least two LH stimulatory areas. One of the latter is located in the ventromedial hypothalamus and probably controls the baseline LH release. The other is in or near the supraoptic nucleus and seems to be the one responsible for the ovulatory peak release of LH. The higher levels of estrogen and progesterone noted above can act by suppressing both of these stimulatory centers, but the supraoptic one is probably more sensitive; thus the ovulatory surge can be shut off while reasonable FSH and LH secretion is maintained provided the estrogen and progesterone levels are not too high.

Furthermore, if the physician gives estrogen and progesterone before ovulation, there is no ovulatory surge of LH despite a normal basal secretion of LH (providing the estrogen and progesterone are not given in particularly large amounts). This is how the oral contraceptives ("the pill") work.

The hypothalamic influences which determine whether or not LH is secreted are integrated by the median eminence. Here, through a catecholamine-mediated mechanism, the release of the LH-releasing factor (LH-RF) into the pituitary portal vein may be raised or lowered. If LH-RF is released, LH secretion will be stimulated.

LH-RF was first postulated in 1941, with little evidence at the time to support its existence. We know now that:

1. LH-RF activity is present in hypothalamic extracts, in pituitary portal blood, and in the blood of hypophysectomized rats.
2. LH-RF is a small polypeptide, with a molecular weight of about 1200 to 2500.
3. Electric stimuli to appropriate hypothalamic areas cause the release of LH-RF in less than three minutes. LH secretion then increases after about one hour.

During the luteal phase, after ovulation, LH secretion continues but at a lower level than at the ovulatory peak or during the follicular phase. LH stimulates increased secretion of estrogen and probably also of progesterone. Conversely both estrogen and progesterone are involved in the inhibition of LH secretion. Once more, the usual pattern of negative feedback control is varied so that two end-organ hormones control the release of one tropic hormone.

As with FSH, there is a further complication in understanding the control of LH secretion. Increased LH secretion may directly inhibit LH-RF release, thus decreasing LH secretion without the intervention of the steroid hormones. Exactly where this short-circuit feedback system fits awaits additional work.

LUTEOTROPIN-PROLACTIN.    The control of luteotropin-prolactin secretion seems to be clearly different from that of FSH and LH. The normal influence of the hypothalamus via the median eminence is to stimulate FSH and LH secretion (despite the presence of inhibitory areas) and to inhibit luteotropin secretion. For example, the ventromedial hypothalamic area mentioned above, which increases LH release when stimulated, inhibits luteotropin release at the same time. Furthermore, the median eminence mediates the process by secreting a *luteotropin-inhibiting factor* (or prolactin-inhibiting factor or PIF) which is probably different from LH-RF. In man, the concept that the hypothalamus is generally inhibitory to prolactin secretion is supported by the occasional occurrence of galactorrhea when the connections of the hypothalamus to the pituitary are broken, as in section of the pituitary stalk.

Despite all this, there are areas of the hypothalamus above the median eminence which can stimulate luteotropin release, e.g., posterior hypothalamus and supraoptic nucleus, and some workers, on little evidence, have proposed a luteotropin-releasing factor. Once again, although the main hypothalamic influence is inhibitory under the usual circumstances of normal ovarian cycling, what the pituitary actually does depends on the net result of hypothalamic stimuli and circulating hormones.

We have already noted stimuli affecting prolactin secretion via the *central nervous system:* suckling, which increases prolactin output during lactation; uterine-cervical stimulation, which does the same to maintain luteal function; and the smell (of a strange male), which inhibits prolactin secretion in the mouse, thus blocking implantation.

Probably the most important hormone affecting prolactin secretion is *estrogen,* which, even at levels that inhibit FSH and LH, is a *stimulus to luteotropin* secretion and therefore to *progesterone* secretion by the corpus luteum. Estrogen may well act at several levels:

1. On the hypothalamus to directly stimulate luteotropin secretion, probably by decreasing the secretion of PIF.
2. On the hypothalamus to inhibit FSH and LH secretion, thereby indirectly allowing more luteotropin secretion.
3. On the pituitary to directly stimulate luteotropin-prolactin secretion (this has been shown in vitro).

4. On the corpus luteum, where estrogen seems to be able to stimulate progesterone secretion directly.

Most of the evidence favors the first two mechanisms in vivo, although there is no reason why all four could not be operating at the same time.

During the luteal phase of the ovarian cycle, then, luteotropin may support the corpus luteum, aided in turn by the estrogen secreted by the same corpus luteum. Luteotropin, or perhaps the basal levels of LH known to be present, stimulates progesterone and estrogen secretion by the corpus luteum.

How is luteotropin-prolactin secretion shut off? During the menstrual cycle, perhaps fairly high levels of estrogen and progesterone in combination will shut it off. However, that high enough levels are ever reached in vivo is not certain. If prolactin secretion is truly increased in pregnancy, when plasma estrogen and progesterone are at their peak, it seems unlikely that there is any negative feedback of estrogen and progesterone on luteotropin-prolactin secretion; since we are not sure what happens to luteotropin-prolactin secretion in pregnancy, this is speculative.

Another possibility is that the secretion of estrogen and progesterone is *necessary* to maintain luteotropin secretion. Their withdrawal, as the corpus luteum decreases in function at the end of the luteal phase, may cause luteotropin secretion to drop. This last thesis of course begs the question of why the corpus luteum fails. Here may be the place where a luteolytic factor is important. As noted above, in a number of species the nonpregnant uterus seems to be luteolytic, allowing the corpus luteum to exist for only a certain number of days. In the rat, some work suggests that luteotropin itself may be luteolytic, the prolongation of luteal function by luteotropin leading ultimately to its own destruction.

Finally, luteotropin-prolactin may shut off its own secretion by stimulating (in rats, at least) the secretion of prolactin-inhibiting factor (PIF) by the hypothalamus. The result, of course, is a drop in secretion of prolactin by the pituitary.

In any case, luteotropin secretion probably does fall, and this condition is associated with a limitation of the life-span of the corpus luteum, laying the groundwork for another cycle to begin.

Much of the discussion of the control of luteotropin and corpus luteum function may be applicable only during early pregnancy or pseudopregnancy in animals such as the rat, or not at all in humans (most of the work is on animals and practically none on humans). At the moment, this point simply cannot be resolved with any degree of confidence. The broad outline is there, but until a good assay for human plasma luteotropin-prolactin can be devised, much fuzziness of detail will remain.

During lactation, the cessation of prolactin secretion is probably related to lack of suckling; thus its control under these circumstances is almost entirely neural and not hormonal. While lactation continues, the high prolactin secretion is associated with low FSH and LH secretion, an example of the reciprocal control of the hypothalamus over FSH/LH and prolactin secretion.

Once again, as with FSH and LH, the usual concept of negative feedback is altered, in this instance almost beyond recognition.

### Clinical Aspects

An immense number of clinical points might be discussed now, but this is not yet the proper place. It is self-evident that many abnormalities may result from slight changes in the hormones here under discussion. A few points are of interest (see also pp. 75, 154–155).

*Poor ovarian function* means poor secretion of estrogen and progesterone and usually poor production of ova. Not only is there sterility, but the vaginal smear is atrophic and poorly cornified. The ovary does not respond to administered gonadotropins (FSH and LH). The plasma and urine contain excessive gonadotropin as the pituitary attempts to drive the deficient ovary. With these findings, the ovary is the culprit, and the pituitary is clearly not at fault. The only therapy is estrogen replacement, with or without progesterone. Nothing can be done about ovum production, and sterility persists. The *menopause* is the most commonly seen type of ovarian failure, but the same thing happens in uncommon diseases such as *Turner's syndrome*, a genetic disease in which the patient lacks one of the normal X chromosomes and has short stature, congenital anomalies, and atrophic ovaries.

On the other hand, a patient may have poor estrogen production with the usual abnormal vaginal smear, yet have normal ovaries. If one can show that gonadotropin secretion is low, and that estrogen is secreted after the administration of gonadotropins (e.g., FSH and LH), then the fault lies somewhere in the hypothalamic-pituitary area. Patients such as this have received worldwide publicity in the past few years because, when given appropriate human gonadotropins (those from other species will not work), they can ovulate, form corpora lutea, and even carry a normal pregnancy to term with the birth of normal children. One of the problems slowly being corrected is that often the dose of gonadotropin is too high and multiple births result.

Either kind of ovarian failure usually causes amenorrhea (absent menses) and infertility. These are the patients' complaints to which the physician must be attuned.

The opposite problem, the woman who is fertile but does not want to become pregnant, also has a hormonal solution, commonly known as "the pill." The oral contraceptives are a mixture of an estrogen and a fairly high dose of a progestin. Referring to the above control mechanisms, one can see how this combination inhibits LH secretion, particularly the ovulatory peak, thus blocking ovulation and conception. Depending on the dosage and kind used, the oral contraceptives may block general FSH and LH secretion; they may also act directly on the ovary to inhibit ovulation or on the uterus to block implantation or to inhibit the motility of the spermatozoa. In humans, the effect on the ovulatory peak of LH is the likely mechanism of action since plasma LH drops after oral contraceptives are given. During pregnancy, of course, oral contraceptives are unnecessary, but after birth they must be resumed within two to five weeks or pregnancy may occur again.

## The Testis and Reproduction in the Male

It is said that no woman ever produced a child without the cooperation of a man.
—PLUTARCH, *Moralia*

Like the ovary, the testis is essential for the existence of the species but not for that of the individual. It makes spermatozoa and secretes hormones.

### Spermatogenesis

The production of spermatozoa is the primary sex characteristic in males. However, it does not seem to be grossly cyclic and so differs from ovulation in females.

Since the testis must be at least 1° C. less than the central body temperature to produce spermatozoa, the testes in mammals must descend into the scrotal sac. There are exceptions, such as the whale, but in general sperm production requires a *descended testis*. Descent in humans normally occurs before birth and requires testosterone, which in this instance is probably supplied by the fetal testis under the influence of maternal HCG. After birth, testosterone secretion drops to a low level, to increase again only at puberty.

If the testes are *not* in the scrotum, there will be a poor germinal epithelium and poor spermatogenesis. Furthermore, while the Leydig cells (which secrete testosterone) appear normal histologically, taken as a whole the testis tends to secrete less testosterone than it should.

At puberty, FSH stimulates tubular growth in the testis and stimulates meiosis in the tubular cells destined to become spermatozoa. FSH is therefore required for spermatogenesis. "FSH" is, of course, a misnomer in males because there are no follicles to stimulate, but since there is no evidence to show that the molecular structure or action is different in males, the same name and abbreviation are used to avoid confusion.

LH is required as well but plays a secondary role in tubule development; its principal job is to stimulate testosterone secretion. Testosterone appears to maintain the tubules, support spermatogenesis, and stimulate maximal development of the final product, the spermatozoa. Whether testosterone does this directly, by stimulating gonadotropin secretion (i.e., FSH), by enhancing the action of FSH on spermatogenesis, or all three, is not certain. Testosterone also helps by developing the prostate and seminal vesicles so that they can supply the carrier of the spermatozoa, the seminal fluid. Again, "LH" is a misnomer in the male; there is nothing to luteinize. Originally, no one was positive that the pituitary hormone that stimulated the Leydig cell was the same as LH, and it was in fact given a different name, interstitial cell–stimulating hormone (ICSH). All now agree that it is identical to LH; the latter is therefore used for clarity.

The function of the spermatogonia and the Leydig (interstitial) cells is reasonably plain. Just what the Sertoli cells of the tubules do is not at all clear. Some have thought, but without much evidence, that they have a kind of nutritive or supportive function. Recent work suggests that they support spermatogenesis by secreting a local "hormone" and that this process depends on FSH.

In any case, both FSH and LH are needed for complete spermatogenesis and effective seminal emission. Testosterone alone, in normal amounts, does not increase sperm production and, if present in excess, decreases LH and FSH secretion. The result would be decreased spermatogenesis. Estrogens secreted by the testis may also play a supportive role in spermatogenesis.

There is controversy over whether the FSH-stimulated tubules have any feedback control over FSH or LH secretion. None has been clearly demonstrated experimentally. However, some such feedback mechanism has been proposed to explain patients with poor tubules, normal Leydig cells, and high gonadotropin (FSH and LH) excretion. If the Leydig cells are secreting normal amounts of testosterone, one would expect normal levels of FSH and LH. With high gonadotropin secretion, one is tempted to look to the tubules. Perhaps they secrete something which is missing when tubular function is poor and which, when missing, allows a higher secretion of gonadotropin in the manner of a classic negative feedback system. Therefore, a separate tubular secretion (inhibin) has been postulated (though never isolated) which has no known action except to inhibit gonadotropin release. Recent work with aspermatogenic guinea pigs lends a measure of support to this idea since these guinea pigs appear to secrete extra FSH. If, however, work in rats suggesting that tubules make testosterone in the absence of Leydig cells is borne out, then inhibin may in fact be testosterone and the testosterone-LH feedback system may still be generally applicable (see p. 197).

Full development of spermatozoa in human testicular tubules takes about two months. Even then, however, they are not fully fertile until they have spent 10 more days in the epididymis. Here they acquire motility and a certain degree of "stickiness."

Before emission, there must be some secretion by the prostate and seminal vesicles. This secretion, the *seminal fluid* or semen, acts as a carrier for the spermatozoa. Again, testosterone is needed; without it, the seminal vesicles and prostate atrophy and make little or no fluid.

While it is true that the seminal fluid is not absolutely necessary for good spermatozoal function and fertility, it does seem to enhance fertility although no one is precisely sure how it helps. Many things in the semen have been measured, such as fructose, sorbitol, citrate, acid phosphatase, fibrinolysin, and prostaglandin. Only prostaglandin appears to have any connection with increased fertility in that it may speed the spermatozoa through the uterus to the fallopian tube.

The seminal fluid also contains proteins. Since the proteins of one individual differ from those of another, and since foreign proteins are usually immunologically rejected on repeated exposure to the protein, females (in largely monogamous species) might be expected sooner or later to "reject" seminal fluid. One can see how this reaction might cause infertility. Precisely this mechanism has been offered to explain infertility in some women, but in general humans are fortunate because the protein components of seminal fluid are normally found in women as well as men and immunologic rejection of male seminal fluid by the female is not a common occurrence.

When finally ejected, human seminal fluid contains 60,000,000 to 100,000,000 sperm per milliliter in a total volume of 3 to 4 ml. Only one of this multitude is needed for fertilization. Although a high concentration of spermatozoa does seem to be associated with better fertility, no one really knows what all the other spermatozoa do.

### Hormones of the Testis

Besides the speculative inhibin, the hormones include *testosterone,* $\Delta^4$-androsten-3,17-dione (which has little if any hormonal activity in man), and some *estrogen*. The principal activity is due to testosterone, a most potent androgen.

Androgenic activity was first shown in testicular extracts in 1927, and testosterone itself isolated in 1935. Hormonal activity had been suspected long before; probably the first experimental demonstration of hormonal activity of any kind was that of Berthold in 1849 when a grafted testis caused typical masculine comb growth in a castrated rooster.

Testosterone is secreted by the *Leydig* or interstitial cells of the testis, described by Leydig in 1850. Some testosterone (in the rat) may be secreted by the testicular tubules but probably not much. The adrenal gland also secretes testosterone, and ACTH increases this secretion. However, the adrenal normally secretes relatively little since the plasma testosterone is normal in men who have had their adrenals removed and since without testes the male secondary sex characteristics may fail to appear.

The estrogen secreted in the male, probably estradiol, may be made by the Leydig cells or by the Sertoli cells of the tubules. Clinical evidence supports the Leydig cells. In the disease testicular feminization, what appears to be a fairly normal-looking woman is actually a genetic male who has testes, not ovaries. Testosterone is secreted but has no masculinizing effect. The important point here is that in these patients the normal development of the feminine habitus and breasts seems to be due to estrogen. The gonads—which in these patients are testes—show many Leydig cells and poor tubules. In all likelihood the Leydig cells are the source of the estrogen. Some of the estrogens found in the male may come from the adrenal gland, but at least 80% comes from the testis.

BIOSYNTHESIS AND SECRETION. Referring back to Figure 20, note that there are two main pathways to $\Delta^4$-androstenedione, the immediate precursor of testosterone. One is via progesterone and the other via dehydroepiandrosterone (DHEA). Which is the more important is not clear, though certain workers lean toward the DHEA pathway (Fig. 48). Some have even raised the question of whether cholesterol is an obligatory intermediate. It may not be essential, but most testosterone synthesis does seem to be via cholesterol. The final step in testosterone synthesis, from $\Delta^4$-androstenedione to testosterone, involves only a reduction of the 17-keto to a 17-hydroxyl group. Some of the testosterone may come from DHEA by a different route, with $\Delta^5$-androsten-3,17-diol as the intermediate, but it is hard to say how important this pathway is. The small amount of estrogen is presumably made from testosterone by a pathway similar to that in the ovary (see Fig. 42).

The immediate stimulus to the secretion of testicular hormones is LH. LH stimulates the growth of the interstitial cells and the secretion of testosterone. When FSH and LH are both present—as is usually the case—testosterone secretion is better than with LH alone.

LH stimulates the secretion of estrogen just as it does the secretion of testosterone. In fact, after an injection of LH or HCG there is a proportionately greater rise in estrogen secretion than in testosterone secretion, a finding that has been used as a clinical test for the integrity of testicular hormonal secretion.

How does LH stimulate testosterone secretion? An increased blood flow to the testis can increase testosterone secretion, but LH increases secretion in the absence of an increased blood flow. LH increases amino

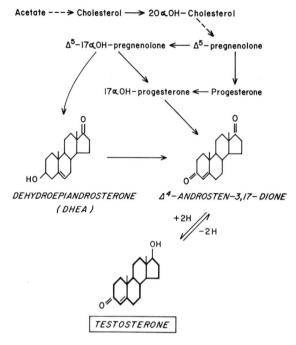

FIG. 48. Biosynthesis of testosterone.

acid uptake and amino acid conversion to protein in the testis. Since blocking these effects also blocks the effect of LH on increasing testosterone synthesis, protein synthesis is necessary for LH to stimulate testosterone secretion. Presumably LH stimulates a rise in the activity of specific enzyme(s) concerned with testosterone synthesis.

More than this, however, LH acts on the testis to increase the conversion of (see Figs. 20, 48):

1. Acetate to cholesterol.
2. Acetate to testosterone.
3. Cholesterol to 20α-OH-cholesterol.
4. Cholesterol to pregnenolone.
5. 17α-OH-pregnenolone to 17α-OH-progesterone.
6. 17α-OH-pregnenolone to testosterone, although there is other evidence controverting this effect.
7. 17α-OH-progesterone to Δ⁴-androstenedione.

There are almost too many possible sites of action for LH, all with some experimental backing. Perhaps LH acts at more than one site; which one is rate-limiting, however, is not settled. The strongest evidence points to items 3 and 7 above, the conversion of cholesterol to

20α-OH-cholesterol or of 17α-OH-progesterone to Δ⁴-androstenedione. Presumably, LH increases the enzymes concerned; this has been definitely shown for action 7 in a testicular microsomal preparation.

Whether cyclic AMP plays any role here is not clear, but it would not be surprising if within a short time it were shown to mediate the effect of LH. In fact, some new work with rabbit testes in vitro suggests just that.

Some of the testosterone secreted by the testis may not be wholly synthesized there. The human testis can convert DHEA and Δ⁴-androstenedione infused into the spermatic artery to testosterone, which is secreted into the spermatic vein. Thus, compounds from the adrenal gland could be precursors of plasma testosterone.

Approximately 4 to 9 mg of testosterone are secreted each day in men and 0.2 to 0.5 mg in women. The secretion rate of estradiol in men is about 20 µg per day, and of estrone 25 µg per day.

TESTOSTERONE AND ESTROGEN IN THE BLOOD. In human plasma, testosterone circulates bound to a specific testosterone-binding protein and to albumin—and to the latter even when metabolized and conjugated. Its plasma half-life is 11 to 90 minutes, depending on which stage of equilibrium is considered. Circulating blood levels are:

*Before Puberty*

| | |
|---|---|
| Boys | 0.04 µg/100 ml |
| Girls | 0.02 µg/100 ml |

*In the Normal Adult*

| | |
|---|---|
| Men | 0.6 µg/100 ml |
| Women | 0.05 µg/100 ml |

In men, there is a slight diurnal variation, the plasma level dropping to about 0.4 µg/100 ml at night.

The fact that elevated levels are found in the virilized female supports the idea that testosterone is the androgenic agent involved.

17-Ketosteroids are present in plasma, including Δ⁴-androstenedione, but there seems to be no difference in the levels in men and women. Thus the idea that testosterone is the significant androgen in normal humans is further supported.

A small amount of estrogen is found in normal male plasma: 2 mµg/100 ml of estradiol and 6 mµg/100 ml of estrone.

METABOLISM OF TESTICULAR HORMONES. Many tissues, e.g., liver and muscle, can reversibly convert testosterone to Δ⁴-androstenedione. As noted before with other hormones, this type of redox reaction may act as a local control mechanism of testosterone's action since Δ⁴-androstenedione is at best a weak androgen. Elsewhere, the prostate can reduce it to dihydrotestosterone. But most is metabolically inactivated by the liver.

The liver converts testosterone and $\Delta^4$-androstenedione to other compounds by the same mechanisms by which hydrocortisone is reduced to THF and then conjugated. Here, the reduced compounds are androsterone and etiocholanolone, which are conjugated mainly as glucuronides. These two compounds, plus DHEA and DHEA sulfate, are the principal compounds making up the *urinary 17-ketosteroids* or 17-KS. A small amount of testosterone is conjugated directly to glucuronide and sulfate; for example, there is about 0.1 μg/100 ml of testosterone sulfate in normal male plasma.

The urinary 17-KS are often measured as an index of androgen secretion. As noted in the discussion of the adrenal gland, this is only a very rough measure of androgenicity or of testicular function. Two-thirds of the 17-KS come from the adrenal, largely as DHEA and DHEA sulfate. Of the one-third coming from the testis, only about half derives from testosterone, the remainder being metabolites of $\Delta^4$-androstenedione. Since such a small part of the urinary 17-KS is derived from testosterone, it is apparent that major changes in testosterone secretion can occur in the absence of much change in 17-KS excretion, and vice versa. The average normal adult 17-KS excretion is 14 mg per day for men and 10 mg per day for women.

While about 30% of secreted testosterone appears in the urine as 17-KS, only about 1% is found unchanged. Nevertheless, when measured, the urine testosterone provides a better separation between normal and abnormal people than the urine 17-KS and is a closer reflection of actual androgen activity. Normal men show a decrease in urine testosterone as they get older, but it never drops to the levels found in women or prepubertal males. The normal amount of testosterone in the urine in adults is 40 to 100 μg per day for men and 3 to 8 μg per day for women.

The estrogens are also metabolized and conjugated, the conjugates appearing in the urine.

ACTIONS OF TESTOSTERONE.   The "male hormone" actually has two major though interrelated actions: It is *androgenic*, that is, it causes the appearance of those secondary sex characteristics found in the male, and it is *anabolic* in the sense that it increases net protein synthesis by the body. The latter property has for years been attractive to drug companies who have been (and are) searching for something that is anabolic and not androgenic, and therefore useful in women as well as men. Whether any of the many synthetic analogues (the "anabolic steroids") that have been produced actually have more anabolic and less androgenic effect than testosterone is a difficult question to answer; most of the evidence is simply not conclusive. Most of the problem revolves around the central issue—also unresolved—of whether these properties are due to two separate actions or are in fact manifestations of a single action.

*Anabolic Action.*   The anabolic activity of testosterone is best seen in its effects on muscle, although it has similar effects on, for example, liver and kidney. Grossly, there is an increase in muscle mass and strength. On a biochemical level there is an increase in amino acid incorporation into protein due to an effect on DNA which results in an increased synthesis of RNA. Presumably, the "anabolic steroids" act the same way.

Other related and important actions, not well defined biochemically, are:

1. Stimulation of *bone growth* in the presence of growth hormone. This may be due to stimulation of growth hormone secretion, and together, testosterone and growth hormone are largely responsible for the pubertal growth spurt.
2. Later on, the *closure of bone epiphyses,* thus ending any further increase in height. This action in boys is the same as estrogen's action in girls. Here, testosterone is more like thyroxine than growth hormone.
3. Stimulation of *red cell production,* which may explain in part the higher hematocrit in men. Testosterone does not seem to increase the secretion of erythropoietin (see p. 19) but may enhance the red cell response to it.

*Androgenic Action.*   The androgenic action of testosterone results in the secondary sex characteristics that appear at puberty, when males have a rising testosterone level. These characteristics are fairly obvious and consist of:

1. *Growth and function of genitalia* other than the testes: penis, scrotum, prostate, seminal vesicles.
2. *Increased hair growth* of typical pattern: beard, chest, and abdominal hair; "diamond-shaped" pubic hair; and "male pattern" baldness. Since the genetic and ethnic background of the individual has a major influence on hair growth, the amount of hair and the secretion of testosterone do not necessarily correlate well when one individual is compared with another.
3. *Direct effects* on the *central nervous system* to cause more aggressive behavior in general, and increased sexual desire (libido) and activity in particular. These changes also require testosterone exposure in utero for optimal development. As in females, the hypothalamus is the critical area: an implant of testosterone into a castrated rat's hypothalamus (but not elsewhere) causes male

sexual behavior without any other androgenic effects. There may also be an effect on the spinal cord, through which testosterone seems to enhance penile erection.

4. Increased *muscle* mass and strength and increased *skeletal growth* (see above: these are perhaps better considered anabolic).
5. Changes in *fat distribution*. Men have less subcutaneous fat than women, and testosterone may have a fat-mobilizing effect.
6. Deepening of the *voice* due to laryngeal growth.
7. Increased oil production (sebum) by *sebaceous glands*. Thus, one sees acne only after puberty, and it is generally worse in men.

*Mechanism of Action.* Compared with that of estrogen, testosterone's mechanism of action has not been as extensively studied. Other than the biochemical changes in muscle noted above, most of the research has been done on the prostate and seminal vesicles. Testosterone localizes to the seminal vesicles and prostate in a matter of minutes after being injected and binds to a protein. It is not clear whether the binding protein is in the nucleus or cytoplasm of the cell; perhaps both types of binding are important. Within 15 minutes most of the testosterone bound to nuclear protein is converted to *dihydrotestosterone* (DHT) or 5α-androsten-17β-ol-3-one. From both biochemical and clinical evidence, it now seems likely that DHT is what actually causes the effects attributed to testosterone. In this instance, then, *the hormonal effect occurs only after the circulating hormone is metabolized to something else at the site of action.*

As in muscle, testosterone stimulates amino acid incorporation into protein. Different experiments have shown that this might be due to a rise in the activity of DNA polymerase and nuclear RNA polymerase, or to a rise in mRNA synthesis, in sRNA synthesis, or in the rate of transfer of amino acids from sRNA to the ribosomes. Perhaps all of these are important.

The growth of the prostate and seminal vesicles is rather sensitive to androgens and, in experimental animals, can be used for assaying androgen activity. Prolactin may enhance this growth; if so, it is about the only known action of prolactin in the male mammal.

CONTROL OF TESTOSTERONE SECRETION. The classic negative feedback system should involve testosterone and luteinizing hormone (LH). The expected findings would be that a rise in testosterone decreases LH secretion and a decrease in testosterone stimulates LH secretion. This relationship appears to hold in fact at physiologic levels of testosterone, both in rats and in adult men.

As we have seen before, the control system is actually more complex. More than the pituitary and testis is involved. Ultimate control of gonadal hormones, in males as well as females, depends upon the hypothalamus. For example, testosterone implanted into the hypothalamus decreases testosterone secretion. In all likelihood the negative feedback control of LH by testosterone is mediated by the hypothalamus and LH-releasing factor (LH-RF).

There is a diurnal variation in plasma testosterone that may depend on parallel variations in the secretion of LH, but the only work done on this problem does not show any observable change in plasma LH at differing times of day. As noted before, there is no monthly (or other) variation in the secretion of testosterone as there is for the ovarian hormones. This absence may be due to testosterone itself; testosterone appears to inhibit directly a natural cyclicity of the hypothalamus.

The testosterone-LH negative feedback relationship generally holds; however, other findings tend to complicate matters somewhat:

1. Testosterone in small amounts may stimulate FSH release.
2. Estrogen in small amounts, and possibly small amounts of testosterone, can lead to an increased LH secretion and thus a further output of estrogen and testosterone, probably via the hypothalamus and median eminence.
3. Testosterone at a high enough level, which can probably be reached in vivo, inhibits both FSH and LH secretion, although LH secretion is more sensitive and is inhibited first.
4. Estrogen at appropriate levels also inhibits both FSH and LH secretion.
5. Epinephrine can inhibit testosterone secretion, and the pineal may also play a role; neither of these has as yet a firm physiologic role.

So both estrogen and testosterone are probably involved in the damping of LH secretion. Whether effects on FSH are found under normal circumstances is not clear, but with the new radioimmunoassays for FSH and LH, this problem should be solved fairly soon. In summary, the resulting normal values for adult men are:

| | |
|---|---|
| Plasma testosterone | 0.6 µg/100 ml |
| Plasma estradiol | 0.002 µg/100 ml |
| Plasma FSH | 0.19 mU/ml |
| Plasma LH | 2.9 mµg/ml |

### Clinical Aspects

Poor or excessive testosterone production is paralleled by low or high testosterone levels in urine or plasma. The masculinized woman has too much testosterone and the hypogonadal man too little; in general, either plasma or urine levels or secretion (production) rate can be used to assay the patient.

If testosterone secretion is deficient, usually spermatogenesis is also impaired, as one might guess from the above. The reverse is often not the case, and poor spermatogenesis may be found in the presence of normal or slightly low testosterone levels.

With poor sperm production, if the tubules are damaged (one tells this by biopsy) there is little that will help. On the other hand, if they simply look inactive, particularly if low plasma or urine gonadotropins suggest pituitary deficiency, treatment may improve spermatogenesis. Both testosterone and HCG have been used with occasional successes; more rational would be treatment with an FSH-like hormone (Pergonal); this is effective, but too little has been done to allow conclusions to be drawn.

When deficient testosterone production is the problem, primary damage to the producing cells (Leydig) indicates that only the administration of testosterone by the physician will be of help. If, on testing, one can show that LH (or HCG) will cause a rise in testosterone levels, then the Leydig cells are functionally intact and the fault must lie in deficient gonadotropin secretion. Therapy is the same, administration of testosterone, although it is possible that sufficient human gonadotropin may be available in the future both to remedy this problem and to stimulate spermatogenesis.

Excessive secretion of testosterone is hard to recognize in men unless it occurs in a boy before puberty. In women, however, it causes readily observed changes that are often most distressing (see pp. 74, 155 for some examples).

## Bibliography

### General

Christian, J. J., and Davis, D. E.   Endocrines, behavior, and population. *Science* 146:1550, 1964.

Christian, J. J., Lloyd, J. A., and Davis, D. E.   The role of endocrines in the self-regulation of mammalian populations. *Recent Progr. Hormone Res.* 21:501, 1965.

Masters, W. H., and Johnson, V. E.   *Human Sexual Response.* Boston: Little, Brown, 1966.

Young, W. C. (Ed.).   *Sex and Internal Secretions* (2 vols.) (3d ed.). Baltimore: Williams & Wilkins, 1961.

### Development and Puberty

Adams Smith, W. N., and Peng, M. T.   Inductive influence of testosterone upon central sexual maturation in the rat. *J. Embryol. Exp. Morph.* 17: 171, 1967.

Donovan, B. T., and Van der Werff ten Bosch, J. J.   *Physiology of Puberty.*
Baltimore: Williams & Wilkins, 1965.

Levine, S., and Mullins, R. F., Jr.   Hormonal influences on brain organization in infant rats. *Science* 152:1585, 1966.

### Estrogen and Its Action

Baird, D. T.   A method for the measurement of estrone and estradiol-17β
in peripheral human blood and other biological fluids using $^{35}$S pipsyl
chloride. *J. Clin. Endocr.* 28:244, 1968.

Bjersing, L., and Carstensen, H.   Biosynthesis of steroids by granulosa cells
of the porcine ovary in vitro. *J. Reprod. Fertil.* 14:101, 1967.

Brecher, P. I., and Wotiz, H. H.   Competition between estradiol and estriol
for end organ receptor proteins. *Steroids* 9:431, 1967.

Eren, S., Reynolds, G. H., Turner, M. E., Jr., Schmidt, F. H., Mackay, J. H.,
Howard, C. M., and Preedy, J. R. K.   Estrogen metabolism in the human:
II. Studies in the male using estradiol-17β-6,7-$^3$H. *J. Clin. Endocr.* 27:
819, 1967.

Gorski, J., Noteboom, W. D., and Nicolette, J. A.   Estrogen control of the
synthesis of RNA and protein in the uterus. *J. Cell. Comp. Physiol.* 66
(Suppl. 1):91, 1965.

Jensen, E. V., Suzuki, T., Kawashima, T., Stumpf, W. E., Jungblut, P. W.,
and DeSombre, E. R.   A two-step mechanism for the interaction of estradiol with rat uterus. *Proc. Nat. Acad. Sci. U.S.A.* 59:632, 1968.

Means, A. R., and Hamilton, T. H.   Early estrogen action: Concomitant
stimulations within two minutes of nuclear RNA synthesis and uptake of
RNA precursor by the uterus. *Proc. Nat. Acad. Sci. U.S.A.* 56:1594, 1966.

Ryan, K. J., and Smith, O. W.   Biogenesis of steroid hormones in the human
ovary. *Recent Progr. Hormone Res.* 21:367, 1965.

Szego, C. M., and Davis, J. S.   Adenosine 3′,5′-monophosphate in rat
uterus: Acute elevation by estrogen. *Proc. Nat. Acad. Sci. U.S.A.* 58:1711,
1967.

### Ovulation and Oral Contraceptives

Döcke, F., and Dörner, G.   Facilitative action of progesterone in induction
of ovulation by oestrogen. *J. Endocr.* 36:209, 1966.

Espey, L. L.   Ultrastructure of the apex of the rabbit graafian follicle during the ovulatory process. *Endocrinology* 81:267, 1967.

Hellman, L. M.   FDA Report on the Oral Contraceptives. Washington:
U.S. Govt. Printing Office, 1966.

Inman, W. H. W., and Vessey, M. P.   Investigation of deaths from pulmonary, coronary, and cerebral thrombosis and embolism in women of
child-bearing age. *Brit. Med. J.* 2:193, 1968. (Hazards of oral contraceptives.)

Palka, Y. S., and Sawyer, C. H.   The effects of hypothalamic implants of
ovarian steroids on oestrous behaviour in rabbits. *J. Physiol.* (London)
185:251, 1966.

## Luteal Phase and Progesterone

Fink, G., Nallar, R., and Worthington, W. C., Jr.   The demonstration of luteinizing hormone releasing factor in hypophysial portal blood of prooestrous and hypophysectomized rats. *J. Physiol.* (London) 191:407, 1967.

Gáti, I., Doszpod, J., and Preisz, J.   LTH production and steroid excretion during the menstrual cycle. *Acta Physiol. Acad. Sci. Hung.* 32:115, 1967.

Hansel, W.   Luteotrophic and luteolytic mechanisms in bovine corpora lutea. *J. Reprod. Fertil.* Suppl. 1, p. 33, 1966.

Marsh, J. M., and Savard, K.   The stimulation of progesterone synthesis in bovine corpora lutea by adenosine 3',5'-monophosphate. *Steroids* 8: 133, 1966.

Neill, J. D., Johansson, E. D. B., Datta, J. K., and Knobil, E.   Relationship between the plasma levels of luteinizing hormone and progesterone during the normal menstrual cycle. *J. Clin. Endocr.* 27:1167, 1967.

## Fertilization

Doak, R. L., Hall, A., and Dale, H. E.   Longevity of spermatozoa in the reproductive tract of the bitch. *J. Reprod. Fertil.* 13:51, 1967.

Dukelow, W. R., Chernoff, H. N., and Williams, W. L.   Properties of decapacitation factor and presence in various species. *J. Reprod. Fertil.* 14: 393, 1967.

## Pregnancy and Lactation

Arai, Y., and Lee, T. H.   Double-antibody radioimmunoassay procedure for ovine pituitary prolactin. *Endocrinology* 81:1041, 1967.

Beck, P., and Daughaday, W. H.   Human placental lactogen: Studies of its acute metabolic effects and disposition in normal man. *J. Clin. Invest.* 46:103, 1967.

Diczfalusy, E.   Endocrine functions of the human fetoplacental unit. *Fed. Proc.* 23:791, 1964.

Griss, G., Keck, J., Engelhorn, R., and Tuppy, H.   The isolation and purification of an ovarian polypeptide with uterine-relaxing activity. *Biochim. Biophys. Acta* 140:45, 1967.

Grosvenor, C. E., and Mena, F.   Effect of auditory, olfactory and optic stimuli upon milk ejection and suckling-induced release of prolactin in lactating rats. *Endocrinology* 80:840, 1967.

Josimovich, J. B., and MacLaren, J. A.   Presence in the human placenta and term serum of a highly lactogenic substance immunologically related to pituitary growth hormone. *Endocrinology* 71:209, 1962.

Kanematsu, S., and Sawyer, C. H.   Effects of intrahypothalamic and intrahypophysial estrogen implants on pituitary prolactin and lactation in the rabbit. *Endocrinology* 72:243, 1963.

Lockwood, D. H., Stockdale, F. E., and Topper, Y. J.   Hormone-dependent differentiation of mammary gland: Sequence of action of hormones in relation to cell cycle. *Science* 156:945, 1967.

Meites, J., and Nicoll, C. S.   Adenohypophysis; Prolactin. *Ann. Rev. Physiol.* 28:57, 1966.

Minaguchi, H., and Meites, J.   Effects of suckling on hypothalamic LH-releasing factor and prolactin inhibiting factor, and on pituitary LH and prolactin. *Endocrinology* 80:603, 1967.

Wilber, J. F.   Alterations of endocrine function in pregnancy. *Med. Clin. N. Amer.* 52:253, 1968.

Yoshinaga, K., and Adams, C. E.   Luteotrophic activity of young conceptus in the rat. *J. Reprod. Fertil.* 13:505, 1967.

## Seminiferous Tubules and Testosterone

Heller, C. G., and Clermont, Y.   Kinetics of the germinal epithelium in man. *Recent Progr. Hormone Res.* 20:545, 1964.

Lacy, D.   Seminiferous tubule in mammals. *Endeavour* 26:101, 1967.

Lipsett, M. B., Wilson, H., Kirschner, M. A., Korenman, S. G., Fishman, L. M., Sarfaty, G. A., and Bardin, C. W.   Studies on Leydig cell physiology and pathology: Secretion and metabolism of testosterone. *Recent Progr. Hormone Res.* 22:245, 1966.

Menon, K. M. J., Dorfman, R. I., and Forchielli, E.   Influence of gonadotrophins on cholesterol-side chain cleavage reaction by rat-testis mitochondrial preparations. *Biochim. Biophys. Acta* 148:486, 1967.

Vande Wiele, R. L., MacDonald, P. C., Gurpide, E., and Liberman, S.   Studies on the secretion and interconversion of the androgens. *Recent Progr. Hormone Res.* 19:275, 1963.

## Clinical

Bardin, C. W., and Lipsett, M. B.   Testosterone and androstenedione blood production rates in normal women and women with idiopathic hirsutism or polycystic ovaries. *J. Clin. Invest.* 46:891, 1967.

Crooke, A. C., Butt, W. R., Bertrand, P. V., and Morris, R.   Treatment of infertility and secondary amenorrhoea with follicle-stimulating hormone and chorionic gonadotrophin. *Lancet* 2:636, 1967.

Engel, E., and Forbes, A. P.   Cytogenetic and clinical findings in 48 patients with congenitally defective or absent ovaries. *Medicine* (Baltimore) 44:135, 1965.

# 10. The Pancreatic Endocrine Secretions and Diabetes Mellitus

## INSULIN

Diabetes mellitus, which means an excessive flow of sweet urine, was noted in written records as early as 1500 B.C. At first, however, it was not clearly separated from other causes of a large urine flow. The distinction was undoubtedly made several times in the last thousand years but is not adequately recorded. Although the word *diabetes* came into the English language in 1562, it was not until 1674 that Thomas Willis, an English physician, noted and described the sweet taste of the urine. Thus a clear distinction between diabetes mellitus and diabetes insipidus ("tasteless diabetes") was made.

Dobson (1776) demonstrated sugar in the urine of diabetic patients, and Chevreul (1815) showed that the sugar was glucose. By 1877 Claude Bernard had demonstrated that the excess urinary glucose was in fact secondary to a high blood glucose.

That the pancreas had something to do with all this was one of many theories proposed by Cawley in 1788. One hundred years later, in 1889, von Mering and Minkowski proved it when, after removing a dog's pancreas, they found that diabetes mellitus appeared. In 1900 Opie focused attention on the islets of Langerhans as the site of the disorder and the probable origin of a substance which prevented diabetes mellitus.

The search began. What was the pancreatic substance that prevented diabetes mellitus? Active extracts causing hypoglycemia were made as early as 1908 (Zuelzer) but they proved too toxic (or perhaps simply too much was given) and the project was dropped. In 1911 Scott had an active pancreatic extract that seemed to be safe, but the idea was not followed up, largely because of lack of money and a place to do the work. In 1921 Banting and Best were able to make an extract of pancreas which reduced the hyperglycemia of a pancreatectomized dog, was not toxic, and allowed the dog to continue living. The substance was named *insulin*, a name originally proposed by de Meyer (1910). On January 11, 1922, the extract was given to a 14-year-old boy dying of diabetes. He recovered; Banting and Best achieved worldwide fame and received the Nobel Prize a few years later. The "discovery of insulin" is generally dated, then, 1921.

## Chemistry

Animal insulin was crystallized in 1924 (Kimball and Murlin) and in 1926 (Abel). After 10 years of work, Sanger in 1955 reported its amino acid sequence and primary molecular structure, and, in 1963 it was completely synthesized de novo in the laboratory by Katsoyannis in Pittsburgh. In 1965 Chinese workers in Shanghai and Peking made enough synthetic insulin to form characteristic crystals. Finally, in 1965 Zahn in Aachen, Germany, and in 1966 Katsoyannis at Brookhaven, Long Island, reported the synthesis of human insulin, the first synthesis of a human protein. Synthetic insulin is still not widely available for experiments because of the relatively poor yield from a most complex procedure; further work should enhance the yield and make the process largely automatic.*

Insulin consists of two peptide chains, the A chain and the B chain. The A chain has 21 amino acids, is acidic, and has an N-terminal glycine. The B chain has 30 amino acids, is basic, and has an N-terminal phenylalanine. The chains are connected by two disulfide bridges (Fig. 49).

The molecular weight is about 6000 and varies from species to species because of variation in amino acid composition. The rat has two different types of insulin molecules in the same animal.

The *biosynthesis* of insulin is still being investigated. Older work suggests that the A and B chains are made separately and then joined at the disulfide bridges, just as in the chemical synthesis of insulin. A glutathione-insulin transhydrogenase may be the enzyme responsible for the disulfide linkage. Some exciting new work indicates that a single peptide molecule containing 84 amino acids, folded upon itself and having both A and B chains already linked by disulfide bridges, is a precursor of insulin. This precursor, called *pro-insulin*, is found in the pancreas and circulates in the blood; enzymatic removal of a 33 amino acid peptide from the middle of the pro-insulin molecule leaves the 51 amino acids of insulin with the A and B chains joined as we know them. Combining this information, one may speculate that after a long peptide is formed, it folds upon itself; enzymes form the disulfide bridges, break off part of the peptide, and convert the original peptide to insulin.

For *insulin activity* the disulfide bonds are essential. Despite wide variations in amino acid composition, insulins from different species have good activity when injected into animals of other species; there is little species specificity. In fact, there can be a difference in as many as 23 of the 51 amino acids without much change in activity. Furthermore, up to five or six of the amino acids of the B chain can be re-

*Merrifield, R. B. The automatic synthesis of proteins. *Sci. Amer.* 218:56, 1968.

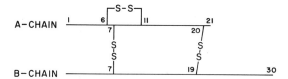

Fɪɢ. 49.   Schematic structure of insulin molecule. Numbers indicate the position of various amino acids in the peptide chains.

moved and activity will still be present. The secondary (probably spiral) and tertiary structures are probably important in insulin action and antibody formation but are not well known or understood at present; fortunately the synthetic chemists do not have to worry about them because the secondary and tertiary structures form spontaneously when the insulin molecule is put together (Dixon and Wardlaw, 1960). The true functional unit is also not certainly known; some investigators think that insulin circulates in the blood—and may be biologically active—as larger dimers, tetramers, or hexamers, with molecular weights of 12,000 to 36,000.

### Functional Anatomy and Secretion

The human pancreas has about 1,000,000 islets. They total about 1 g in weight. Between 60% and 80% of the cells are β-cells, and it has been shown by the binding of specific anti-insulin antibodies that insulin is in the β-cell. Each β-cell has about 1.7 μU of insulin, and the entire pancreas about 200 units (how many β-cells are there per islet?).

Insulin as usually prepared has 24 units/mg, and 1 unit then equals 40 μg of insulin. The unit is an arbitrary quantity, determined usually by bioassay; it is necessary to be aware of it, though bioassays are no longer widely used, because preparations of insulin are still standardized in terms of the arbitrary unit, because patients with diabetes mellitus are always treated in terms of units of insulin, and because even the results of the modern radioimmunoassay are recorded in units.

In the β-cell, the endoplasmic reticulum forms tiny sacs inside which form insulin granules. These sacs then lose their RNA and act as storage vesicles. When the blood glucose rises, the sacs move to the periphery of the cell and insulin is released to the blood stream. It is not certain whether the insulin dissolves first or whether the granule is discharged intact or both. Within 30 minutes after glucose administration, there are less granules and more empty sacs in the β-cells (Fig. 50).

About 25 to 50 units, or 1 to 2 mg, are secreted each day into the

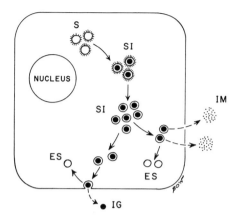

FIG. 50.  Insulin granules in a pancreatic islet cell and two possible modes of release of insulin from the cell.  S = sacs with RNA;  SI = sacs with insulin granules, some of which have lost the RNA; IM = insulin molecules; IG = insulin granule; ES = empty sacs.

pancreatic vein of humans, but about half of this never gets beyond the liver. Thus, about 1 mg is actually secreted to the peripheral blood.

### Plasma Levels

The first assays capable of detecting insulin in plasma were bio-assays. One assay, using the rat diaphragm, tests the ability of the unknown sample to increase the uptake or oxidation of radioactive glucose. Another, more sensitive, bioassay uses rat adipose tissue; the unknown is assayed for its ability to increase the oxidation of glucose to $CO_2$. The amounts of insulin detected, we now realize, are too high—particularly with the assay using adipose tissue—when compared with those found by the newer radioimmunoassay. Most workers now accept the latter assay and feel that the bioassays measure other things besides insulin. The radioimmunoassay can detect as little as 1 μμg (1 picogram) of insulin, or 0.025 μU.

Normal fasting levels in man are 20 μU/ml (range 0 to 70) with one variant of radioimmunoassay; with another the value is 7 μU/ml (range 0 to 15). So even with this fairly specific method the amounts noted are not absolute but are subject to variation due to differences in technique. Fasting levels are increased in patients with acromegaly, hyperthyroidism, obesity, and insulin-secreting tumors, and, surprising as it may seem, in many diabetics. The last finding, the high levels of insulin in some diabetic patients, is discussed later.

The plasma *half-life* is about 30 minutes in humans. Insulin is mostly metabolized to inactive products, but some does pass through capillaries to other fluid compartments intact. Insulin is found, for instance, in the spinal fluid, the bile, and the urine and probably crosses the placenta. Renal failure, as one might predict, slows clearance of insulin from the blood.

The circulating form of insulin in the plasma is a problem that has aroused great controversy. Is what we extract from the pancreas the same as what circulates in the blood? Probably the overall molecular structure is different, since extracted insulin causes antibody formation even in the animal species from which it was extracted. Once in the plasma, is insulin always in the same form? We have already mentioned that insulin may exist as a polymer; some new work suggests that some of the circulating insulin is a larger molecule than expected (perhaps pro-insulin), particularly during fasting.

Moreover, many workers, using principally some form of bioassay, have proposed that some of the plasma insulin is bound to something that limits its action on muscle, but still allows it to act on adipose tissue, and that prevents its reaction with insulin antibodies. This material is variously called "bound," "complexed," "atypical," or "nonsuppressible" insulin, or, perhaps better, "insulin-like activity" (ILA). Purification of ILA is difficult since many procedures apparently degrade the molecule. Some ILA was thought to be a protein with a molecular weight of about 6000; actually this particular ILA is a considerably larger molecule, with a molecular weight of at least 50,000 to 70,000, and it accounts for only about 5% of the total ILA in plasma. The remainder (over 90%) is a different substance, with a molecular weight of 100,000 to 150,000. ILA may be formed by the liver as insulin passes from the pancreas to the systemic blood stream. On the other hand, some investigators feel that, while this material exists, it is not made in the liver and it is as effective on muscle as on adipose tissue. Other workers object to the whole idea. With the radioimmunoassay, no insulin appears to be bound, and when the ILA is purified, the immunoassay shows no evidence of either insulin or its A or B chain in the ILA. Furthermore, the pancreatectomized dog still has "complexed insulin" in its blood several days after the operation, long past the time when insulin should have been completely metabolized. All of which supports the idea that ILA or "bound" or "complexed" insulin is in fact not insulin at all; it has even been suggested that this substance is only an artifact of the isolation procedure.

Insulin *antagonists* in the plasma have also been described. Usually this term refers to some serum factor, not an antibody, which inhibits insulin action. One such, associated with albumin, is probably an artifact of the isolation method and not physiologically active. The A and B chains of insulin have been proposed as antagonists of insulin; their role is not settled. Synthetic A chain, when injected, does not seem to antagonize insulin's action, but radioimmunoassay shows that diabetics have more isolated A chains circulating in the blood than do normal people. The B chain is equally controversial, one experiment showing that it does not inhibit insulin's action on muscle and another that, when combined with albumin, it does and causes hyperglycemia.

There are likewise insulin antibodies, which are always formed to a greater or lesser degree when insulin is given to patients, but the antibodies do not usually seem to antagonize insulin to any great degree.

Whether any of these factors or antagonists have anything to do with insulin action is not certain. A major problem is that most of these phenomena were described in terms of a bioassay rather than using combined bioassay and radioimmunoassay methods. At present, physiologic meaning cannot be assigned to any of the factors, but it is conceivable that they are of some importance in the development of diabetes mellitus.

### General Action of Insulin on Glucose Transport

Insulin is typically thought of as a hormone that controls the entry of glucose into muscle cells. While true, this is by no means a complete description of what insulin does; it has profound effects on other tissues than muscle and, as we shall see, has important actions on fat and protein metabolism.

In 1939, Lundsgaard suggested that insulin may act by *increasing cell permeability to glucose.* Beginning in 1949, Levine and his associates established in a series of papers that insulin did exactly that, particularly in muscle. While not the only effect of insulin on glucose metabolism, it is probably the most important since this step is the rate-limiting one under most circumstances. The affinity for glucose of the glucose uptake system of muscle is not changed; only the velocity of glucose entry into the cell is increased. The increase in cell permeability is actually in both directions, but once in the cell, glucose is rapidly phosphorylated. Since glucose-6-phosphate is not able to get out of the cell (muscle), the glucose is effectively trapped inside and the net effect is an increased glucose uptake. This action of insulin is relatively specific, working for some but not all sugars.

*Anoxia* and *exercise* seem to mimic insulin and also increase glucose permeability. The response to exercise explains why a diabetic needs less insulin while exercising. In a sense this is a humoral phenomenon, for a factor has been isolated from exercising muscle which increases glucose uptake by muscle by acting at the same site as insulin, yet it is not insulin. Nevertheless, insulin's presence is needed for this factor to work; in the total absence of insulin, no such effect is seen.

The specific mechanism by which insulin gets glucose into the cell is unknown. At least two processes are involved. The first is *insulin binding* to the cell membrane, perhaps by sulfhydryl groups since without intact disulfide bridges insulin loses its activity. The second is the actual *increase in glucose transport*, in which changes in the phospholipids or lipoproteins of the cell membrane are probably important. One theory is that insulin reduces the activity of a cellular inhibitor of glucose transport that is normally present.

Insulin does not affect glucose transport in all tissues. This effect is easily seen in muscle, adipose tissue, and connective tissue, but *not* in red blood cells, renal tubules, intestinal mucosa, or, perhaps most important, in the liver or central nervous system. Clearly, such tissue differences are of physiologic importance.

The *central nervous system* is a particular case in point. Like the renal medulla, it is generally *dependent* upon *glucose* alone for its energy supply (although some ketone bodies may be utilized in special circumstances), yet it is *not* affected by insulin in the usual sense wherein insulin causes a rapid increase in glucose uptake. Insulin may have a slower effect on the brain; total glucose uptake is not affected, but insulin can perhaps lower the threshold for glucose entry into brain cells.

Some work, however, suggests that certain areas of the brain, in particular the hypothalamus, do respond to insulin. The evidence on this point includes some interesting examples of using the abnormal physiology of disease to throw light on normal physiology:

1.  Under normal circumstances, hyperglycemia decreases growth hormone secretion, and hypoglycemia increases it. These responses are mediated by the hypothalamus. In diabetes mellitus, however, a high blood glucose can be associated with a high plasma growth hormone level. The elevated growth hormone suggests that, despite the high blood glucose, not much glucose is getting into the cells of the hypothalamus to shut off the secretion of growth hormone. Since the diabetic lacks insulin, this suggests that when insulin is present it enhances the transfer of glucose into hypothalamic cells.
2.  In diabetes, there is a decreased uptake of glucose in the cells of the satiety center of the hypothalamus (see p. 262), the suggestion again being that insulin normally enhances glucose uptake by these cells.
3.  Insulin injected in the cerebrospinal fluid (CSF) lowers the concentration of glucose in the CSF without much effect on the blood sugar, thus insulin may directly stimulate glucose uptake by the spinal cord.

### Actions of Insulin on Specific Tissues

A great amount of effort has been spent over the years in defining the actions of insulin on specific tissues. As already mentioned, these actions are not only on carbohydrate metabolism, as might be thought from the above discussion, but also on fat and protein metabolism. We now take up these actions, in order, as they relate to muscle, adipose tissue, and liver.

MUSCLE. Insulin binds to muscle, and its effect persists even if insulin is removed from around the muscle.

*Carbohydrate Metabolism.* As noted, *glucose transport* into the cell is increased, a process requiring neither protein synthesis nor mRNA synthesis. *Potassium uptake* is also increased, an effect which is used clinically to decrease dangerously elevated potassium levels in the serum of patients. The potassium effect was thought to parallel the glucose effect, but in fact it occurs later in time and may occur at low levels of insulin which do not affect glucose uptake. It is, then, a separate action of insulin on muscle.

Once inside the cell, glucose has several pathways open to it. Insulin has several effects here, too, all of which *do* require protein synthesis, though probably not mRNA synthesis. Therefore, these effects are a qualitatively different action of insulin, and probably a different, or perhaps secondary, mechanism is involved.

There is an increased incorporation of *glucose into glycogen*. The key enzyme for this, glycogen synthetase, exists in two forms. The form dependent on glucose-6-phosphate for its activity has a relatively low capacity for making glycogen; the form independent of glucose-6-phosphate is much more active. The two are called the D and I forms (dependent and independent). Insulin causes a specific increase in the more active or I form of glycogen synthetase (the D to I transformation) and thus an increase in glycogen synthesis. Insulin may also stimulate glycogen formation without affecting the forms of glycogen synthetase through some as yet unknown mechanism. Cyclic AMP does the reverse, stimulating the conversion of the I to D form. It is possible then that insulin lowers the concentration of cAMP in muscle and thus increases the D to I conversion, but tests in one experiment did not reveal a lower cAMP. Confirmation is needed.

One also sees an increase in the overall oxidation of glucose to $CO_2$, some of which may be secondary simply to an increased glucose uptake, but there is more to it than that. While glucose conversion into glycogen is increased, insulin directs even more glucose into the *glycolytic pathway*. Precisely how this is done is uncertain, but it is probably related to the demonstrable increase in the activities of *phosphofructokinase*, which catalyzes an irreversible reaction in muscle, and in *pyruvate kinase* (see Fig. 52). Apparently the pyruvate is made so fast that it cannot be completely utilized, and there is release of lactate from the insulin-stimulated muscle.

*Fat Metabolism.* There is less intracellular release of free fatty acids from muscle triglyceride because insulin decreases the lipolysis of triglyceride.

*Protein Metabolism.*   Insulin has major significant effects on muscle protein metabolism, as one might expect from the above changes in enzyme activity. The actions are independent of the effect on glucose transport but are probably responsible for the effects of insulin on intracellular glucose metabolism.

Along with a decrease in plasma amino acids, insulin *increases* the *uptake of amino acids* into muscle and their *incorporation* into muscle protein by ribosomes. Not all amino acids are affected in the same way. This action is different from a similar action of growth hormone, since the latter exerts its effect on a different spectrum of amino acids. However, there is no *net* protein synthesis unless growth hormone is present. Furthermore, there is evidence to suggest that insulin is required for growth hormone or testosterone to affect protein synthesis. These points are not completely clarified because many of them depend on in vitro observations where the incubation conditions can cause major changes in the results. For example, some investigators have claimed that insulin does not stimulate amino acid incorporation into protein when the proper control experiment is done in vitro.

In any case, assuming that the effect on protein synthesis occurs in vivo, mRNA synthesis is not required although it may occur and enhance further protein synthesis later on. The best guess at the moment is that insulin somehow directly stimulates ribosomal protein synthesis, perhaps by enhancing the transfer of amino acids from tRNA to protein, by increasing polysome formation from the ribosomes, or by increasing the synthesis of ribosomal RNA. Growth hormone and testosterone appear to act as synergists; growth hormone and insulin work together to give optimal protein synthesis.

ADIPOSE TISSUE.   Many of the effects on adipose tissue are similar to those on muscle. As in muscle, insulin binds to adipose tissue, but in this case the insulin effect can be reversed, in vitro at least, by washing the adipose cells. The difference between adipose tissue and muscle seems to be that adipose tissue inactivates insulin faster; thus a continuous supply of exogenous insulin is necessary for a persistent insulin effect.

*Carbohydrate Metabolism.*   As in muscle, insulin *increases glucose transport* across the cell membrane. In this instance insulin may act both by increasing the maximum velocity of glucose transport and by increasing the affinity of glucose for the transport system. Surprisingly enough, actinomycin D both inhibits the binding process (which is not dependent on RNA synthesis) and increases glucose utilization; this is another example in which one must use caution in the interpretation of experiments with actinomycin. An intact cell membrane is necessary for glucose transport; perhaps insulin affects it by changing the phospholipid-protein structure and allowing increased glucose (and amino acid) entry into the cell.

Following this, hexokinase activity and glucose-6-phosphate (G-6-P) content increase. Again, as in muscle, the G-6-P can go to glycogen or be broken down to other things. Insulin increases the conversion of *glucose* to *glycogen* and at the same time decreases glycogen breakdown. The former is mediated by an increase in the D to I form of glycogen synthetase and probably does not involve changes in cAMP. Puromycin, however, does not block the two effects of insulin on glycogen metabolism; presumably, then, protein synthesis is not involved and they may be due to direct (allosteric?) effects of insulin on the glycogen synthetase and phosphorylase enzyme systems.

Along the other pathway, glucose breakdown, insulin increases overall *glucose oxidation* to $CO_2$. This effect occurs at levels of insulin as low as 1 $\mu U/ml$ and, in this instance, probably does result from a drop in cAMP content. Whether there are the same changes in enzymes as in muscle is not certain. A bioassay for insulin is based on the amount of $CO_2$ generated by the rat epididymal fat pad; for the most part the assay has been replaced by the newer immunoassay.

*Fat Metabolism.* Fat metabolism, needless to say, is well studied in adipose tissue. The general tendency of insulin is to *increase* adipose tissue *fat*, which is mostly triglyceride, by a variety of mechanisms (Fig. 51).

Insulin increases the uptake of fatty acids by adipose tissue just as it does the uptake of glucose. *Lipogenesis*, the synthesis of fatty acids, is increased at levels of insulin as low as 1 $\mu U/ml$ (in vitro). Thus, inside the adipose cell, there is a greater conversion of glucose, amino acids, and pyruvate to fatty acids (Figs. 51, 52). Under some circumstances as much as 45% of the glucose entering under the influence of insulin is converted to fat. mRNA synthesis is generally required here, although apparently not for the incorporation of pyruvate into fatty acids. Just what reaction(s) of the many between glucose and long-chain fatty acid is stimulated is not clear. For example, insulin need not stimulate the synthesis of acetyl-CoA into fatty acid but may act instead to increase the supply of acetyl-CoA. It could enhance the activity of citrate cleavage enzyme, which may be the main source of acetyl-CoA in the cytoplasm, the locus of fatty acid synthesis; some workers, however, have not been able to find any citrate cleavage enzyme in human adipose cells although the enzyme is clearly present in the adipose tissue of rats. More work is needed here. Another possibility: Insulin may in some way stimulate the production in the cytoplasm of more of the TPNH needed to synthesize fatty acids; again, the answer lies in the future. For further discussion of insulin and lipogenesis in liver, see pp. 215–217 and Figure 52.

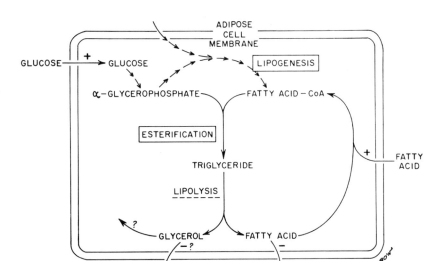

FIG. 51. Overall view of fat metabolism in an adipose cell. Processes stimulated by insulin are enclosed in boxes or indicated by +; those probably inhibited by insulin are underlined with a broken line or indicated by a −.

Two other reactions are affected by insulin, the net result being increased fat in the adipose tissue. One is the *esterification* of fatty acids with glycerophosphate to form triglycerides, which is *increased*, and the other is the *lipolysis* of triglycerides to fatty acids and glycerol, which is *decreased*. The two are probably separate reactions.

Much research, however, indicates that insulin acts to increase esterification but not directly to inhibit lipolysis. This idea hinges on the absence of glycerokinase in adipose tissue, and the argument runs as follows:

1. Since adipose tissue apparently lacks glycerokinase, then any glycerol formed by breaking down triglyceride cannot be phosphorylated to glycerophosphate. The glycerol cannot be used again to form new triglyceride—a process requiring glycerophosphate—but must stay in the adipose tissue or be released to the plasma.

2. If insulin inhibits lipolysis, one would expect not only less fatty acids to come out of the adipose tissue but also an equal inhibition of glycerol release.

3. Since in some experiments the release of glycerol was not inhibited when insulin was added, although the release of fatty

acids was, it is a reasonable conclusion that insulin stimulates esterification but does not inhibit lipolysis.

However, other work suggests that (1) adipose tissue does have glycerokinase but it is hard to demonstrate, (2) glycerol release can be inhibited by insulin, and (3) insulin probably lowers both adenyl cyclase activity and cAMP content in adipose tissue. Since lipolysis is usually directly related to levels of cAMP, this recent work makes it reasonable to say that insulin inhibits lipolysis and that it does so by lowering cAMP. That is not to say it has no effect on esterification; in all likelihood insulin both stimulates esterification and inhibits lipolysis.

It must be admitted, however, that agreement on this point is far from universal. Several workers have good data supporting the original idea—i.e., insulin stimulates esterification but does not inhibit lipolysis—and are unable to confirm the antilipolytic action.

The effect on lipolysis is rapid and may occur even before an increase in glucose uptake is seen. As one would predict, the overall effect of insulin on adipose tissue is to store fat and lessen the release of free fatty acids. In the blood, the net result is a *decrease* in the *plasma free fatty acids* and also in plasma triglycerides.

So striking is the effect of insulin on fatty acid release that some workers have suggested that the decreased lipolysis itself induces insulin's effects on glucose uptake and its conversion to $CO_2$, glycerol, and fatty acids. However, insulin retains its effects on glucose metabolism in adipose tissue "ghosts," a special preparation of adipose cells from which all the lipid has been removed. Without triglyceride there obviously can be no effect on lipolysis, so inhibition of lipolysis per se does not cause insulin's effect on glucose metabolism.

Cyclic AMP plays a key role in adipose tissue (see Fig. 31); insulin drops the level of cAMP, thereby causing some of its effects on fatty acid metabolism. Whether the effects on glucose are secondary to a drop in cAMP concentration is at the moment speculative.

Finally, insulin may actually induce a type of *lipase* in adipose tissue, but it is a lipase that remains inactive until insulin's effect is gone.

*Protein Metabolism.* Insulin increases amino acid incorporation into adipose tissue protein. This effect is independent of the one on glucose transport since the former is blocked by puromycin and the latter is not.

LIVER. *Carbohydrate Metabolism.* Here the liver is strikingly different from muscle and adipose tissue. Insulin has no effect on glucose transport into the liver cell, which seems to be freely permeable to glucose without insulin. Nevertheless, insulin does have significant effects on intracellular glucose metabolism.

Despite the lack of effect on glucose transport, there is an increased glucose uptake, but this is a slow response taking several hours, as opposed to the rapid effect on muscle. It is due to a specific increase in glucokinase activity; insulin seems to act as a permissive agent, allowing glucose to actually induce the increase in enzyme activity.

The general pattern seen in muscle and adipose tissue is now repeated in the liver; insulin *increases the disposition of glucose-6-phosphate* along the several paths open to it.

1. More glucose can be incorporated into glycogen, on account of a change in glycogen synthetase from the D to the I form that happens within 10 minutes after insulin is given. Some research suggests that the increased synthetase activity is dependent on mRNA synthesis because it is blocked by actinomycin D, but the effect is rapid enough to make one wonder whether it might not be a more direct effect.
2. At about the same time (10 minutes) there is a drop in active phosphorylase, which also tends to increase the glycogen content of liver.
3. Insulin acts as a permissive agent in the induction of glucose-6-phosphate dehydrogenase (G-6-PD) by G-6-P, thereby increasing glucose entry into the hexose monophosphate shunt.
4. There is increased glucose utilization along the glycolytic pathway, with increases in the activity of phosphofructokinase and pyruvate kinase (see Fig. 52).

Finally, insulin reduces the amount of glucose made by the liver—*decreased gluconeogenesis*—with an observable drop in the enzyme converting oxaloacetate to phosphoenolpyruvate, phosphoenolpyruvate carboxykinase. It also, late in the game, decreases the activity of glucose-6-phosphatase, the enzyme responsible for getting glucose out of the liver and into the blood stream. Whether these enzyme effects are directly due to insulin or are secondary to some other effect of insulin is not clear.

For some years it was widely debated whether or not net glucose output by the liver was affected by insulin. There now seems little question that *insulin decreases net glucose output* by the liver into the blood. All the effects noted on hepatic glucose metabolism would suggest that this is an obvious conclusion, but many of these effects observed in special preparations might well not apply in vivo. Furthermore, actual measurement of hepatic glycogen content shows that it is not always increased after insulin administration. The question was settled by measuring differences in glucose concentration in blood going into and out of the liver, which is a fairly complex problem in technical and physiologic design. The reason why hepatic glycogen is not always increased is probably that glycogen content is to some degree a result of glycogen synthesis, glycogen breakdown, gluconeo-genesis, and glycolysis, processes which may be variably affected by insulin so that there may or may not be a rise in the amount of glycogen.

In liver, as in muscle and fat, the changes in glucose metabolism seen with insulin may be due to a drop in cAMP concentration. There is some evidence to support this idea, but the data are not convincing as yet.

*Fat Metabolism.* Insulin causes the liver to take up more fatty acids from the blood and to *increase lipogenesis* from glucose or pyruvate. As in adipose tissue, lipogenesis of the usual long-chain fatty acids is basically a cytoplasmic, not a mitochondrial, process. Because it is an easier tissue to work with, lipogenesis has been more carefully studied in the liver than in adipose tissue. The mechanisms may or may not be similar in both tissues, but evidence to date does not show any major discrepancies between the two (except for the problem of whether or not human adipose tissue has any citrate cleavage enzyme), and what applies to liver may well apply to adipose tissue.

With glucose as the starting point, lipogenesis should logically occur when glucose passes down the glycolytic pathway to pyruvate, where-upon the pyruvate should be converted to acetyl-CoA and the latter in turn to fatty acids. However, the process is not that simple. The reaction pyruvate $\rightarrow$ acetyl-CoA does not readily occur in the cyto-plasm; it is largely a mitochondrial reaction. Moreover, the acetyl-CoA in the mitochondria has a difficult time diffusing into the cytoplasm; it can cross the mitochondrial membrane into the cytoplasm only after it is converted, for example, to citrate. We also know that something from the mitochondria, in addition to acetyl-CoA, specifically stimu-lates fatty acid synthesis in the cytoplasm. Candidates for that "some-thing" are acylcarnitine (fatty acid–carnitine) and citrate itself. These compounds may stimulate lipogenesis either by acting as substrates or by enhancing the activity of the enzymes of lipogenesis; the latter is the more likely.

The facts then, qualified by the usual problems of transferring in-formation from experiments done with broken cells to the intact animal, seem to be as follows (see Fig. 52):

1. Pyruvate from glycolysis enters the mitochondria and is con-verted to acetyl-CoA.
2. Acetyl-CoA then combines with oxaloacetate to form citrate, catalyzed by citrate synthetase.
3. In the presence of malate, citrate passes through the mitochon-drial membrane into the cytoplasm.
4. In the cytoplasm, citrate is probably the main source of the acetyl-CoA used in lipogenesis. Citrate, CoA, and ATP are cata-

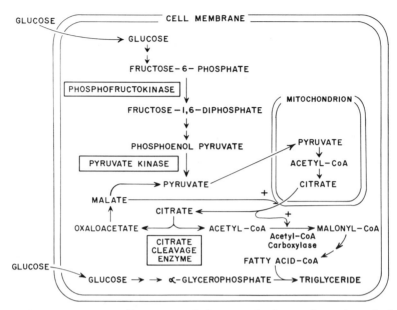

FIG. 52. Lipogenesis (formation of fatty acids from glucose) and the formation of triglyceride. Enzymes thought to be stimulated by insulin are enclosed in boxes. Stimulation of a process is shown by +.

lyzed by citrate cleavage enzyme to acetyl-CoA, oxaloacetate, and ADP. The cleavage enzyme may be active only during active formation of ATP and when fatty acid synthesis is high. Here is an effect of insulin: It seems to increase the activity of citrate cleavage enzyme.

5. Acetyl-CoA is then converted to malonyl-CoA, catalyzed by acetyl-CoA carboxylase.
6. TPNH is required for acetyl-CoA to be converted to fatty acids; perhaps its formation, too, is enhanced.

In addition to "secreting" citrate as a source of acetyl-CoA, the mitochondria seem to make something that directly enhances lipogenesis. As noted, the "something" could be acylcarnitine or citrate. Acylcarnitine is known to increase fatty acid synthesis. One might speculate that it acts by stimulating either acetyl-CoA carboxylase or citrate cleavage enzyme. Or it may simply be another good substrate for the formation of cytoplasmic acetyl-CoA. Citrate also stimulates fatty acid synthesis above and beyond the increase seen with acylcarnitine and therefore probably by a different mechanism. It has been shown to enhance directly the activity of acetyl-CoA carboxylase in addition to being converted to acetyl-CoA.

The problem is that while it seems clear that something from the mitochondria stimulates lipogenesis, probably by directly stimulating acetyl-CoA carboxylase, and that both citrate and acylcarnitine have such an effect, no one knows whether the mitochondrial material is in fact either of these substances. There is a question, for example, whether the liver contains enough citrate to actually stimulate acetyl-CoA carboxylase. It is also not known whether insulin affects any part of the mitochondrial mechanism.

Insulin therefore increases glycolysis (see p. 214) and increases citrate cleavage, either or both of which could indirectly result in increased lipogenesis. There may be more direct effects of insulin beyond the formation of acetyl-CoA—for example, on acetyl-CoA carboxylase—but nothing is known of them.

Figure 52 briefly outlines the action of insulin on lipogenesis with the stimulated enzymes in boxes. Most of the pyruvate kinase may actually be in the mitochondrion, but this is not certain. As mentioned, many of these details of lipogenesis in the liver may well apply to adipose tissue.

Whether a drop in hepatic cAMP concentration accounts for the effect of insulin on lipogenesis is speculation, but an experiment to find out will undoubtedly be done soon.

In addition to affecting lipogenesis, insulin probably decreases fatty acid oxidation by hepatic mitochondria and, under some circumstances, increases the uptake of triglycerides by liver and the hepatic content of triglycerides. The overall effect is therefore to make and keep fat in the liver to a certain degree.

*Protein Metabolism.* As in other tissues, insulin *stimulates amino acid uptake* by the liver. Some of the net amino acid uptake may be a result of decreased breakdown of protein, but the whole effect is not explained this way. Insulin also enhances amino acid *incorporation into protein*. These actions are dependent on mRNA synthesis, as are the actions noted above requiring the synthesis of various enzymes.

To sum up, the *overall effect of insulin* on the body is to diminish the use of fatty acids as an energy source and increase their storage in adipose tissue, while enhancing the use of glucose for energy but allowing for storage of glucose not needed immediately, both in the liver as glycogen and fat and in adipose tissue as fat. At the same time, the burning of amino acids for energy is inhibited and their incorporation into protein enhanced. Hence the so-called protein-sparing effect of carbohydrate.

The *action of insulin* has obviously been intensively investigated. It has such a wide spectrum of different effects that positing a single action is difficult. At the time when only one effect was known, it was easy to say what that was. Now, the multitude of effects has changed things. One thought is that, since insulin affects the cell membrane in some tissues, a kind of chain reaction might be set up throughout the entire cell involving the "internal cell membrane" or endoplasmic reticulum. All the other effects could conceivably derive from this. This seems a reasonable idea since intact cells—and therefore cell membranes—are usually necessary to show an action of insulin. Or one could postulate an effect directly on the cell nucleus and its DNA, changing nuclear RNA synthesis; however, the cell membrane actions would be hard to explain in this way. Perhaps there are many effects, and insulin may act on the cell membrane, the ribosome (or endoplasmic reticulum), and the nucleus, all at the same time or in sequence. A general diminution of cAMP concentration in tissues may, if consistently demonstrated, be a key to much of the confusion.

Since the control of insulin secretion involves glucagon, the next hormone to be discussed, the factors controlling the secretion of both insulin and glucagon are taken up later (pp. 222, 223).

## Glucagon

Commercial insulin is a pancreatic extract, not a pure, synthesized protein. Other pancreatic material besides insulin is necessarily carried along when the extract is made. Injection of these "insulin" extracts sometimes causes a transient *rise* in *glucose* before the expected drop. The substance responsible for this effect was observed in 1923 by Kimball, Murlin, and others, and was named *glucagon*. For many years glucagon was regarded as a curiosity which, although it had many physiologic effects when injected, played little or no role in glucose metabolism in the body. This attitude is changing, largely because glucagon can now be measured in the plasma.

*Pancreatic glucagon* is a single-chain polypeptide with 29 amino acids (3485 mol. wt.) and has been completely synthesized in the chemical laboratory (Wuensch, 1968). It is made by the pancreatic α-*cells* in the islets of Langerhans—possibly by only some of these, the so-called $\alpha_2$-cells. The human pancreas contains about 3.7 µg of glucagon per gram of pancreas. In addition to some of the "pancreatic" glucagon, the duodenum and jejunum contain a similar though not identical substance which can tentatively be called *gastrointestinal* or *GI glucagon*. This material has about twice the molecular weight of pancreatic glucagon; the jejunum contains about 300 mµg per gram according to one report. Other hyperglycemic substances can be extracted from many other tissues; little is known of their chemistry or significance.

## Plasma Levels of Glucagon

With the advent of the radioimmunoassay, glucagon could be measured in plasma for the first time. The actual values found in published papers vary rather widely; in the fasting state the reported level of plasma glucagon has ranged from 0.05 mμg/ml to 8.0 mμg/ml or more.

The differences among workers have caused a good deal of uncertainty in the minds of many, particularly after the material from the small intestine—GI glucagon—was described. GI glucagon crossreacts with glucagon in the immunoassay, which makes it hard to know exactly what one is measuring when doing the immunoassay. Plasma samples could contain varying amounts of pancreatic glucagon and GI glucagon, yet give the same value for glucagon content in the assay. For example, bioassay of a large volume of plasma, using a method that does not detect GI glucagon, suggests that the level of pancreatic glucagon in plasma is actually less than 0.1 mμg/ml. Compare this to the values found in the immunoassay noted above, and the cause for concern is clear. Obviously what is needed is an assay that is both highly sensitive and capable of measuring each type of glucagon independently. Recent work suggests that an immunoassay can be developed for both pancreatic and GI glucagon; in the next year or two the assay may be perfected and we will be able to talk of glucagon with more confidence. In the meantime, we must use the data at hand and make reasonable guesses as to whether we are dealing with pancreatic or GI glucagon. The only exception occurs when the measurements are made on plasma taken directly from the pancreatic or mesenteric veins; the measurement is not easy to make in humans but has been done in several animal experiments, and the results where pertinent are noted below.

The plasma half-life of injected pancreatic glucagon is less than 10 minutes.

## Actions of Glucagon

With the exception of the effect on insulin secretion (see p. 221), all the actions of glucagon discussed here refer to the pancreatic hormone.

CARBOHYDRATE METABOLISM. The principal and most rapid action is to *raise the blood glucose.*

*In the liver,* glucagon increases *glycogen breakdown* in a matter of 1 to 2 minutes and thus increases the blood glucose. The liver is ideally located since glucagon from the pancreas must come first to the liver before being diluted in the peripheral circulation. In the liver, glucagon stimulates *adenyl cyclase* to make more cAMP, which in turn increases the amount of *active phosphorylase*. Active phosphorylase then catalyzes the breakdown of glycogen (glycogenolysis), and more glucose is released to the blood. Blood glucose levels rise only transiently (because of stimulation of insulin secretion) unless glucagon secretion continues.

There is some recent evidence to suggest that the action of glucagon on glycogenolysis may actually be slightly different. While active phosphorylase increases, it may not be a rate-limiting enzyme in the first place. If not, then an increase in phosphorylase would not explain the action of glucagon. Perhaps glucagon somehow *increases* the *exposure of glycogen* to the phosphorylase. Hydrocortisone plays a supportive role in the glycogenolysis.

Glucagon also increases the rate of *gluconeogenesis*, largely from liver protein, plasma amino acids, and pyruvate. This process, however, takes longer; while glycogenolysis is apparent in a few minutes, gluconeogenesis increases only at one-half hour. As with glycogenolysis, hydrocortisone plays a permissive role in glucagon's stimulation of gluconeogenesis. Once again cAMP is involved; glucagon stimulates the production of cAMP, but the cAMP cannot act on gluconeogenesis unless hydrocortisone is present. Hydrocortisone somehow allows cAMP to enhance the conversion of pyruvate to phosphoenolpyruvate on the way to glucose (see Fig. 54).

Increased gluconeogenesis would make more glucose available for either glycogen synthesis or release to the blood. Since glucagon *decreases* the active form of *glycogen synthetase* in about 10 minutes and also *decreases glucokinase* activity, it seems clear that the net effect of glucagon on both glycogen and glucose metabolism is to increase the hepatic output of glucose.

*In the periphery,* although it increases the blood glucose, glucagon does not inhibit glucose uptake by muscle. In fact, *glucose uptake* by muscle is probably *increased.* This may be a direct effect, or it may be secondary to a glucagon- or glucose-induced rise in insulin secretion. Muscle glycogen content can be increased. Further, in the body as a whole, glucagon causes an increase in glucose oxidation to $CO_2$ along with the expected increase in oxygen consumption.

FAT METABOLISM.   Glucagon is not without effects on fat metabolism. In vitro, glucagon *stimulates free fatty acid release* from adipose tissue. Yet, in vivo, the plasma free fatty acid level is lower after glucagon is given, as are the serum triglycerides. Probably glucagon *stimulates fatty acid uptake and catabolism* by other tissues—e.g., the liver and muscle—more than it stimulates lipolysis, so that plasma free fatty acids are decreased in the face of higher utilization.

In the liver there is indeed an increased *fatty acid oxidation*, and more fatty acids are converted to *ketone bodies* (acetoacetate and β-hydroxybutyrate) while at the same time there is more storage of fatty acids as triglycerides. The resulting increase in *acetyl-CoA* increases pyruvate carboxylation, and the increase in *acyl-CoA* decreases pyruvate decarboxylation; the outcome of all this is a further enhancement of gluconeogenesis. Finally, fatty acid synthesis from acetate is less. Again, glucagon acts to supply glucose where needed and allow fat to be used where it can.

PROTEIN METABOLISM.   In general, effects on protein metabolism have been observed only with high doses of glucagon. The *net effect* on the body is *protein loss*. One sees total weight loss as well as decreased weight of muscle and liver. Less amino acids get into muscle protein; in fact, muscle releases more amino acids to the blood. Nevertheless, the level of plasma amino acids is lower, probably because the liver takes them up faster than muscle releases them. In the liver the amino acids are metabolized, resulting in an increase in gluconeogenesis, in urea production by the liver, and in urinary urea. Along with this, there is a net decrease in liver protein synthesis. The presence of growth hormone, strangely enough, may be necessary for these actions on protein metabolism.

OTHER ACTIONS OF GLUCAGON.   Other effects are not well understood, and their role in normal physiology is unclear. They include, for example, a hypocalcemic effect, a stimulatory effect on cardiac contraction, and a stimulatory effect on the secretion of growth hormone from the pituitary and catecholamines from the adrenal medulla.

Do these actions of pancreatic glucagon have physiologic significance? The question was debated for many years, as mentioned above, but I thought it settled when the data on the radioimmunoassay of glucagon were published. Now that we know of GI glucagon as well as pancreatic glucagon, the question becomes pertinent again and the solution awaits an assay specific for pancreatic glucagon. In the meantime, a rational approach would be to regard as physiologic the effects of pancreatic glucagon on glucose and fatty acid metabolism. The effects on protein catabolism may well occur only at levels of glucagon not found in the body.

INSULIN SECRETION.   There seems little doubt that oral doses of glucose stimulate a transient rise in glucagon secretion, if enough glucose is given. Glucose administered intravenously has no such effect. The rise in plasma glucagon is probably due to GI glucagon, a thesis supported by extensive work with dogs using the radioimmunoassay as the main analytic tool. The facts are:

1. After glucose given orally, glucagon in the portal vein rises from 0.6 to 1.0 mμg/ml and falls to normal by two hours.

2. Pancreatectomy does not eliminate the rise in glucagon in the portal vein.
3. The pancreatic vein contains little of this glucagon; it is, however, found in the mesenteric veins.

A most important finding is that GI glucagon stimulates insulin secretion but does *not* have any of the other classic actions of glucagon; i.e., it does not stimulate the breakdown of glycogen or raise the blood glucose.

For the moment then, GI glucagon can be regarded as something that increases insulin secretion and does nothing else. Perhaps pancreatic glucagon stimulates insulin secretion, too. It does so when injected into an animal, but this effect may not occur with the amounts of glucagon actually found in the plasma. Conceivably, pancreatic glucagon could directly stimulate an adjacent β-cell without a change in its level in plasma or, in vitro, in the surrounding medium.

### Control of Glucagon Secretion

Just about all the evidence bearing on the control of glucagon secretion depends on the radioimmunoassay of glucagon in blood. Because of the problems with the assay and the discrepancies among different workers noted before (p. 219), much of what follows may have to be changed as new research is done.

*Glucose taken by mouth*, as already noted, results in a rapid, transient *rise in plasma glucagon*, which in turn stimulates insulin secretion. All the evidence to date suggests that this glucagon is *GI glucagon;* the main evidence is the work with dogs just noted and other work showing that a rise in blood glucose actively inhibits pancreatic glucagon secretion.

*Amino acids taken orally* also *increase plasma glucagon.* Amino acids injected into a vein do the same thing; for example, arginine injected into humans increases glucagon in the peripheral plasma from 0.05 to 0.3 mμg/ml in a few minutes. Here the glucagon is *pancreatic glucagon* (in the dog's pancreatic vein the level rises from 1.0 to 2.5 mμg/ml after intravenous administration of amino acids) and not GI glucagon. However, one can also detect a rise in glucagon in the dog's pancreatic vein *after* an oral dose of amino acids but *before* there is any increase in the level of plasma amino acids. This means that somehow the pancreas knows the amino acids are coming before they get there; there must be something like GI glucagon to mediate this effect. So far, the best candidate is the well-known gastrointestinal hormone, *pancreozymin,* the secretion of which is known to be stimulated by amino acids and which is also known to stimulate pancreatic glucagon secretion.

While glucose given by mouth stimulates the secretion of GI glucagon, a *rise in blood glucose,* as just mentioned, *inhibits* the secretion of *pancreatic glucagon.* For example, an elevated blood glucose drops the glucagon level in the dog's pancreatic vein from 2.5 mμg/ml to 1.9 mμg/ml in only 5 minutes.

*Hypoglycemia, fasting,* and perhaps growth hormone are *stimulators of pancreatic glucagon secretion.* A drop in blood glucose to less than 60 mg/100 ml causes the glucagon level in the dog's pancreatic vein to rise from 2.5 mμg/ml to 6.0 mμg/ml in 30 minutes. With fasting the data are not as clear. Most measurements of glucagon in human peripheral plasma show an increase with fasting, but agreement is not universal. Here the rise may again be due to the mild hypoglycemia seen in the fasting state. The slow fall in blood glucose may explain why the rise in plasma glucagon, when it occurs, takes a day or two to become apparent. There are reported levels of plasma glucagon in fasting humans as high as 15 to 20 mμg/ml. Much of the problem in deciding whether or not plasma glucagon rises during fasting is, as we have said, technical, but it may be due in part to the plasma *free fatty acids* (FFA). Plasma FFA increases during fasting and they also appear to *inhibit glucagon secretion;* a high rise in plasma FFA may blunt a rise in glucagon that might otherwise have occurred.

In any case, it does make excellent teleologic sense for plasma glucagon to be elevated during fasting. Such an elevation would enhance glycogen breakdown and gluconeogenesis, thus helping to keep up the blood glucose, a highly desirable effect. It might also help mobilize the FFA from adipose tissue needed as a source of energy. Finally, it may be here that pancreatic glucagon acts to stimulate mildly the secretion of insulin; plasma insulin is low during fasting, but one might speculate that it would fall away to nothing, thereby causing diabetes mellitus, were it not for pancreatic glucagon.

Whether the central and autonomic nervous systems play a significant role in regulating glucagon secretion is not known—another good area for speculation, experiments, and integration of the nervous and endocrine systems.

## CONTROL OF INSULIN SECRETION

### Glucose: A Direct Stimulus to Insulin Secretion

The main determinant of insulin secretion is the *level of blood glucose.* Insulin does not suppress its own secretion; there is no self-regulation. The control of insulin secretion by blood glucose is a classic example of a *negative feedback* control mechanism. A rise in blood sugar above a critical level of about 80 to 100 mg/100 ml stimulates the pancreatic islets to secrete insulin; for example, the plasma insulin rises fivefold one hour after the eating of 100 g of glucose. The insulin, of course, lowers the blood glucose, removing the stimulus to insulin secretion, and the plasma insulin falls to its formerly low level. The liver may somehow act as a sensor for increased need of insulin whenever the glucose content of the portal vein rises.

Glucose—and a few other sugars: fructose, mannose, and ribose—acts directly on the pancreas to stimulate insulin secretion since the same thing happens in vitro when glucose is added to pieces of pancreas. Calcium must be present, and the concomitant entry of sodium into the β-cell along with the glucose seems to be important. Once in the β-cell, glucose itself is apparently *not* the stimulus; the glucose, to be effective, must be metabolized at least to glucose-6-phosphate and perhaps further. The process requires oxygen, but synthesis of neither insulin nor any other protein is immediately required. Glucose-stimulated insulin secretion is probably mediated by a β-adrenergic receptor and by an increase in cAMP, although exactly what compound is the stimulant and precisely where it acts are not known. Finally, there is a rapid release of insulin from the granules stored in the β-cells (see Fig. 50).

Glucose does increase insulin synthesis as well as secretion; the point is that the two effects are separate. Newly synthesized insulin is released later on if necessary.

### Factors Affecting Blood Glucose: Indirect Stimuli to Insulin Secretion

Since the level of blood glucose is the controlling factor in regulating insulin secretion, it is clear that practically anything affecting carbohydrate metabolism will affect insulin secretion. A simple negative feedback system involving only glucose and insulin is then a convenient abstraction; in fact anything that affects blood glucose belongs in the control system.

*Growth hormone* does not stimulate insulin release in vitro except at high concentrations of glucose, but it can raise plasma insulin in vivo. Some of this action is due to an inhibition of glucose uptake by muscle and adipose tissue causing a temporary rise in blood glucose and a resulting secondary rise in plasma insulin. There is also, however, a direct effect on the pancreas whereby growth hormone sensitizes the adenyl cyclase system to glucose stimulation. The result would then be more cAMP formed in response to a given glucose load and so more insulin secreted. Growth hormone also has effects on the liver which would raise the blood sugar: an increase in both fructose-1,6-diphosphatase and glucose-6-phosphatase. Note that after growth hormone the blood sugar can rise only slightly since the insulin response to an elevated blood sugar is rapid. In effect, then, in the presence of growth hormone more insulin is needed to keep the blood glucose down to normal. Growth hormone would be *diabetogenic* (cause diabetes mellitus) only when insulin failed to rise enough and the blood sugar remained elevated. This happens in some animals—for example, the dog.

A rise in plasma *free fatty acids* tends to inhibit insulin's stimulation of glucose transport and phosphofructokinase activity (in muscle). Less glucose gets into the cell, the blood glucose tends to go up, and there is more insulin secretion. This effect, however, may not be present at the usual levels of free fatty acids present in plasma.

*Thyroxine* tends to raise the blood sugar by affecting liver enzymes as growth hormone does, and thus stimulating glucose release from the liver. *Hydrocortisone* also increases the glucose output of the liver (see Chap. 5) and may raise the blood sugar by another effect, an inhibition of peripheral insulin-induced glucose uptake (it is not yet certain that this is a direct effect on muscle or adipose tissue). *Glucagon* causes a rapid increase in blood glucose as a direct result of glycogen breakdown in the liver. It also has a direct effect on insulin secretion (see Glucagon, above, and p. 226).

On more of an emergency basis, *epinephrine* stimulates a rapid rise in blood glucose. While this was classically thought to be due to a direct stimulation of glycogenolysis in the liver, recent evidence suggests that some other mechanism is involved. Epinephrine at levels present in plasma does not increase glycogen breakdown in vitro, yet there is no question that it raises the blood sugar. Perhaps epinephrine acts on the central nervous system to increase sympathetic nerve activity; one can imagine direct sympathetic stimulation either to the liver, resulting in glycogen breakdown, or to the pancreas, resulting in glucagon secretion with the same end result. Such speculation—which is all it is—may not be necessary since epinephrine can raise the blood sugar by other means. Epinephrine (1) decreases insulin-stimulated glucose uptake by muscle (though apparently not by fat) and (2) actually inhibits insulin secretion by the pancreas, an α-adrenergic effect.

All these factors (growth hormone, free fatty acids, thyroxine, hydrocortisone, glucagon, and epinephrine) tend to raise the blood sugar and therefore to stimulate insulin secretion. Some, of course, can directly stimulate insulin secretion (growth hormone, glucagon) and one (epinephrine) can directly inhibit it. The net effect depends on the state of the organism; if blood sugar is low to begin with, a rise in blood sugar may not lead to more insulin secretion if the critical level is not exceeded. Removal of any of these factors tends to lower blood glucose and, again depending on circumstances, may lower insulin secretion. All of them, in addition to insulin, are probably involved in maintaining the blood glucose at what we call a normal level.

### Other Direct Stimuli to Insulin Secretion

Our convenient abstraction of a simple negative feedback relationship between blood glucose level and insulin secretion must be further modified because there are direct stimuli to insulin secretion other than glucose.

A *rise* in the level of plasma *amino acids* increases insulin secretion whether the blood glucose is elevated or not. Some glucose, however, must be present. In this instance cAMP may not be involved. Since the same thing happens after eating protein, the rise in plasma insulin seen after a usual meal is due in part to glucose and in part to amino acids.

*Nervous stimuli* may be important though their role is not at all clear. Efferent *vagal* stimuli may slightly increase the amount of insulin in the pancreatic vein, perhaps enough to affect hepatic glucose metabolism but not enough to lower the circulating blood glucose. The effect is probably not a consistent one because some workers find no such increase after vagal stimulation. The *sympathetic nervous system* may also affect insulin secretion. We have mentioned the effect of epinephrine; stimulation of α-adrenergic receptors by epinephrine inhibits insulin secretion. β-Adrenergic stimulation does just the opposite and stimulates insulin secretion, probably mediated by increased cAMP. Since the pancreatic β-cell appears to be adrenergically innervated, appropriate sympathetic stimuli may be more important than we now suspect.

Both *pancreatic* and *GI glucagon* are stimulators of insulin secretion, as discussed before, and both may act as such in vivo under appropriate circumstances. Other gastrointestinal hormones, including gastrin, secretin, and pancreozymin, increase plasma insulin when injected. Whether they do so physiologically is uncertain; there is a great similarity in the molecular structures of glucagon and secretin, and recent work suggests that secretin and pancreozymin may be physiologic stimulators. The mechanism of action of glucagon on insulin secretion is probably different from that of glucose and β-adrenergic stimuli. Propranolol, a β-adrenergic blocking agent, does not block (or at best only partially blocks) the effect of glucagon while it does block the effects of glucose and β-adrenergic stimuli. Therefore, glucagon does not act via a β-adrenergic receptor, but glucose and, of course, β-adrenergic stimuli do. Nevertheless, cAMP may still be a mediator for the stimulation of insulin secretion by glucagon.

*Hydrocortisone* may also have a direct effect on insulin secretion; the response is relatively slow. Once again, an increase in cAMP is probably involved; in this instance, however, the rise in cAMP may result from a drop in phosphodiesterase rather than from a rise in adenyl cyclase (see Fig. 4). *Growth hormone*, as mentioned above, can directly stimulate pancreatic secretion of insulin, probably by sensitizing the adenyl cyclase system to glucose. Clinically, patients with a deficiency of growth hormone alone do not secrete insulin easily in response to glucose, evidence that growth hormone is required for normal insulin secretion in the normal person.

### Inhibition of Insulin Secretion

The secretion of insulin is less, as expected, when there is a *low blood glucose*. The two physiologic states in which this is the situation are *exercise* and *fasting*. In addition, epinephrine (or any α-adrenergic stimulus) inhibits insulin secretion; physiologically, this is the case with any *acute stress*.

Exercise increases the removal of glucose from the blood, a process mediated by a specific *muscle factor* that increases muscular uptake of glucose. The drop in blood glucose may be responsible for the lower plasma insulin. Insulin cannot drop too low, however, since its presence is necessary for the muscle factor to work. This phenomenon explains why a diabetic requires less insulin during exercise than when his activity is less. During fasting, the body shifts more to fatty acids as fuel with a drop in blood glucose, glucose utilization, and plasma insulin; a drop in plasma insulin below 6 to 8 μU/ml actually enhances fatty acid release. Since one sees increased epinephrine secretion during exercise and perhaps during fasting as well as during an acute stress, some of the lower plasma insulin seen in exercise and fasting may be due to epinephrine and not simply to changes in blood glucose.

Other findings that are not well integrated are the inhibition of insulin secretion by angiotensin II and an unexplained diurnal variation in plasma insulin unrelated to the level of blood glucose.

Viewed in broad perspective, then, insulin secretion is actually controlled by a host of factors, most related to blood sugar, some related to dietary glucose, and others unrelated to carbohydrate metabolism.

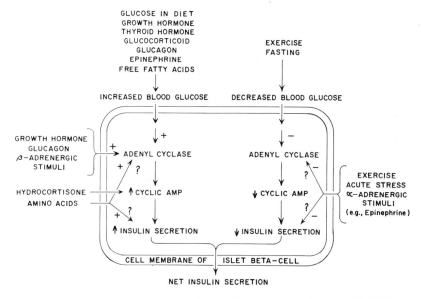

FIG. 53.   Insulin secretion as a resultant of several stimulants and inhibitors, mediated in large part by changes in cyclic AMP. Exact site of some effects is uncertain and is shown by split arrows with question marks. + indicates stimulation; − indicates inhibition.

The undefined role of the nervous system in the control of insulin secretion may be the "sleeper" in our present understanding of it (Fig. 53).

## DIABETES MELLITUS

About 3,000,000 people in the United States have diabetes mellitus —roughly 1.7% to 1.9% of the population. It is more common in women than in men. The dimensions of the public health problem are emphasized by the fact that almost half these people do not know they have it and are discovered only when large populations are tested routinely. Oddly enough, there are more men than women among the "newly discovered" diabetics. The widespread extent of the disease is one of the reasons so much effort has been put into understanding insulin and glucose metabolism.

### Diagnosis

Diabetes mellitus, as the name indicates, is often detected because excess glucose is found in the urine (the normal daily glucose output in urine is about 65 mg). Many diabetics do not have excess urinary glucose, however, but do have a high blood glucose. This elevation may be evident in the fasting state, or it may be seen only after a glucose meal (the glucose tolerance test). Diabetes mellitus is now defined as an *abnormally high blood glucose,* either while fasting or after a glucose tolerance test. In the latter case, the diabetic patient is said to have a "diabetic curve" or "poor glucose tolerance."

The diagnosis is not always as clear-cut as the last statement would make it seem. The interpretation of an elevated blood glucose is often difficult in pregnant patients and in patients over the age of 50 or 55. *Pregnant women* all have some resistance to the action of insulin, probably due to the large amount of human placental lactogen (HPL) in the blood, and may have an abnormal glucose tolerance test without having true diabetes mellitus. *Older patients,* male or female, have an increasingly higher incidence of poor glucose tolerance as they get older. The incidence becomes so high in the seventh and eighth decades of life that it is difficult to believe that all these people are truly diabetic. Probably they are not, but if not, the difficulty in diagnosing diabetes mellitus is obvious.

### Basic Cause

Diabetes is *due to the lack of enough insulin* to get glucose speedily out of the blood and into tissues. The problem is more complex than a simple lack of insulin since many diabetics have a normal or even elevated plasma insulin (see p. 229, on adult type).

Insulin deficiency is not all there is to this disease, making the situation more complex.

1. Diabetes tends to appear in the same family more often than expected, and, although not well understood, a strong *genetic* factor is involved. Possibly the diabetic is homozygous for a recessive gene. One could say that the insulin deficiency has a genetic basis.
2. Moreover, in diabetes mellitus, there is widespread *vascular damage* especially to small vessels (capillaries and arterioles), which may well be a separate defect from insulin deficiency. In fact, some research suggests that the early capillary lesion— a thickening of the basement membrane—actually causes diabetes mellitus. There is no clear evidence that the vascular damage is helped by insulin, despite improvement in the blood sugar. The vascular problem causes more illness and kills more patients than the results of absolute insulin deficiency, namely, ketoacidosis or hyperglycemia.
3. Finally, since injections of growth hormone can cause diabetes in some animals, *growth hormone* may cause human disease. There is scattered evidence to support this idea but it is not too solid.

Because of the variety of possible causes, it would surprise no one if what we call diabetes mellitus turned out to be several different diseases all of which happen to have a high blood glucose.

### Types of Diabetes Mellitus and the Defects in Insulin Secretion

Spontaneous diabetes mellitus is that which is not due to some other obvious cause such as Cushing's syndrome or acromegaly. It is usually divided into the juvenile (or "brittle" because it is harder to control) and the adult types.

The *juvenile type* usually occurs before the age of 30 in a person of normal weight. The disease is more severe, and the plasma insulin is low. This type of diabetes is clearly due to an absolute insulin deficiency and therefore almost always requires insulin treatment.

Most patients have diabetes of the *adult type*. The patient is older and often obese. The fasting insulin level is usually normal or elevated. However, the normal person responds to a glucose load with a prompt rise in plasma insulin; the adult diabetic responds somewhat more slowly, reaching a peak only after two to three hours, and often secretes *more* total insulin than a normal person given the same load of glucose.

It seems that there is something more to diabetes than absolute deficiency of insulin, a suggestion made some years ago (Houssay, 1929; Long and Lukens, 1936), and that the "something" is largely found in adult-onset diabetes mellitus. There are at least two principal defects. First, the elevated blood sugar despite normal amounts of insulin indicates *resistance to insulin;* second, the slow response of plasma insulin to a glucose load shows that the *islet cells* are *responding sluggishly*. The second defect could be a special case of the first, if it could be shown that glucose entry into the islet cell was insulin sensitive and that, in adult diabetes, the islet $\beta$-cell was resistant to insulin. To date, this point has not been resolved. Another possibility is that the pancreas in adult diabetes makes an *abnormal insulin;* for example, pro-insulin instead of insulin might be secreted. If in fact this is so, it might be possible to explain the puzzling elevated insulin levels. Pro-insulin reacts partly like insulin in the usual immunoassay but has little of its biologic effect. Thus, there might be high levels of "insulin" but little of it would be biologically effective. In this situation we cannot really speak of insulin resistance. We should await data using an assay that can distinguish pro-insulin from insulin; to date, limited work has not shown any excess of pro-insulin in diabetic patients. Barring this explanation, insulin resistance has to be accounted for in some other way.

INSULIN RESISTANCE. The resistance to insulin in adult-type diabetes is not absolute; the blood glucose becomes normal when the patient receives insulin by injection. Many ideas have been offered in an attempt to explain why the plasma insulin in this type of diabetic is not doing its job. At one time or another, excess growth hormone, hydrocortisone, and glucagon have been proposed as the cause of diabetes. Except in special cases of pituitary or adrenal disease, no good evidence is available to support any of these proposals in the large majority of diabetics. There is some work suggesting that growth hormone may make insulin resistance worse once insulin secretion is deficient, but this doesn't explain the original defect.

Some say that, while the adult diabetic has insulin, most of it is "complexed" insulin (see p. 206). Complexed insulin is said to be inactive on muscle but active on adipose tissue; thus the relative lack of effective insulin and the obesity are both explained at once. It is true that diabetic adipose tissue can take up more glucose than normal, and this action might partly explain the obesity. However, the problems of complexed insulin have been discussed above; most recent work suggests that "complexed," or "bound," or "nonsuppressible" insulin are all the same thing, that it is not insulin, that it may well be an artifact of the isolation procedure, and that in any event it shows no difference in activity between muscle and adipose tissue. The issue is still unsettled, and someone may yet show that complexed insulin, whatever it is, is responsible for adult-onset diabetes mellitus.

It has been postulated too that insulin is bound to an antibody and is therefore inactive, but there is still no explanation of why the antibody was there in the first place, since exogenous insulin is the only known stimulus to its production. Some sort of immunologic disorder might be at the root of the problem. Nevertheless, the combination of insulin with antibody does not seem to hinder greatly its biologic effect.

Another idea is that an insulin antagonist, which is produced endogenously for unknown reasons and which may possibly be the A or B chain of insulin, partially inhibits insulin's action. Although A and B chains have been synthesized and can now be measured in plasma by immunoassay, no one is certain what they really do, if anything (see pp. 206–207).

Although the plasma half-life of insulin is prolonged in the treated diabetic, suggesting slower metabolism and perhaps a poor effect of insulin on tissues, none of these proposed explanations of insulin resistance have as yet been conclusively related to the patient with diabetes. All have involved an abnormal factor in the blood. Conceivably, the fault may be in the tissues themselves, e.g., the muscle cell membrane; there is, however, practically no evidence to support this idea—another question awaiting solution by new research.

A fruitful area for attacking the problem of insulin resistance is obesity. Since the obesity of the adult diabetic remains as poorly explained as the insulin resistance, there is no complete answer. However, it is a fact that obese patients have insulin resistance; their plasma insulin is higher than normal for a given level of blood glucose even when they are not diabetic, i.e., when they have a normal glucose tolerance test. When diabetes—abnormal glucose tolerance—occurs in an obese patient, he may have more insulin in his plasma than the normal person, but it now seems fairly clear that many of these patients are still deficient in insulin *when compared with the obese patient without diabetes.* Insulin resistance may therefore be associated with diabetes but actually be due to obesity. Some patients with obesity lose the insulin resistance and their diabetes improves when they lose weight; it is reasonable to attribute at least part of the problem to the insulin resistance of obesity. Nevertheless, we still do not know why diabetes appears, and the cause of the insulin resistance is as obscure as ever. One suggestion is that resistance occurs because there are simply too many adipose cells in the obese person for the amount of insulin available—clearly a speculative answer.

SLUGGISH β-CELLS. Although β-cells do seem to be sluggish and there may be something wrong with the transmission of the hyperglycemic signal to the β-cell, little is known about this condition as a possible cause of diabetes. It could equally be a result of whatever causes diabetes, simply reflecting the fact that the pancreas is slowly becoming exhausted.

So we do not know why insulin resistance appears or why the β-cells respond slowly. We do not know which of the two occurs first or whether they both appear together. If nothing else, it should be clear that diabetes mellitus is not a simple problem and many aspects of it await solutions.

*Symptoms and Biochemical Changes in Diabetes
Mellitus*

The classic symptoms of severe diabetes mellitus are *weight loss, hunger, thirst,* and a *large urine volume.* These can generally be explained by the known results of the lack of insulin: high blood glucose, elevated free fatty acids and triglycerides in the plasma, and decreased protein synthesis. Of course, most diabetics do *not* present this classic picture but have a milder variant of the disease or even have no symptoms at all. A high blood glucose may be all that is found.

The following discussion is based on what happens when insulin is totally lacking. Most patients with diabetes mellitus have some insulin and do not have such severe changes. The changes are nevertheless there, but in milder degree.

CARBOHYDRATE METABOLISM.    Glucose does get into muscle in diabetes; in fact, the amount of glucose uptake and utilization is probably not much less than normal unless the diabetes is severe. The difference is that the process is slower and occurs at a higher level of blood glucose.

The *lack of insulin* causes a high blood glucose by not only *impeding glucose uptake* by tissues such as muscle and fat but also by *increasing gluconeogenesis and glucose output by the liver.* This would be expected from what we know of insulin's actions on the liver but it certainly does not help the diabetic hyperglycemia. We have a great deal of information on the biochemical changes in various tissues in diabetes, particularly in the liver, in regard to both gluconeogenesis and (as we shall see) ketogenesis. Some of the work is difficult to synthesize into a complete and understandable framework either because the experimental results are contradictory, or because the work was done under highly artificial circumstances in vitro where relevance to the living animal is uncertain, or both. Therefore, although this discussion is based on known experimental facts, their pertinence to reality outside the laboratory may be open to question.

Since insulin enhances, in the *liver,* glucose conversion to glucose-6-phosphate and the latter's metabolism to glycogen and down the glycolytic pathway, removal of insulin should increase glycogen breakdown, increase gluconeogenesis, and enhance the breakdown of glucose-6-phosphate to glucose, which then enters the blood stream. For the most part, this is exactly what happens.

*Gluconeogenesis* is increased from lactate and pyruvate and from several amino acids. Lactate, for example, can be converted to glucose in 75 seconds. There is good evidence that gluconeogenesis is specifically stimulated by a higher concentration of free fatty acids—which, as we shall see, is characteristic of diabetes. The stimulatory effect of fatty acids is not accepted by all; one experiment showed that an increase in acetyl-CoA may not of itself increase gluconeogenesis, and another that perfusion of liver with free fatty acids also did not increase gluconeogenesis. Other workers accept the idea but feel that the effect is rather indirect. The weight of evidence is that free fatty acids increase gluconeogenesis but by an uncertain mechanism. The high level of plasma free fatty acids may also be responsible for the increased *glycogenolysis*.

Figure 54 shows the general pathway of hepatic gluconeogenesis and glucose release in somewhat more detail than before (see Fig. 26). One can see how increases in the boxed compounds and enzymes and decreases in the underlined ones tend to *enhance gluconeogenesis*, increase *glycogen breakdown*, and help *increase hepatic output of glucose*.

The amino acids (some of which are more directly converted to oxaloacetate), lactate, and pyruvate are the precursors for the glucose resulting from gluconeogenesis. Free fatty acids, via acetyl-CoA, may enter the pathway to glucose, but most investigators feel that there is no net conversion of fatty acid to glucose, and therefore we can focus our attention on what happens to amino acids, lactate, and pyruvate. In general, these precursors must first be converted to oxaloacetate. Oxaloacetate is thus a key compound; there is an increase in its formation and in its conversion to phosphoenolpyruvate (PEP) along with a rise in activity of pyruvate (PYR) carboxylase and PEP carboxylase. Whether or not there is a rise in the actual concentration of oxaloacetate has not been completely settled; probably there is not; in fact, the concentration of oxaloacetate is lower in most reported experiments.

Acetyl-CoA is at least as important as oxaloacetate. The concentration of acetyl-CoA is higher in a diabetic liver than in a normal one. Most of it comes from the breakdown of the huge influx of fatty acids from the plasma. It, or in part its precursor, acyl-CoA, is important because it is a likely mediator of the enhancement of gluconeogenesis by free fatty acids noted above (p. 232). For example, acetyl-CoA (or acyl-CoA) probably causes the fall in activity of PYR decarboxylase and the rise in activity of PYR carboxylase; the result is a greater conversion of PYR to oxaloacetate with less conversion to acetyl-CoA. Acetyl-CoA (or acyl-CoA) also causes a greater overall conversion of PYR to PEP; whether this effect is secondary to the one just mentioned or is due to a separate effect on the conversion of oxaloacetate to PEP is not clear. Nevertheless, there *is* a shift in the metabolism of oxaloacetate so that more goes to PEP (as mentioned above) and less to citrate (see Fig. 54). The latter effect, less incorporation of oxaloacetate into citrate, may in part be due to a lower concentration of oxaloacetate, but it is also due to an inhibition of citrate synthetase. Acyl-CoA is the inhibitor, and it acts by decreasing

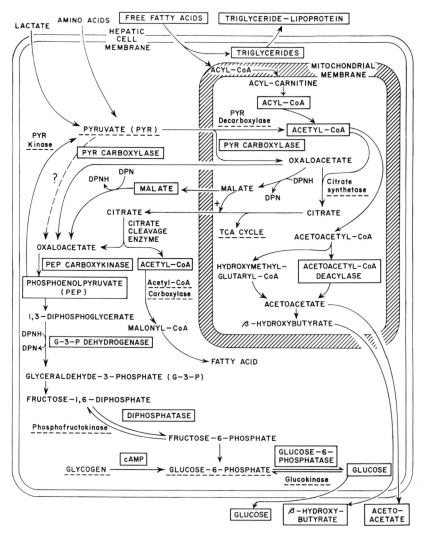

FIG. 54.   Gluconeogenesis and its enhancement by a hepatic influx of free fatty acids. Also shown is the relationship of the influx of fatty acids to the synthesis of fatty acids (lipogenesis) and to the synthesis of acetoacetate and β-hydroxybutyrate (ketogenesis). The former is depressed and the latter increased. The compounds or enzymes that are increased in concentration or activity in severe diabetes (or starvation) are enclosed in boxes; those that are decreased are underlined with a broken line. Since many of the concentrations and activities are known only for whole liver, some of the labeling showing changes inside and outside the mitochondria is speculative. Many aspects are simplified, particularly the entry of amino acids into the scheme. Note that malate enhances the exit of citrate from the mitochondrion. + indicates stimulation.

A complex diagram but the processes are complex; careful examination and correlation with the text will improve understanding.

234

the affinity of the enzyme for oxaloacetate. Acetyl-CoA also inhibits PYR kinase, preventing the recycling of PEP to PYR and shunting it toward glucose. PEP in turn inhibits glucokinase, again increasing net glucose output.

Despite the observed changes in enzyme activities and in the amount of acetyl-CoA, it is possible that these changes are not critical. The enzymes might not be rate-limiting in vivo and it *is* possible to show increased gluconeogenesis without a rise in acetyl-CoA provided there is a rise in the oxidation of fatty acids. Since this oxidative process generates DPNH and since gluconeogenesis requires DPNH (see Fig. 54), perhaps the connecting link between the two processes is simply the generation of the necessary DPNH.

In any case, the overall scheme makes reasonable sense, whether all or only some of it applies in vivo. There are still, however, major problems in completely understanding carbohydrate metabolism in the diabetic liver. For example, sometimes the glycogen content of the liver is increased rather than decreased. One may speculate that gross hyperglycemia or increased plasma cortisol overcomes the effect of insulin lack, or that glycogen formation is increased even more than glycogen breakdown, but no one really knows.

Other serious problems, perhaps more critical, are (1) the question of citrate metabolism, (2) the question of oxaloacetate metabolism, and (3) the question of the mitochondrion's role in gluconeogenesis and in ketogenesis (pp. 239–241).

*Citrate Metabolism.*    If insulin increases the activity of *citrate cleavage* enzyme, then lack of insulin should decrease the enzyme's activity. This is not indicated in Figure 54 because the available information is not clear-cut. There is probably less *citrate synthetase* activity, as shown in Figure 54, but some work has shown no such decrease. A decrease in activity is more common a finding than no drop at all, but truth in biochemistry is not found by comparing the number of scientists on one side of a question with that on the other. Similarly, there is no agreement on the *citrate content* of the diabetic liver; some find it low, others find it high, and still others find no change. For example, within a few months of each other in 1968, two papers on the citrate content of the diabetic liver appeared; one said it was high, the other said low. Since citrate is the form in which acetyl-CoA and some oxaloacetate are transported out of liver mitochondria to the cytoplasm, citrate metabolism is of obvious importance. A low cytoplasmic level of citrate, for example, would help explain the decreased lipogenesis that occurs (p. 240), although this might also be due to the increase in acyl-CoA.

*Oxaloacetate Metabolism.*    Although the general direction of oxaloacetate metabolism in the diabetic liver is reasonably clear, as discussed above, there is disagreement on the *oxaloacetate content.* Some work indicates that there is more oxaloacetate, but most investigations show there is less.

*The Mitochondrion.* If all the changes noted above occurred at the same site in the cell, enhanced gluconeogenesis in the diabetic liver would not be too hard to explain. However, some of the changes occur in the *mitochondrion,* where the fatty acids are oxidized and where acetyl-CoA, citrate, and some DPNH are made; others occur in the *cytoplasm,* the site of the later steps in gluconeogenesis. How events inside and outside the mitochondrion relate to each other, what substances go in and out of the mitochondrion, and what controls their exit and entry are therefore vital questions; unfortunately, they are questions with only a few answers.

For example, PYR carboxylase is probably limited to the mitochondrion. If so, PYR cannot be directly converted to oxaloacetate in the cytoplasm; the conversion must take place in the mitochondrion. The oxaloacetate must somehow find its way back to the cytoplasm before it can contribute to gluconeogenesis because the enzyme that converts oxaloacetate to PEP, PEP carboxykinase, is found mostly in the cytoplasm.

The oxaloacetate may go directly back to the cytoplasm without hindrance, but some evidence suggests that it does not do so fast enough to account for the observed amount of gluconeogenesis. Some oxaloacetate combines with acetyl-CoA to form citrate which goes to the cytoplasm fairly readily, but, as we have said, citrate synthesis is relatively inhibited and this would not be an effective way of delivering oxaloacetate to the cytoplasm. The formation of citrate is, however, one of the few ways of getting acetyl-CoA to the cytoplasm since acetyl-CoA cannot cross the mitochondrial membrane. Since acetyl-CoA affects cytoplasmic lipogenesis as well as gluconeogenesis, the regulation of citrate passage across the mitochondrial membrane is important in understanding the metabolism of acetyl-CoA as well as of citrate. We know little about this regulation except that malate enhances it.

Perhaps a more effective means of getting oxaloacetate out of the mitochondrion is to convert it to *malate,* which then goes through the membrane to the cytoplasm. This would enhance gluconeogenesis in two ways: (1) After the oxaloacetate changes to malate in the mitochondrion, the malate goes into the cytoplasm and there changes back to the oxaloacetate necessary to make glucose. (2) The conversion of oxaloacetate to malate in the mitochondrion requires the use of some of the DPNH generated by the oxidation of fatty acids; the malate then acts as a hydrogen carrier, with the hydrogen being used in the cytoplasm to generate there some of the cytoplasmic DPNH needed for gluconeogenesis (see Fig. 54).

We need more agreement on the levels of acetyl-CoA, oxaloacetate, malate, citrate, and DPNH in the diabetic liver. We need more information about the distribution of these substances between mitochondria and cytoplasm, about their transport from one to the other, and about the effects of hormones—particularly insulin—on all these processes. A better understanding of mitochondrial transport systems may hold the key to many of these problems.

A final note: Underlying the whole discussion of enhanced gluconeogenesis in the diabetic liver has been the tacit assumption that all the changes are directly due to the lack of insulin. This may not be true. The changes are real, insofar as they are established, but they may stem from the large influx of fatty acids to the liver rather than directly from the effects of insulin lack on the liver. Furthermore, the plasma of the severely ill diabetic probably has high levels of hormones such as hydrocortisone, glucagon, growth hormone, and epinephrine. All four can directly stimulate gluconeogenesis, although precisely how is not clear. The last three stimulate glycogen breakdown as well, thereby increasing the hepatic output of glucose. These three hormones can also stimulate lipolysis and increase the flow of fatty acids to the liver; so even the hormonal effects on gluconeogenesis may be secondary to the influx of fatty acids. Further work is necessary to settle these points. For the moment, a reasonable position would be to assume that gluconeogenesis is directly stimulated by changes in hormones, including the fall in insulin, and is also indirectly stimulated by the rise in plasma free fatty acids.

The picture we now have as shown in Figure 54 is, then, a reasonable but not complete exposition of gluconeogenesis in the diabetic liver. In essence, the same changes occur in fasting and starvation (see p. 258).

LIPID METABOLISM.   Although a high blood glucose is the hallmark of diabetes mellitus, most of the biochemical abnormalities are more directly due to changes in lipid metabolism. In the severely ill diabetic, there is a *rise* in *plasma free fatty acids*, a large *fatty liver*, a *rise* in *plasma triglycerides* which causes the serum to appear milky or *hyperlipemic*, and a *rise* in *plasma ketone bodies* which results in *ketosis* and *metabolic acidosis*.

What causes these abnormalities in lipid metabolism? Their ultimate cause, of course, is the lack of insulin, and most of them result from the effect of this deficiency on *adipose tissue*. Without insulin the adipose tissue makes less fat from glucose and releases more free fatty acids into the blood.

*Increased Plasma Free Fatty Acids* (*FFA*).   There is a massive outpouring of FFA from adipose tissue. Several things are awry in diabetic adipose tissue (see Fig. 51 and imagine a reversal of the effects of insulin indicated).

First, there is a lower conversion of glucose to fat or *decreased lipogenesis*. Referring to Figure 52 and assuming it applies to adipose tissue, we see that insulin deficiency might inhibit lipogenesis by lowering, for example, glucose entry into the cell, the activity of phosphofructokinase (PFK), and/or the activity of citrate cleavage enzyme. Experiments with insulin-deficient adipose tissue as well as muscle have shown less glucose-6-phosphate, less PFK, and more citrate, thus supporting this scheme. However, the inhibition of PFK may not be a direct effect of insulin lack; rather, it may be due to the increased citrate.

Second, fatty acid incorporation into triglycerides becomes difficult —*decreased esterification*. Poor entry of glucose into the cell and less PFK causes a fall in the synthesis of α-glycerophosphate, which is necessary for the conversion of fatty acids to triglycerides. In addition, insulin deficiency may decrease the activity of the enzymes involved in esterification. So whatever fatty acids are there tend to leak out into the plasma.

Third, there is an *increased lipolysis* of the triglycerides already in the fat cell. This is at least in part directly due to insulin deficiency; as noted before, insulin probably decreases lipolysis and its removal increases lipolysis. Some of the rise in triglyceride breakdown, however, may simply be due to a lack of available carbohydrate. If less glucose gets into the cell, in some way this seems to enhance lipolysis; insulin corrects the defect in the presence of glucose, but so does glycerol without insulin, since glycerol is a carbohydrate that does not need insulin to get into the cell. Finally, the lower utilization of glucose by the body stimulates those mechanisms which actively mobilize fatty acids; in man, growth hormone and glucagon may take part and, in the acute situation, perhaps epinephrine/norepinephrine.

The overall result is an increased plasma level of free fatty acids. Some of the fatty acid is used as fuel, particularly since glucose is not being used efficiently. A good deal, however, goes to the liver, where the fatty acids are normally converted to triglycerides; the triglycerides may be stored as such or be released to the blood as lipoproteins.

In diabetes, both modes of handling triglycerides are exaggerated. One sees a large, fatty liver and hyperlipemia.

*Fatty Liver.*   Triglyceride cannot get out of the liver unless it is in the form of a lipoprotein particle. The lipoprotein particle contains newly synthesized protein and phospholipid. Without insulin, the liver has difficulty in incorporating amino acids into protein and incorporating fatty acids into phospholipids; it has a harder time making lipoproteins. Thus triglycerides cannot easily get out of the liver, and when this situation is combined with a high influx of free fatty acids from the plasma, the end result is a large liver stuffed with fat.

*Hyperlipemia.* The defect in lipoprotein synthesis is, however, only a relative one. The total output of triglycerides by the liver is higher than normal; the trouble is that it should be even higher in order to avoid the fatty liver. Enough lipoprotein is released to cause hyperlipemia, or high plasma triglycerides. Logically, of course, hyperlipemia could be due as much to diminished removal of lipoproteins from the plasma as to increased input into the plasma by the liver. Studies show that both factors are involved. Diabetic skeletal and cardiac muscle seems to take up higher than normal amounts of triglyceride from plasma and use it as an energy source. Yet the uptake of triglycerides by adipose tissue, and perhaps liver, is lower than normal, and so is the overall clearance of lipoproteins from the blood. The poor clearance is probably due to a decrease in the lipoprotein lipase of adipose tissue, an enzyme required for clearance of triglycerides from blood. Hyperlipemia is, therefore, a result of a high output of triglycerides by the liver and a poor clearance of triglycerides from the blood.

*Ketogenesis and Ketosis.* Much of the fatty acid reaching the liver is not converted to triglycerides but catabolized, as it is in peripheral tissues. Some of the triglyceride is also broken down. Under normal conditions the resulting acetyl-CoA is eventually oxidized to $CO_2$ and a small amount of ketone bodies is made. In the liver of the acutely ill diabetic patient, the whole process is accentuated. A huge inflow of fatty acids is activated to fatty acid–CoA (or acyl-CoA), metabolized to acetyl-CoA, and oxidized to $CO_2$. Thus there is an increase in acyl-CoA content, acetyl-CoA content, and fatty acid oxidation by the mitochondria in the diabetic liver.

In addition, there is a vastly increased formation of ketone bodies (acetoacetate, β-hydroxybutyrate, and acetone) by the liver (*ketogenesis*) and more ketone bodies in the plasma (*ketosis*). Ketosis occurs then as a direct result of the influx of fatty acids; whether it is a necessary result is not so clear since the correlation is not particularly good between the amount of fatty acids entering the liver and the amount of ketone bodies produced.

Just why is ketogenesis increased? Why doesn't the extra acetyl-CoA simply go through the tricarboxylic acid (TCA) cycle or enter some other pathway? Many studies have been done attempting to answer this question. The findings allow a fairly satisfactory explanation although the problems noted before of interpreting experiments done in vitro remain. The critical thing seems to be what happens to the extra acetyl-CoA. The three principal pathways open to it are (1) resynthesis back to fatty acid, (2) combination with oxaloacetate to form citrate, and (3) formation of ketone bodies, e.g., acetoacetate (see Fig. 54). Taking these one by one:

1. Resynthesis in the cytoplasm of acetyl-CoA to fatty acid is inhibited. For a while it was thought that not enough of the TPNH needed for lipogenesis was available. It seems, though, that TPNH is not a limiting factor. The critical factor is *acetyl carboxylase*, the enzyme that converts acetyl-CoA to malonyl-CoA; in the diabetic liver the activity of this cytoplasmic enzyme is decreased.

There are several possible reasons for the diminished acetyl carboxylase, all with some experimental basis. It may be due to an increase in free fatty acids, an increase in fatty acid–CoA (acyl-CoA), a decrease in acylcarnitine from mitochondria, a decrease in the amount of citrate reaching the cytoplasm, or various combinations of these. Particularly interesting is a possible mechanism involving both acyl-CoA and citrate. An excess of acyl-CoA decreases the activity of citrate synthetase, the mitochondrial enzyme responsible for converting oxaloacetate to citrate. A lower concentration of citrate in the cytoplasm might then result. Acetyl carboxylase has a filamentous structure, at least in some species. When this structure is broken, enzyme activity is lost. Experiments have shown that citrate (or other multicarboxylic acids) induces aggregation of the inactive monomer form of the enzyme to the active polymer and maintains the filamentous structure. A lack of citrate secondary to excessive acyl-CoA is an attractive idea as an explanation for diminished acetyl carboxylase.

However attractive the idea, we have already noted the disagreement among researchers over the concentration of citrate and the activity of citrate synthetase in the diabetic liver. Perhaps the defect is one of transport of citrate from mitochondria to cytoplasm or perhaps it is not related to citrate at all; for example, acyl-CoA may directly inhibit acetyl carboxylase, and, in diabetic adipose tissue, lipogenesis is decreased in the presence of increased citrate. In any case, acetyl carboxylase activity is less, and less acetyl-CoA is converted to fatty acids.

2. Combination of acetyl-CoA with oxaloacetate to form citrate is probably diminished as well. Some experiments show not only a decrease in citrate synthetase but also a decrease in the affinity of oxaloacetate for the enzyme. Less acetyl-CoA goes through the TCA cycle, and much of the oxaloacetate winds up as glucose.

3. That leaves ketogenesis as a relatively open pathway for acetyl-CoA. Ketogenesis is a mitochondrial process. Along with the accentuation of this pathway, there is an increase in the enzyme, acetoacetyl-CoA deacylase, which converts acetoacetyl-CoA to acetoacetate. Some workers feel that most of this enzyme is found in the mitochondria;

others consider it mostly cytoplasmic and think that it is not increased in diabetes. This enzyme may not, in fact, be too important because recent work indicates that most acetoacetate derives from hydroxy-methylglutaryl-CoA (see Fig. 54). Whatever the exact mechanism, and it may be that both these mechanisms are significant, the end result is an increased production of acetoacetate, β-hydroxybutyrate, and acetone, all of which spill over into the blood and cause ketosis.

It should be remembered that these changes are not absolute, like turning a faucet off and on, but are rather ones of degree. The TCA cycle operates, but on a relatively lower level; the ketogenic pathway is always there, but in diabetes it is accentuated.

*Metabolic Acidosis.* Ketosis, of course, can occur only if the liver puts more ketone bodies into the blood than are removed by the other tissues. Ketone bodies *are* normally metabolized by tissues such as muscle and may sometimes be an essential source of energy. The problem in diabetes is that more are produced than can be used. Insulin deficiency causes a double fault here: Not only does it increase hepatic production of ketone bodies but it also causes a relative inhibition of their utilization by muscle.

All of which might not be so bad except for the fact that acetoacetate and β-hydroxybutyrate are relatively strong acids and too much of them lowers the pH of the blood, causing acidosis and all its effects on respiration, the central nervous system, and tissues in general. The acidosis caused by the ketone bodies, along with the grossly elevated plasma free fatty acids, inhibits glucose utilization even more than the lack of insulin per se, worsening an already precarious situation.

PROTEIN METABOLISM.   The acutely ill diabetic has a negative nitrogen balance, and net protein synthesis is thus decreased. From what we now know of insulin's actions, this is not surprising. However, not much else is known about protein metabolism in the diabetic except for the defect in lipoprotein synthesis just noted and the fact that amino acid incorporation into the protein of muscle is less.

## Treatment

For all but the mild cases, *insulin* is a specific. Of all the endocrine therapies, this has saved more lives than any other. Note, however, that insulin is not a cure and that once insulin is required it must often be given for life. The adult obese diabetic who has only a mild case may benefit from simply weight loss and a proper diet. Weight loss in these patients improves the insulin resistance mentioned before but does not abolish it.

If more therapy is needed in these milder cases, the sulfonylurea drugs, especially *tolbutamide*, are often useful. These drugs seem to increase the insulin output by the pancreas by direct stimulation, so they are useful only in patients with a pancreas capable of producing insulin. Treatment of the complications of diabetes mellitus (vascular disease, ketoacidosis, and so forth) is a complex subject which will not be discussed here.

## OTHER CLINICAL ASPECTS OF PANCREATIC HORMONES

*Spontaneous hypoglycemia*, the opposite of diabetes, is relatively rare. Hypoglycemia is, of course, most commonly caused by an overdose of insulin and is therefore seen in the diabetic. This is the so-called insulin reaction, and to cope with it diabetics taking insulin usually carry with them candy or something else with sugar in it. On the other hand, actual spontaneous hypoglycemia can be a presenting sign of diabetes mellitus, a seeming paradox due to the prolonged secretion of insulin mentioned in the discussion of adult-type diabetes above. An unusual cause of hypoglycemia, but a curable one, is the *islet-cell tumor of the pancreas*. Such a tumor makes too much insulin and must be considered in any patient with a low blood glucose.

*Glucagon excess and deficiency* are not widely recognized as diseases, but glucagon deficiency may be an uncommon cause of hypoglycemia and glucagon excess may be caused by rare tumors of the pancreas.

The *glucose tolerance test*, widely used to diagnose mild diabetes mellitus, is needed because the fasting blood glucose in such patients is often normal. Basically, one gives the patient 50 to 100 g of glucose orally or intravenously. If the oral test is done, which is usually the case, the blood glucose will rise and should fall back to normal at the end of two hours. If it stays up, the glucose tolerance test is abnormal, glucose tolerance is said to be decreased, and the patient is usually told he has diabetes mellitus. As we have said, in pregnancy and in older patients, one should be somewhat cautious in making the diagnosis.

## BIBLIOGRAPHY

### Insulin

Batchelor, B. R.   Insulin-like activity. *Diabetes* 16:418, 1967.

Brooker, W. D., Lech, J. J., and Calvert, D. N.   Insulin inhibition of hormone and theophylline induced glycerol release in isolated adipocytes. *Europ. J. Pharmacol.* 1:278, 1967.

Buse, M. G., and Buse, J.   Effect of free fatty acids and insulin on protein synthesis and amino acid metabolism of isolated rat diaphragms. *Diabetes* 16:753, 1967.

Coore, H. G., and Randle, P. J.   Regulation of insulin secretion studied with pieces of rabbit pancreas incubated in vitro. *Biochem. J.* 93:66, 1964.

Debons, A. F., Krimsky, I., Likuski, H. J., From, A., and Cloutier, R. J. Gold thioglucose damage to the satiety center: Inhibition in diabetes. *Amer. J. Physiol.* 214:652, 1968.

Floyd, J. C., Jr., Fajans, S. S., Conn, J. W., Knopf, R. F., and Rull, J. Insulin secretion in response to protein ingestion. *J. Clin. Invest.* 45:1479, 1966.

Froesch, E. R., Bürgi, H., Müller, W. A., Humbel, R. E., Jakob, A., and Labhart, A.   Nonsuppressible insulin-like activity of human serum: Purification, physicochemical and biological properties and its relation to total serum ILA. *Recent Progr. Hormone Res.* 23:565, 1967.

Katsoyannis, P. G.   Synthetic insulins. *Recent Progr. Hormone Res.* 23:505, 1967.

Katsoyannis, P. G., and Schwartz, I. L. (Eds.).   Symposium on insulin. *Amer. J. Med.* 40:651, 1966.

Levine, R.   Insulin—the biography of a small protein. *New Eng. J. Med.* 277:1059, 1967.

Meek, J. C., Doffing, K. M., and Bolinger, R. E.   Radioimmunoassay of insulin A and B chains in normal and diabetic human plasma. *Diabetes* 17:61, 1968.

Porte, D., Jr.   Beta adrenergic stimulation of insulin release in man. *Diabetes* 16:150, 1967.

Porte, D., Jr., Graber, A. L., Kuzuya, T., and Williams, R. H.   Effect of epinephrine on immunoreactive insulin levels in man. *J. Clin. Invest.* 45:228, 1966.

Richards, D. W.   Effect of pancreas extract on depancreatized dogs: Ernest L. Scott's thesis of 1911. *Perspect. Biol. Med.* 10:84, 1966.

Rubenstein, A. H., Cho, S., and Steiner, D. F.   Evidence for proinsulin in human urine and serum. *Lancet* 1:1353, 1968.

## Glucagon

Sokal, J. E.   Glucagon—an essential hormone. *Amer. J. Med.* 41:331, 1966.

Sokal, J. E., Ezdinli, E. Z., Schiller, C., and Dobbins, A.   Basal plasma glucagon levels of man. *J. Clin. Invest.* 46:778, 1967.

Unger, R. H., Ohneda, A., Valverde, I., Eisentraut, A. M., and Exton, J. Characterization of the responses of circulating glucagon-like immunoreactivity to intraduodenal and intravenous administration of glucose. *J. Clin. Invest.* 47:48, 1968.

## Diabetes Mellitus

Beaser, S.   Oral treatment of diabetes mellitus. *J.A.M.A.* 187:887, 1964.

*Diabetes Fact Book.* Washington: U.S. Govt. Printing Office, 1961.

Exton, J. H., and Park, C. R.   Control of gluconeogenesis in liver: I. general features of gluconeogenesis in the perfused livers of rats. *J. Biol. Chem.* 242:2622, 1967.

Falconer, D. S. The inheritance of liability to diseases with variable age of onset, with particular reference to diabetes mellitus. *Ann. Hum. Genet.* 31:1, 1967.

Hamwi, G. J., and Danowski, T. S. (Eds.). *Diabetes Mellitus: Diagnosis and Treatment*, vol. 2. New York: American Diabetes Association, 1967.

Kalkhoff, R. K., Hornbrook, K. R., Burch, H. B., and Kipnis, D. M. Studies of the metabolic effects of acute insulin deficiency: II. Changes in hepatic glycolytic and Krebs-cycle intermediates and pyridine nucleotides. *Diabetes* 15:451, 1966.

Kalkhoff, R. K., and Kipnis, D. M. Studies of the metabolic effects of acute insulin deficiency: I. Mechanism of impairment of hepatic fatty acid and protein synthesis. *Diabetes* 15:443, 1966.

O'Sullivan, J. B., Williams, R. F., and McDonald, G. W. The prevalence of diabetes mellitus and related variables—a population study in Sudbury, Mass. *J. Chronic Dis.* 20:535, 1967.

Singer, D. L., and Hurwitz, D. Long-term experience with sulfonylureas and placebo. *New Eng. J. Med.* 277:450, 1967.

Start, C., and Newsholme, E. A. The effects of starvation and alloxan-diabetes on the contents of citrate and other metabolic intermediates in rat liver. *Biochem. J.* 107:411, 1968.

Weber, G., Lea, M. A., and Stamm, N. B. Inhibition of pyruvate kinase and glucokinase by acetyl CoA and inhibition of glucokinase by phosphoenolpyruvate. *Life Sci.* 6:2441, 1967.

Williams, R. H. (Ed.). *Diabetes.* New York: Hoeber, 1960.

# 11. Growth: Growth Hormone and Other Hormones

Growth is the only evidence of life.

—JOHN HENRY, CARDINAL NEWMAN, *Apologia pro Vita Sua*

"GROWTH" is a vague thing. It is easy to look at something and say that it has grown, but it is not easy to decide how best to measure growth. Should one measure the increase in *length*, in *weight, number of mitoses*, or in *protein synthesis*? Growth hormone was isolated using the first two of these ways of measuring growth, yet biochemical investigations concentrate on the last; all seem to be correlated in a gross way, but there is no proof that all are equivalent. In man, *height* is generally used to measure growth. This is, of course, directly related to skeletal height and depends on the growth of *bone,* particularly the long bones of the legs.

## NONENDOCRINE FACTORS AND GROWTH

People may be either too tall or too short. Those who are *too tall* may have an endocrine abnormality, but one must be careful because the patient may simply be at one end of the normal distribution curve. Most basketball players, for example, are perfectly normal. People who are *too short* may also have some endocrine disease, particularly in this well-fed country. Nevertheless, most people who seem overly tall or short are normal; they simply represent the extremes of the normal range.

In many countries where data have been collected over a long period, it seems clear that the average height of adults is slowly increasing. Norway is a classic example, with data going back to 1741, but records over the last 100 years in the United States and over 50 years in Japan, for instance, show the same trend.

Good *nutrition* is usually offered as the reason for the increase in average height. There is no question that poor nutrition stunts growth and has more serious consequences such as smaller brain size and poor cerebral function; moreover, the food supply and general nutrition do seem to have improved in several countries over the course of time. Chronic illness also stunts growth; perhaps better general health as well as nutrition has played a role in the increase in average height. Today, on a worldwide basis, poor nutrition may very well be the

245

most common cause of poor growth. Whether poor nutrition causes endocrine deficiencies that are the immediate cause of poor growth is not settled; bad nutrition may lead, for example, to deficient secretion of growth hormone in some instances.

The *genetic constitution* is as important in determining human growth as the state of nutrition and the endocrine glands. The short Pygmy and the tall Watusi show that the genetic determinants may be racial or tribal, while the fact that tall parents tend to have tall children and short parents short children points out the importance of family background. Part of the Pygmy's problem may be hormonal; he may respond poorly to growth hormone or may secrete a form of growth hormone that is inactive. Since hormonal deficiencies may be genetically determined, endocrine and genetic factors may both be responsible for short stature. For example, some patients have a deficiency of growth hormone that is genetically controlled and is passed on from generation to generation. Other genetic diseases directly cause short stature that is not due to a hormonal deficiency. Turner's syndrome, for instance, is a disease of phenotypic females who are short and lack functioning ovaries; these patients are missing an entire X-chromosome. The short stature is due to the lack of the usual double dose of genes present on the short arm of the X-chromosome. They have a normal secretion of growth hormone. Although the syndrome is rare, it serves to show that genes need not act hormonally to affect growth and that short stature can occur despite the presence of normal amounts of growth hormone.

## HORMONES AND GROWTH

Even if the growth disturbance is hormonal in origin, one cannot assume that the cause is primarily a disturbance of *growth hormone*, particularly when short stature is the problem. Normal growth requires the proper amount, neither too much nor too little, of thyroxine, hydrocortisone, and insulin, in addition to growth hormone. At puberty, the normal pubertal growth spurt can occur only if the proper gonadal hormone, testosterone or estradiol, is present.

For example, deficient thyroxine causes short stature because the bones do not increase in length fast enough. Still, growth hormone plays a role because hypothyroidism both diminishes growth hormone secretion and impedes the action of the growth hormone that is secreted. Excessive hydrocortisone stunts growth—also possibly because of an inhibition of growth hormone secretion.

When too little androgen is present in a pubertal male, the pubertal growth spurt does not occur and the bony epiphyses remain unfused.

Slow, continued growth of the long bones continues longer than usual, and final height may be increased. On the other hand, excessive androgen, though causing an initial growth spurt, fuses the bony epiphyses, and if this should occur before normal puberty is reached, the boy will eventually be short. Once again, the growth spurt induced by testosterone at puberty (before the epiphyses fuse) may be due to growth hormone rather than directly to testosterone, since patients with normal but delayed puberty seem to have a mild deficiency in growth hormone secretion which can be corrected by giving testosterone.

## GROWTH HORMONE, BODY GROWTH, AND PROTEIN SYNTHESIS

Growth hormone is therefore a major determinant of both height (or length) and growth of tissues in mammals. It is in fact an absolute requirement for both types of growth. As we have mentioned, the problem of whether growth hormone is separate from prolactin in man is not completely settled, although it seems clear in the rat that the two are separate. The secretion rate of growth hormone in humans has been estimated at 0.4 to 1.0 mg per day, but other estimates are as high as 5 mg per day.

The *plasma levels* of growth hormone in the fasting state (0 to 5 m$\mu$g/ml) tend to be higher in women, probably because of the estrogen they secrete. Perhaps more important, the plasma levels in the newborn child are higher than in the mother, and older children have higher levels some hours after eating than do adults. The higher levels in children suggest that the level of plasma growth hormone *is related to the growth rate* of the individual under some circumstances.

How does growth hormone stimulate growth? This is a difficult problem to attack experimentally because height and weight change slowly. If one is trying to isolate a specific effect of growth hormone, it will be hard to recognize it as a direct effect unless it occurs soon after administration of growth hormone or can be shown in vitro. The in vitro systems available are useful for only a few hours. Thus, whether studying growth hormone in vivo or in vitro, we need to study some short-term effect and hope that it is significantly related to the long-term effects on height and weight seen in the intact animal.

Most workers have therefore studied *protein synthesis*. In vivo, protein synthesis may not always lead to growth, but its analysis may be more pertinent to an understanding of what growth hormone does in the adult, nongrowing animal, and, from a practical point of view, it is approachable in the laboratory.

*Action of Growth Hormone on Protein Synthesis*

In the intact animal, injected growth hormone causes a net retention of nitrogen. This is probably due to increased protein synthesis since there is no evidence of decreased protein breakdown. One can observe it only after one to two days. The earliest effect observed in man related to protein metabolism is a drop in blood urea, which can be seen at 6 to 24 hours and implies that amino acids are being converted to protein rather than oxidized for fuel.

A logical tissue to study in vitro is *muscle*, which contains much of the body's protein. Growth hormone binds tightly to muscle, and then comes an increase both in uptake of amino acids and in amino acid incorporation into protein, two independent actions of growth hormone. There need not be any RNA synthesis for growth hormone to act in this way. Nevertheless, later on there is an increase in RNA synthesis, RNA content, and RNA-mediated protein synthesis which reflects a prolonged effect of GH. In contrast to testosterone, which increases the template activity of DNA, growth hormone increases RNA synthesis by increasing RNA polymerase activity. Growth hormone and testosterone, therefore, have additive effects on protein synthesis in muscle. Not all muscular growth is due to growth hormone, however; the muscular growth occuring after prolonged exercise happens even in the absence of growth hormone.

In the *liver*, growth hormone increases both the incorporation of amino acids into protein and the synthesis of albumin. Here the effect does seem to require nucleolar RNA synthesis, with an associated increase in the template activity of mRNA, in ribosomal RNA, in the ability of the ribosomes to synthesize protein, and eventually in the number of ribosomes. There is no increase in amino acid activation or transport by sRNA.

Effects can be seen in other tissues as well. For example, in the kidney there is a higher uptake of amino acids and in fibroblasts an increase in collagen synthesis.

*Insulin* is probably a critical requirement for optimal stimulation by growth hormone of protein synthesis in general and of muscle development in particular. This point is of interest, since insulin itself increases protein synthesis (see p. 210).

Since, as we shall see later, growth hormone tends to diminish total body fat, the increase in body weight after its administration is best explained by its effect on protein synthesis. In all likelihood the effect on protein synthesis also explains the increase in height seen in children. Growth hormone, perhaps through an indirect in vivo mechanism involving a poorly defined "sulfation factor," stimulates the growth and protein synthesis of the cartilaginous bony epiphyses, but only if they are not fused. Thus, height increases because of growth hormone but stops increasing once androgens and/or estrogens have caused the epiphyses to fuse. What slows down net protein synthesis as adulthood is reached is a mystery. Presumably the secretion of growth hormone is slowed, but this has not been proved.

## Growth Hormone and the Metabolism of Electrolytes, Fat, and Carbohydrate

Growth hormone was isolated and purified on the basis of its effect on growth. Many other actions might have been present but were not tested. We know now that the substance we call growth hormone has, in fact, several other important effects.

### Electrolytes

In humans, many electrolytes are affected. There is retention in the body of phosphate, potassium, sodium, and calcium. *Phosphate* retention may be secondary to the increased cell mass that goes along with protein synthesis, but there is also an increased renal capacity for resorbing phosphate (an increased $TmPO_4$). *Potassium* retention is largely secondary to increased cell mass. *Sodium* retention, on the other hand, is not well explained and occurs despite an increased glomerular filtration rate (GFR); there may be a direct renal effect of growth hormone or an enhancement of aldosterone's action. *Calcium* retention occurs despite an increased loss of calcium in the urine and is probably due to an even greater calcium absorption from the intestine.

### Fat Metabolism

SHORT-TERM EFFECTS.    A single injection of growth hormone causes at first a brief drop in plasma glucose and in free fatty acids. This is the "insulin-like" effect of growth hormone. Part may be due to a direct stimulation of insulin release, but part is due to a direct action on *adipose tissue*. In adipose tissue, growth hormone initially increases the uptake of glucose, its oxidation to $CO_2$, and its conversion to fatty acids (lipogenesis). In fact, growth hormone, in this early stage of its action, also increases amino acid conversion to fatty acids, which might be termed "liponeogenesis." These actions are probably not mediated by insulin, although they are insulin-like, because the increase in glycogen synthesis seen with insulin does not occur; their physiologic meaning is not clear because naturally secreted growth hormone may not be secreted in amounts large enough to cause these effects.

These short-term effects are not dependent on either RNA or protein synthesis. After two or three hours have passed, the effect on adipose tissue "switches" from an insulin-like pattern to a lipid-mobilizing effect.

LONG-TERM EFFECTS. Several hours after an injection of growth hormone, there is a *rise in plasma free fatty acids*, due to lipolysis of adipose tissue fat, and an increase in fatty acid uptake by muscle. After a while longer, lipogenesis in adipose tissue is decreased, and, in the whole animal, there is a drop in total body fat. All these later effects on fat metabolism are dependent on RNA synthesis, as are the later effects on protein metabolism. The lipolytic response requires thyroxine and hydrocortisone. Growth hormone also seems to increase the sensitivity of adipose tissue to other lipolytic agents, such as catecholamines; growth hormone may then act as a "permissive agent" for lipolysis. It is possible, in fact, that the *entire* effect of growth hormone on lipolysis is to sensitize the process (by acting on adenyl cyclase?) to substances such as the catecholamines.

Just how fat mobilization is related to growth or even protein synthesis is not clear, except that it may be a result of the synthesis of some specific protein in adipose tissue. Fat mobilization is of obvious physiologic importance because during most of the day we depend on fatty acids as our main source of energy. In man, growth hormone may play a major role in supplying this energy source and is perhaps one of the main lipid mobilizer ·.

### Glucose Metabolism

Growth hormone and glucose metabolism are also closely interrelated. For a long time growth hormone has been known to be diabetogenic in some animals; the dog can develop permanent hyperglycemia and even ketosis if enough growth hormone is given. It is not likely that this action plays much of a role in causing human diabetes, and man does not seem to respond as the dog does, but clearly growth hormone influences glucose metabolism.

As further investigation was done, several findings emerged. One is the short-term hypoglycemia mentioned above. Most of the effects, however, are relatively long-term effects and parallel the lipolytic effect on adipose tissue. They include:

1. An increased gluconeogenesis in the liver along with a higher hepatic output of glucose. This is associated, for example, with higher levels of fructose-1,6-diphosphatase and glucose-6-phosphatase (see Fig. 54).
2. A decrease in glucose transport into muscle and adipose tissue, and less phosphorylation of glucose by muscle. This, of course, decreases the hypoglycemic response to a given dose of insulin and may result in an abnormal glucose tolerance test.

3. A rise in free fatty acids after growth hormone is given which may also inhibit glucose uptake by muscle.
4. A *rise in blood glucose*, on the basis of 1 to 3. Normally this is transient because *insulin secretion* is stimulated by the *hyperglycemia* and enhanced directly by *growth hormone* itself. After growth hormone is given, then, the pancreas responds to glucose by putting out insulin faster, and net glucose uptake by the body is approximately normal. Only when the ability to secrete more insulin is lost does hyperglycemia persist.

The *ketosis* that appears in some species with growth hormone is probably secondary to the fatty acid mobilization, via a mechanism similar to that noted for diabetes mellitus.


## CONTROL OF GROWTH HORMONE SECRETION

The hypothalamus contains a growth hormone releasing factor (GH-RF), with a tentative molecular weight of 2000. GH-RF can be found in the peripheral plasma; thus it is actually secreted. The isolated pituitary in vitro secretes little or no growth hormone. In man, pituitary stalk section, severing the connection between the hypothalamus and the pituitary, abolishes the usual growth hormone secretion. It is clear that the *hypothalamus is the mediator* of growth hormone secretion and that GH-RF directly stimulates the secretion, perhaps mediated by cyclic AMP.

Further observations have supported the importance of the *central nervous system* in the regulation of growth hormone secretion. The stress of surgery or of simply getting out of bed in the morning (which is more stressful for some than for others) increases plasma growth hormone levels. More GH-RF is found in the hypothalamuses of young animals, suggesting that the central nervous system plays a role in the growth of the body.

While such stresses act unidirectionally to increase growth hormone secretion, there are *negative feedback* controls. Growth hormone itself may shut off its own secretion by acting directly on the pituitary, perhaps by blocking the stimulatory effect of GH-RF. More important, however, is the fact that the *level of blood glucose varies inversely with the level of growth hormone*. Sudden hypoglycemia causes a marked rise in plasma growth hormone by increasing the secretion of GH-RF; the rise in GH-RF is probably mediated by hypothalamic catecholamines. Fasting in humans drops the blood glucose and also tends to increase plasma growth hormone, though it does not seem to increase plasma growth hormone in rats. Conversely, an elevated blood glucose inhibits growth hormone secretion. Of some interest here is the fact that growth hormone acts on the hypothalamus to increase food intake, particularly of carbohydrate.

Just why this control mechanism should exist is somewhat of a mystery. It has no obvious connection with growth or protein synthesis but it does tend to support the idea that growth hormone is important in glucose metabolism and in maintaining a normal blood glucose.

On the other hand, while a rise in blood glucose blocks growth hormone release, a *rise* in *plasma amino acids* is a *stimulus* to its secretion. Even if the blood glucose is high, arginine or eating a protein meal raises the level of plasma growth hormone. A rise in plasma free fatty acids may inhibit growth hormone secretion, but the evidence is not yet clear on this point.

In trying to understand the regulation of the secretion of growth hormone, perhaps we should not be looking only at growth or only at blood glucose. If one looks at the whole spectrum of metabolic effects of growth hormone, one sees a tendency to raise the blood glucose, to raise plasma free fatty acids, and to lower plasma amino acids (by incorporating them into protein). In turn, there is at least some evidence that each of these effects of growth hormone tends to shut off the secretion of growth hormone: The best evidence, as noted above, is for glucose; there is sketchy evidence for free fatty acid; and, while there are no data for amino acids, the fact that a rise in plasma amino acids stimulates growth hormone secretion makes one suspect that a drop in amino acids might shut off its secretion. The regulator of growth hormone secretion may be a resultant of the plasma levels of glucose, free fatty acids, and amino acids. When the levels of glucose and free fatty acids are up and the level of amino acids is down, less growth hormone might be secreted; when the levels of glucose and free fatty acids are low and the level of amino acids is up, more growth hormone might be released. Various other combinations of the three determinants would affect growth hormone secretion in an intermediate way. Since plasma levels of glucose and free fatty acids often vary inversely rather than in parallel, it might be difficult to predict the exact effect on plasma growth hormone. We would have, then, if this proposal is correct, a control system with a classic negative feedback mechanism wherein the effects of a hormone tend to inhibit the secretion of that hormone. Until more research is done, however, this thought remains enticing but speculative. Superimposed on all this, of course, are the effects of stressful situations noted above.

Other hormones affect growth hormone secretion. Thyroxine is needed for both its synthesis and its secretion, estrogen, glucagon, and epinephrine increase its secretion, and hydrocortisone in excess tends to decrease its secretion.

## Role of Growth Hormone in Adults

In man, both hypoglycemia and fasting stimulate growth hormone secretion, the former quickly and the latter slowly. Both are also followed by fatty acid mobilization. Growth hormone increases plasma free fatty acid levels. These facts strongly suggest that growth hormone is a physiologically significant mobilizer of fatty acids.

Thus, with a carbohydrate load, such as eating a meal, insulin ensures the energy supply, enhances protein synthesis, and enables excess glucose to be stored for future use. Under conditions of carbohydrate lack, growth hormone may mobilize fatty acids for energy and enhance protein synthesis, or at least cut down on protein catabolism.

## Clinical Aspects of Growth Hormone

Excess secretion of growth hormone before epiphyseal fusion causes *gigantism*, which is rare. If this happens after epiphyseal fusion, one sees *acromegaly*, in which only bones without epiphyses continue to grow. Though not as rare, it is still an uncommon disease. Plasma growth hormone levels are elevated to over 10 mμg/ml and characteristically do not suppress after a glucose load.

Deficient growth hormone in childhood causes *pituitary dwarfism*. The patients usually have other pituitary deficiencies as well although there may be an isolated deficiency of growth hormone. This is the only group of short individuals (dwarfism) who can be made to grow with injections of human growth hormone (HGH); since the supply of HGH is small, it is fortunate that pituitary dwarfism is not common. In the adult, growth hormone deficiency has no immediately apparent effects and may not be recognized, probably because in many cases it is only partial and because the proper testing to bring out the defect is not usually done. Growth hormone deficiency can be detected by inducing hypoglycemia with insulin (the insulin tolerance test), by infusing arginine, by injecting vasopressin, or by injecting glucagon, and then measuring the changes in plasma growth hormone. Normally, there is a prompt rise after these stimuli; if the normal rise is not present, there is deficient secretion of growth hormone.

Giving growth hormone to patients who are short but who have growth hormone in the plasma is a waste of time and of growth hormone. GH has also been used in protein catabolic states such as follow a severe burn in an attempt to reverse the catabolic state; it doesn't work.

## BIBLIOGRAPHY

Cheek, D. B. *Human Growth*. Philadelphia: Lea & Febiger, 1968.

Forsyth, I. A. Lactogenic activity of primate growth hormone: A possible role of synergism studied with non-primate growth hormone and prolactin. *J. Endocr.* 31:xxx, 1964

Glick, S. M., Roth, J., Yalow, R. S., and Berson, S. A. The regulation of growth hormone secretion. *Recent Progr. Hormone Res.* 21:241, 1965.

Katz, S. H., Dhariwal, A. P. S., and McCann, S. M. Effect of hypoglycemia on content of pituitary growth hormone (GH) and hypothalamic growth hormone-releasing factor (GH-RF) in the rat. *Endocrinology* 81:333, 1967.

Martin, L. G., Clark, J. W., and Connor, T. B. Growth hormone secretion enhanced by androgens. *J. Clin. Endocr.* 28:425, 1968.

Müller, E. E., Sawano, S., Arimura, A., and Schally, A. V. Blockade of release of growth hormone by brain norepinephrine depletors. *Endocrinology* 80:471, 1967

Raben, M. S. Human growth hormone. *Recent Progr. Hormone Res.* 15:71, 1959.

Roth, J., Glick, S. M., Cuatrecasas, P., and Hollander, C. S. Acromegaly and other disorders of growth hormone secretion. *Ann. Intern. Med.* 66:760, 1967.

Sonenberg, M. (Ed.). Growth hormone. *Ann. N.Y. Acad. Sci.* 148:289, 1968.

# 12. Hormonal Control of Daily Energy Supply

FOR a long time glucose was thought to be the main source of energy for most tissues of the body, probably because more was known about it and also because adipose tissue was regarded as an inactive storage depot. Recently the plasma *free fatty acids*, a minor component of the plasma lipids, have been shown to be a major source of energy for the body and in fact probably supply about two-thirds of the calories burned each day.

During the course of a day we replenish our energy supplies by *eating*, use them up slowly while *fasting*, which is actually most of the day, and use them more quickly while *exercising* or during many kinds of *stress*. The hormones have an important place in all these processes. Some of the hormonal effects discussed below may not in fact occur in all species; for example, glucagon has a direct lipolytic action on adipose tissue from rats but may not be lipolytic (in vitro) on human adipose tissue. Nevertheless, for this discussion it is probably better to avoid the problem of differences between species in order to keep confusion to a minimum.

## EATING

What happens when an ordinary meal is eaten? In the peripheral blood there is a striking rise in glucose, a slight rise in free fatty acids (FFA), a slower rise in triglycerides (often seen as lipemia), and a rise in amino acids. The glucose comes from dietary carbohydrate, the free fatty acids and triglycerides come from dietary fat, and the amino acids come from dietary protein.

### Blood Glucose

The rise in blood glucose sets off a train of hormonal responses. First, a small intestine factor (GI glucagon), released when glucose is absorbed, stimulates insulin secretion. As does glucose itself, it probably acts by direct stimulation of the pancreas. Possibly pancreatic glucagon stimulates insulin secretion locally by simply diffusing to nearby β-cells. Work with isolated pancreatic tissue in vitro, however, shows that glucose *inhibits* the secretion of pancreatic glucagon making this contingency unlikely. It seems reasonably clear, then, that glucose absorption is followed within 20 minutes by a rise in glucagon secretion—mostly GI glucagon—and in insulin secretion. At the same time, the high blood glucose causes a drop in plasma growth hormone.

Once in the systemic circulation, the higher level of insulin and the lower level of growth hormone now work together to enhance peripheral glucose uptake; the glucose is oxidized, supplying energy, or stored temporarily until needed.

More glucose is usually absorbed after eating than is needed for energy at that time. Since little is normally lost to the body in the urine or stool, the excess must be stored. Some is converted to glycogen, particularly in muscle and liver; optimal glycogen synthesis requires both insulin and hydrocortisone. The principal storage form, however, is the triglyceride of adipose tissue, in which the carbon atoms of glucose appear as both glycerol and fatty acid.

The rise in GI glucagon is transient and has little or no effect on glucose storage as fat. Plasma insulin, on the other hand, remains elevated for a somewhat longer time, about two to three hours. Insulin enhances the storage of glucose as triglyceride in several ways:

1. It increases conversion of glucose to fatty acids (lipogenesis) in adipose tissue and liver.
2. It increases conversion of fatty acids to triglycerides (esterification) in adipose tissue and (perhaps) muscle; this may be secondary to an increase in the formation of $\alpha$-glycerophosphate from glucose. The resulting increase in triglyceride synthesis removes from the cytoplasm free fatty acids which might otherwise inhibit lipogenesis.
3. It decreases lipolysis in adipose tissue; a lower concentration of cyclic AMP probably accounts for this effect.
4. It increases the formation of new adipose tissue cells.

It is entirely possible that the actions of insulin on fat metabolism are more important to the organism than its effects on the metabolism of carbohydrate.

In addition, a rise in blood glucose appears to act somehow on the central nervous system to decrease the lipolysis induced by the sympathetic nervous system and norepinephrine. The lower growth hormone level also diminishes any lipolytic tendency.

Insulin acts as well on the major component of blood lipids, the triglycerides, which are found in lipoproteins and chylomicrons. The triglycerides must in large part be hydrolyzed to fatty acids before the fatty acids can be incorporated into the fat of adipose tissue and perhaps liver and muscle. Triglycerides in the blood perfusing adipose tissue are broken down by the enzyme lipoprotein lipase; the fat cell then takes up the fatty acids and reesterifies them into triglycerides. Both eating and insulin increase the activity of lipoprotein lipase in adipose tissue, thus enhancing the storage of serum triglycerides in adipose tissue. A similar mechanism may exist in liver, but it is not as well studied.

Overall, then, glucose metabolism just after eating is regulated by changes in GI glucagon, insulin, growth hormone, and the sympathetic nervous system, all of which act in toto to increase the oxidation of glucose and to store any excess as glycogen and fat.

### Plasma Free Fatty Acids

After most meals plasma free fatty acids rise slightly. The overall effect of the hormonal changes just discussed would lead one to expect a drop, if anything, in plasma free fatty acids. In fact, there is a drop when the meal consists entirely of glucose. However, the normal meal contains fair amounts of fat, and thus plasma free fatty acids as well as triglycerides show a slight rise after eating.

### Plasma Amino Acids

Immediately after eating is the time of peak levels of amino acids as well as glucose. If the amino acids are to be used to synthesize new protein and not diverted to some other use (e.g., gluconeogenesis), they must be used fairly quickly. Like glucose, they stimulate insulin secretion, which in turn lowers their level in plasma and enhances their incorporation into protein, an ideal situation. The amino acids also stimulate glucagon secretion by the pancreas, both by direct action and indirectly by stimulating the secretion of pancreozymin by the intestine (see p. 222).

Unlike glucose, the amino acids stimulate rather than diminish growth hormone secretion. Since plasma growth hormone is usually lowered after a meal, the predominant effect must be that of glucose, but the actual amount of growth hormone suppression is probably the resultant of the amounts of glucose and amino acids absorbed. The rise in growth hormone after amino acids are given makes teleologic sense since some growth hormone in addition to insulin is required for optimal protein synthesis.

## THE TRANSITION PERIOD: POSTPRANDIAL CHANGES

The blood glucose returns to normal about two hours after eating. At this point there is less insulin, less glucagon, and more growth hormone than just after eating. Glucose removal from the blood continues, though less rapidly. FFA release (lipolysis) is still inhibited by the lower level of insulin even though glucose removal from the blood is slowed and more growth hormone is present. The reason is that the inhibition of fatty acid release is more sensitive to insulin than the enhancement of glucose uptake; FFA release is completely blocked by levels of insulin that stimulate little or no glucose uptake. Perhaps the insulin-like action of growth hormone is at work here as well. Although it has not been measured, one would expect protein synthesis from amino acids to continue.

## FASTING

Beyond two hours or so after eating begins the fasting, or early starvation, stage. At present, in the United States, few people have to wait more than a few hours before eating their next meal. Obviously, in many parts of the world and in some parts of the United States this is not the case. Nor was it the case for any human in many less stable earlier societies. For most people in the world now, and for most people in the past, the fasting state is the usual state. And, with three meals a day, even well-fed people spend most of the day in the fasting state, perhaps as much as 16 to 18 of every 24 hours.

Blood glucose and amino acids, after falling from the peak levels seen after a meal, continue to fall more slowly. The blood glucose stabilizes at 60 to 70 mg/100 ml and falls no further. The plasma free fatty acids begin a slow but persistent rise, going from a few hundred microequivalents per liter to 1200 to 1500 µEq/liter.

In this state the blood contains less insulin, more growth hormone, and more pancreatic glucagon. It is likely that sympathetic nervous system activity is increased. The changes in these hormones are small and require sensitive techniques to detect, at least in the early stages of fasting. Consequently there is still some argument about them; for example, some workers feel that insulin levels do not fall, and others think that glucagon levels do not rise.

### Blood Glucose

The blood glucose falls moderately and then drops no further. The drop alone is probably enough to lower insulin secretion and increase the output of growth hormone and epinephrine. Pancreatic glucagon levels also rise after some hours have passed, although precisely why is not clear; perhaps this rise, too, is due to the drop in blood glucose. That the glucose level stops falling is entirely because of the liver, where both gluconeogenesis and glycogenolysis are increased.

At first glycogenolysis accounts for most of the glucose released by the liver. It is increased by glucagon and the catecholamines. Whether circulating catecholamines are involved is not clear; possibly only the catecholamines from hepatic sympathetic nerve endings are important. Some central nervous system effect may play a role here as well, perhaps acting via the sympathetic nervous system to increase glycogenolysis. Although such an effect was described in the mid-nineteenth century by Claude Bernard, it is still poorly defined. Both glucagon and catecholamines probably act by increasing cAMP. Since insulin, if anything, tends to decrease cAMP in the liver, the lower plasma insulin may raise hepatic levels of cAMP somewhat, further enhancing glycogenolysis. Whether or not glucose is released depends, then, on glucagon, the sympathetic nervous system, and insulin and the resulting effect on the concentration of cAMP.

Later on, most of the glycogen is depleted from the liver, and gluconeogenesis supplies the glucose needed by the body. Gluconeogenesis is enhanced by growth hormone, hydrocortisone, glucagon, low levels of insulin, and the high levels of free fatty acids. All the enzymic changes that occur in diabetes mellitus (see Fig. 54) occur here. In fact, the metabolic changes of starvation are very much like those of diabetes with the exception, of course, of the high blood glucose in the latter.

Under these circumstances, glucose is a valuable commodity. The tissues, principally the nervous system, that cannot burn fatty acids must have glucose to survive. The brain can burn ketone bodies but prefers glucose. Most of the hormonal changes that support the blood glucose level also tend to direct what glucose there is away from muscle and toward the brain. The low amount of insulin may act here to direct free fatty acids and amino acids to the liver for gluconeogenesis.

### Plasma Free Fatty Acids

Shortly after eating, the plasma free fatty acids may rise somewhat if the meal is fatty or fall if the meal is mostly carbohydrate. During fasting, they invariably rise, reflecting a switch to fat as the main metabolic fuel. Some of the fatty acids used come from triglycerides in the oxidizing tissue (e.g. muscle), but a great deal of the fatty acids burned comes from adipose tissue triglycerides and appears in the plasma as free fatty acids. Not all of the fat mobilized from adipose tissue is oxidized, but it is the major fuel of the body.

The hormonal changes we have noted (in glucagon, growth hormone, insulin, and sympathetic nervous system) all contribute their bit. Other lipid mobilizers (see p. 30) play an uncertain role at the moment; they are hormones in search of a job. The end result is a rise in plasma free fatty acids and in fatty acid oxidation and a lower respiratory quotient.

The net increase in the output of free fatty acids by adipose tissue results from changes in all three steps controlling the amount of fat. *Lipogenesis* is lower because of more growth hormone, glucagon, and perhaps hydrocortisone. The lower plasma insulin also tends to lower lipogenesis because, among other things, of a lower level of glucokinase. The actions of these hormones on lipogenesis may be direct or they may in part be secondary to increased lipolysis, with fatty acids or acyl-CoA as the actual inhibitor of lipogenesis. *Esterification* of fatty acids to triglycerides is less; there is a drop in the catalytic capacity of the enzyme system involved. Hydrocortisone in plasma and the lower level of insulin contribute to this effect. Finally, *lipolysis* is notably increased. Glucagon and hydrocortisone are known to be lipolytic and may enhance the process; thyroid hormone is also needed. Probably more important are the lipolytic effects of increased growth hormone, increased catecholamines, and a low level of insulin. When plasma insulin drops, for example, more free fatty acids are released. Regarding catecholamines, increased activity of the sympathetic nervous system may directly increase lipolysis, or perhaps the lipase in adipose tissue is just more sensitive to the same amount of catecholamines.

As with glycogenolysis in the liver, lipolysis in adipose tissue can be viewed as a resultant of the hormonal effects on cAMP, with catecholamines increasing cAMP and insulin decreasing it. More catecholamines and less insulin may both allow the content of cAMP to rise and thus stimulate lipolysis. The other hormones mentioned have not been as well studied in this respect, but thyroxine seems to enhance the activity of adenyl cyclase, and growth hormone may act indirectly via cAMP.

The outpouring of fatty acids from adipose tissue supplies much of the body's energy needs, enhances gluconeogenesis, and decreases glucose utilization by muscle, allowing more glucose to go to the central nervous system.

Many of the changes in lipid metabolism, including ketosis, that occur during starvation are identical to those seen in diabetes mellitus; the changes are of lesser degree and the fasting patient usually loses little glucose in the urine. The critical difference, of course, is the absence of insulin in diabetic ketosis and the presence of insulin (though in low amounts) in fasting. If insulin totally disappeared during fasting, ketoacidosis as seen in diabetes would probably develop. The small amount of circulating insulin is therefore of great importance. Recent work indicates that the elevated free fatty acids and ketone bodies in the plasma, as well as the elevated level of glucagon, help maintain the plasma insulin at its fasting level and prevent it from dropping to zero. The insulin in turn modulates the release of free fatty acids to some degree and prevents dangerous ketosis.

While catecholamines, growth hormone, and insulin are at present the best candidates for regulators of fat mobilization during fasting, it must be admitted that the question is not really settled.

*Catecholamine* excretion is probably increased during fasting, and the sympathetic nervous system probably stimulates a tonic release of free fatty acids. However, the fatty acid release during fasting is not inhibited by β-adrenergic blocking agents or by prostaglandin E, both of which do inhibit catecholamine-induced lipolysis. Denervation of adipose tissue does not seem to impair the lipolysis of fasting. Some experiments suggest that, while the sympathetic nervous system plays a role in lipolysis during exercise or stress, it may not be essential to the release of fatty acids during fasting.

*Growth hormone* unquestionably raises the plasma free fatty acids when it is injected, and the general level of plasma growth hormone increases during fasting. However, several findings are of note:

1. Growth hormone levels in plasma during fasting are erratic and correlate poorly with free fatty acid levels, at least during the first day of fast.
2. The free fatty acids in plasma rise during fasting before any detectable change in growth hormone. The rise, of course, does not eliminate growth hormone as a lipolytic agent later on.
3. The hypophysectomized animal (rat, monkey) when fasted mobilizes fatty acids fairly well.
4. Growth hormone often does not stimulate lipolysis in vitro unless large amounts of corticoids are added.
5. Other pituitary factors than growth hormone may be responsible for enhanced lipolysis. Several have been described and include ACTH, "fat-mobilizing substance" (Chalmers), peptides I and II (Astwood), and lipotropin (Li). The physiologic significance of these substances is not settled; however, ACTH is not lipolytic for human adipose cells, and whole pituitary extracts seem to be no more lipolytic than growth hormone alone.

Because of these problems, it has been suggested that the drop in *insulin* is the main determinant of fatty acid release. Perhaps the lipase operating during fasting is different from the one that catalyzes lipolysis after administration of catecholamines. For the moment, it is probably better to think of the hormones we have mentioned acting in concert and to attribute some of the problems to difficulties in assay and interpretation.

### Amino Acids and Protein Synthesis

Net protein synthesis in the body is unlikely during fasting, with increased gluconeogenesis and little gastrointestinal intake of amino acids. The high growth hormone level, rather than causing actual growth of tissues, may be acting to keep nitrogen loss at a minimum by stimulating protein synthesis to as high a level as possible. It might make more sense, teleologically, to minimize protein loss by increasing synthesis rather than by inhibiting breakdown because *different* proteins may be needed in the fasting state and only synthesis of new protein could supply them. Thus, the main roles of growth hormone in the adult may be the mobilization of fat and the minimizing of protein loss, but not growth.

## Appetite

During the fasting state the body somehow recognizes that it cannot go on this way. New calories must come in; food must be eaten. The appetite is increased. Appetite in this sense of recognition of a need for food can also be viewed as subdued or actual hunger.

The signal for changing the appetite is unknown despite the many theories that have been offered, and despite the fact that the hypothalamus is clearly involved in both increasing and decreasing food intake. These theories include the following:

1. Thermostatic theory. Food ingestion raises the body temperature slightly, which in turn decreases the appetite and vice versa. The idea has not much support, although warming the hypothalamus does tend to decrease food intake by animals, and less food is eaten in a hot environment.

2. Glucostatic theory. A high blood glucose or a high arterial-venous difference in glucose concentration probably causes a general decrease in appetite. Glucose seems to selectively affect the ventromedial nucleus of the hypothalamus (the "satiety center") and stimulate it to decrease the appetite and the intake of food. However, rats that are becoming obese can decrease their food intake without having hyperglycemia or a high arterial-venous difference in blood glucose, and hyperglycemia in an obese or diabetic patient need not decrease the appetite.

3. Lipostatic theory. The plasma free fatty acids may regulate appetite. Unfortunately, it is not clear whether FFA's increase or decrease appetite; while an isocaloric diet high in fat may decrease appetite, when most of us are hungry the plasma FFA's are elevated. Perhaps some metabolite of fat or fatty acids is the substance decreasing appetite. Or perhaps one of the hormones that stimulate lipolysis also stimulates appetite; there is some suggestion that growth hormone may do this.

In rats, exercise decreases appetite. After the exercise is stopped, appetite increases again but not until a full day has passed. The delay is difficult to explain by any of the above theories.

At any rate, hunger does occur when food is needed, whatever the mechanism. It is likely that more than one type of stimulus is involved, and perhaps several or all of the proposed theories are correct.

Eating almost any kind of reasonable diet reverses all the changes in appetite and in fat and carbohydrate metabolism.

## EXERCISE AND OTHER STRESSES

So far, we have discussed changes that occur with eating or not eating without reference to the other activities, stresses, and problems of living. For some, eating *is* living but for most there seems more to life than that.

Exercise initially causes a drop in blood glucose and free fatty acids because of a rapid increase in utilization of both. Within 10 minutes lipolysis is increased, eventually to two and one-half times the resting rate, and more fatty acids are sent into the blood from fat. Shortly after, there is a rise in the plasma free fatty acids; they become the principal source of calories, and the respiratory quotient drops to 0.77. Of course, the glycogen and triglycerides in the exercising muscle itself are used as well, but alone they are not enough. The athlete who is better trained is apparently able to release the fatty acids from adipose tissue more easily.

There is a fairly rapid *rise in plasma growth hormone* within 20 to 60 minutes, but it is not as consistent as one might like and appears later than the initial increase in lipolysis. Growth hormone may stimulate continued lipolysis later on, however, if the exercise is prolonged. *Plasma insulin drops,* and perhaps this is important in activating lipolysis. Still, about the only mechanism that appears to account for such rapid lipolysis is the *sympathetic nervous system,* operating in conjunction with the changes in growth hormone and insulin. The sympathetic nervous system (SNS) or circulating catecholamines are probably responsible for both the rapid rise in free fatty acid release and the increased glycogenolysis seen in muscle. The SNS may even stimulate lipolysis of triglycerides in muscle, thus increasing the supply of free fatty acids for muscle without increasing the plasma level.

Norepinephrine from the sympathetic nerve endings is a good stimulant for lipolysis but causes only modest glycogenolysis and glucose release from the liver. If a real emergency is at hand, and a good deal of glucose is needed quickly (for the nervous system as well as muscle), the adrenal medulla and epinephrine secretion are important because epinephrine raises the blood glucose more than does norepinephrine (see pp. 86–88). Catecholamine-induced lipolysis is probably enhanced by thyroid hormone; $T_4$ increases the sensitivity of adipose tissue to catecholamines, and a rise in plasma free fatty acids increases the plasma free $T_4$.

How is the sympathetic nervous system stimulated during exercise? What stimulates growth hormone release? These questions have no clear answers. Growth hormone levels may rise without a prior drop in blood glucose, and other stimuli than exercise have the same effect. Presumably these stimuli are mediated by the central nervous system.

After exercise is stopped, the plasma FFA rises even more for a short time, because lipolysis continues and utilization drops.

Stresses other than exercise (e.g., hypoglycemia, cold, surgery, severe and strong emotions) will stimulate, via the central nervous system, the sympathetic nervous system with a resulting increase in epinephrine and norepinephrine secretion. Many of these stresses have also been shown to increase growth hormone and hydrocortisone in the plasma. The body's reactions to stresses are much the same as during exercise, except that there is no initial rapid utilization of glucose and fatty acids.

Cold, for example, increases the secretion of growth hormone, TSH, ACTH (and therefore cortisol), and catecholamines and elevates the level of free $T_4$ in the plasma. All of these hormones, directly or indirectly, could well enhance lipolysis and thus maintain the body's integrity.

Note that here, as with exercise, the catecholamines help the nervous tissue get its glucose by increasing glycogenolysis, by inhibiting insulin secretion, and by blocking glucose uptake by muscle; and that, while growth hormone is perhaps not essential for lipolysis at the very beginning, it may be crucial if lipolysis is to be sustained.

## OVERVIEW

One may conclude that the level of plasma insulin plays a major role in regulating the changes following the intake of food and that the sympathetic nervous system plays the same role following changes in activity or mental state. Although this is clearly an oversimplification in view of all else that we have discussed, it can serve as a useful mental peg on which to hang much of the information available.

From an evolutionary position, the ability to withstand the stresses of sudden exercise and a sharp increase in glucose utilization while, for example, chasing the next meal, and the ability to store some of the food energy for later use are both to the good. The former permits one to stay alive until the meal is caught and eaten; the latter allows one to stay alive between meals and perhaps devote some time to other pursuits than simply getting the next meal. Thus we progress.

## BIBLIOGRAPHY

Cahill, G. F., Herrera, M. G., Morgan, A. P., Soeldner, J. S., Steinke, J., Levy, P. L., Reichard, G. A., Jr., and Kipnis, D. M.   Hormone-fuel interrelationships during fasting. *J. Clin. Invest.* 45:1751, 1966.

Carlson, L. A.   Lipid metabolism and muscular work. *Fed. Proc.* 26:1755, 1967.

Castelli, W. P., Nickerson, R. J., Newell, J. M., and Rutstein, D. D.   Serum NEFA following fat, carbohydrate and protein ingestion, and during fasting as related to intracellular lipid deposition. *J. Atheroscler. Res.* 6:328, 1966.

Galton, D. J., and Bray, G. A.   Studies on lipolysis in human adipose cells. *J. Clin. Invest.* 46:621, 1967.

Goodman, H. M.   Effects of growth hormone on the lipolytic response of adipose tissue to theophylline. *Endocrinology* 81:1027, 1968.

Hultman, E.   Physiological role of muscle glycogen in man, with special reference to exercise. *Circ. Res.* 20, 21 (Suppl. I):99, 1967.

Lawrence, A. M.   Radioimmunoassayable glucagon levels in man: Effects of starvation, hypoglycemia, and glucose administration. *Proc. Nat. Acad. Sci. U.S.A.* 55:316, 1966.

Paul, P., and Issekutz, B., Jr.   Role of extramuscular energy sources in metabolism of the exercising dog. *J. Appl. Physiol.* 22:615, 1967.

Pinter, E. J., and Pattee, C. J.   Effect of β-adrenergic blockade on resting and stimulated fat mobilization. *J. Clin. Endocr.* 27:1441, 1967.

Pinter, E. J., Peterfy, G., Cleghorn, J. M., and Pattee, C. J.   The influence of emotional stress on fat mobilization: The role of endogenous catecholamines and the β adrenergic receptors. *Amer. J. Med.* 254:634, 1967.

Senft, G.   Hormonal control of carbohydrate and lipid metabolism and drug induced alterations. *Naunyn Schmiedeberg. Arch. Pharm. Exp. Path.* 259:117, 1968.

Seyffert, W. A., Jr., and Madison, L. L.   Physiologic effects of metabolic fuels on carbohydrate metabolism. *Diabetes* 16:765, 1967.

Sukkar, M. Y., Hunter, W. M., and Passmore, R.   Changes in plasma levels of insulin and growth-hormone levels after a protein meal. *Lancet* 2:1020, 1967.

Wertheimer, E., and Shafrir, E.   Influence of hormones on adipose tissue as a center of fat metabolism. *Recent Progr. Hormone Res.* 16:467, 1960.

# 13.  Body Fat and Obesity

Persons who are naturally very fat are apt to die earlier than those who are slender.

—HIPPOCRATES, *Aphorisms*

## BODY FAT AND ITS MEASUREMENT

It is apparent that glucose and fatty acids turn over rapidly. The adipose tissue is highly active and not an inert storage depot. All the triglyceride, however, is not equally involved in the rapid turnover. Adipose tissue can be viewed functionally as a two-compartment system. The first consists of newly made triglycerides which also seem to be the first to break down; the second is made up of the remaining triglyceride (probably most of it) which turns over relatively slowly and may serve as a temporary storage site.

With all the activity in adipose tissue—glucose entry, fatty acid synthesis, triglyceride lipolysis, etc.—it is easily seen that there are many points where metabolism in adipose tissue might be defective. If the net result of a defect, whatever the cause, is an abnormally decreased total body fat, it is called a *lipodystrophy*. If the net result is an increase in body fat, we call it *obesity*. In normal people, between 20% and 40% of total body weight is fat; the percentage is obviously greater in obesity but even in normal people it increases with age.

When measuring body fat, we are concerned principally with adipose tissue. It is true that tissues such as muscle and brain contain fair amounts of lipids. However, when dealing with obesity, the obvious changes are in the adipose tissue, so most of the effort has gone into measuring this tissue alone, a difficult enough problem.

One way of measuring body fat would be to dissect all the fat tissue from the body and weigh it. This direct method is obviously impractical in living people and is quite tedious for more than few cadavers, so other more indirect methods are usually used.

Most of the indirect methods make use of some or all of the following facts:

1. Fat tissue is lighter than the rest of the body.
2. The body as a whole is about 60% water.
3. Adipose tissue is about 15% water, 2% to 3% protein, and most of the rest is fat.
4. The rest of the body—nonadipose tissue or "lean body mass"— is about 70% water, and 15% to 20% protein.

5. Almost all the exchangeable potassium in the body is associated with protein.

Knowing these facts, one can devise various methods of assaying body fat. One may:

1. *Measure body density* (by calculating volume and measuring displacement of water). The lighter the body (i.e., less dense), the fatter it is.
2. *Measure total body water* (using radioisotopes) and compare it with the weight or body density. The less water per unit weight, the more fat there is. At present, the most accurate method of estimating body fat is probably a combination of the measurements of body water and body density.
3. *Measure exchangeable potassium* (using radioisotopes). Since most of the body's potassium is associated with protein, and fat tissue has little protein, the exchangeable potassium reflects mostly the lean body mass. Combined with measurements of body density or weight, body fat can be estimated.

If one is willing to assume that adipose tissue is 15% water and the rest of the body ("lean body mass") is 70% water, one can estimate body fat using only the person's weight and the total body water.

If      $X =$ adipose tissue weight (in kilograms)
   $TBW =$ total body water (in liters)
     $BW =$ body weight (in kilograms)

then                 $0.15\,X + 0.70\,(BW - X) = TBW$

and this rearranges to   $X = \dfrac{0.7\,BW - TBW}{0.55}$

Substituting the values for body weight and total body water, one has the weight of body fat.

These methods, however, are technically not easy or convenient. Furthermore, they are subject to error if the patient is grossly abnormal, e.g., edematous, dehydrated, undergoing weight loss, or markedly obese. In practice, then, for clinical purposes one usually estimates obesity from:

1. The *appearance* of the patient. Surprisingly enough, that ancient tool the eye of the physician is a good judge of obesity.
2. Standard *height-weight tables*, although it is clear that increased weight does not necessarily mean obesity. A well-muscled football player may weigh much more than the tables say he should for his height, but the excess weight is mostly muscle and not fat. What it may be 15 or 20 years later is another story.

3. *Skin-fold thickness,* measured with special calipers, x-ray, or ul-
trasound. The thicker the skin fold—for example, that overlying
the triceps muscle—the fatter you are.

The measurement of skin-fold thickness is probably the best simple
method available that is well standardized and can be used to observe
changes in the individual patient.

## LIPODYSTROPHY

Lipodystrophy, or too little fat, is usually associated with a high
blood glucose and hyperlipemia. There is no good evidence as to the
cause; it could be due to a defect in the adipose tissue or an increase
in fat mobilizers, but nothing is really known about it.

## OBESITY

The complaint of the obese person that "everything I eat turns to
fat" is accurate. The unanswered problem is why it is so in some
people and not in others. Simple overeating has for years been considered the cause of obesity. Fat people who did not lose weight were,
and are, regarded as weak-willed "cheaters" who do not follow their
diet and who are in need of psychotherapy. All this may be true as far
as it goes; however, while overeating is clearly necessary for obesity
to occur, it does not exclude other factors as possible underlying causes
of obesity. To say that the obese eat too much and that the answer is
to eat less is probably an oversimplification. Although eating less is
the only effective treatment, the reason for the overeating is not at
all clear.

Obesity is common. In the United States 30% of the population are
10% or more overweight. In the teen-age group, about 10% are obese.
Since these figures are based on height-weight tables, this is probably
an underestimation of the problem.

Obesity is not healthy. Probably 10% of obese people are diabetic,
and their chances of dying from all causes are 13% greater than those
of their normal-weight colleagues, unless they are over age 55 or so.
The obese person is subject to arthritis, heart disease, lung disease,
and $CO_2$ retention if very obese. Surgery and pregnancy are more
hazardous.

Embarrassment and unhappiness are major problems for the obese
patient, at least in our culture where thinness is more acceptable than
fatness. These are particular problems in teen-agers for obvious reasons; perhaps a more important problem for fat adolescents is that
obesity statistically decreases their chance of getting into college.

Losing weight, once a person is obese, probably improves the survival rate. But then "good eating joins the increasing list of pleasant things that we must avoid in order to live longer, miserably."*

## Possible Causes of Obesity

*Overeating* is, of course, necessary in all cases. It alone without another cause is one possible mechanism. The *type of food* overeaten may be important. Some work with baboons has shown that sucrose in the diet will increase body fat while the same amount of glucose will not. *Psychologic factors* may cause too much eating. Nevertheless, psychotherapy is in large part a failure, perhaps because these factors are not well understood.

Perhaps *appetite* control is awry; the obese person may be always a bit more hungry or a bit less satiable. Note the difference between hunger and satiety. To be abnormally hungry implies that the conscious need for more food comes sooner than one might expect; to be less satiable means that eating comes at a normal time but that an amount of food that would satisfy a normal person and stop him from eating more does not in fact do so. For example, some obese people do not ask for more food at the end of a meal if none is on the table, but they do finish whatever is there no matter how much it is (to a certain limit, of course). Such people are less satiable than normal. When the control of appetite is defective, the resulting obesity is sometimes called regulatory obesity.

*Genetics* may play an important part. The simple fact that a fat person's children are obese is not enough; this could just as easily be due to a common environment. But when four of eight siblings are grossly obese and the other four are normal, it is difficult to see how a common environment could account for the discrepancy. Certainly in rats and mice obesity can have a genetic basis. The association with diabetes mellitus, which has a genetic component, again suggests some genetic basis for obesity.

A *lack of exercise* or a general decrease in activity may be a cause, particularly if food habits stay the same and the intake of food is not proportionately reduced. In rats, regular exercise has been shown to decrease the total body fat. Unknown, however, is why activity decreases, or why food intake does not decrease along with it.

Finally, there might be some *metabolic abnormality* in the regulation of fat metabolism or in the adipose tissue itself, wherein the overeating is a secondary response by the body in an attempt to correct the abnormality. This is the so-called metabolic obesity as opposed to regulatory obesity.

*Astwood, E. B.   Presidential address: The heritage of corpulence. *Endocrinology* 71:337, 1962.

A good deal of attention has been focused on two of these possibilities, the abnormal control of food intake and possible metabolic abnormalities.

ABNORMAL CONTROL OF FOOD INTAKE. As we have said, no one really knows what controls food intake, but we are sure that the hypothalamus has something to do with it (see p. 262). An abnormality in the hypothalamus, however small, might explain obesity.

One might, as noted, divide obese people into two groups: those with poor control of food intake (regulatory obesity) and those with some metabolic abnormality as the prime defect (metabolic obesity). However, until one knows what controls food intake, it is impossible to judge how much overlap there is between the two groups. For example, when a rat with a hypothalamic lesion overeats and becomes obese, it has *regulatory* obesity. However, when the same rat shows a high plasma insulin and its adipose tissue releases free fatty acids poorly, it has *metabolic* obesity. One might be the cause of the other.

Whatever it is that controls caloric intake, it is a fine control indeed. For example, imagine that each day a person retained the number of calories in one small orange and stored them as fat. At the end of 10 years, that person would have 200,000 extra calories as fat. Since one pound of fat tissue has about 3400 calories, the weight gain would amount to 60 pounds.

Yet we know that few people gain this much. The 50 calories in the orange are less than 2% of the average daily caloric intake. The body somehow manages to deal with wide variations in food intake and yet is so finely controlled that the average daily food intake is within 20 to 30 calories of what is needed. The control is good enough to keep body weight reasonably constant in most people. Obviously, small and subtle changes may be at the root of the obesity problem and may therefore be difficult to detect.

Our knowledge of abnormal control of food intake is limited to rather crude information such as the change in satiety mentioned just above. The sort of subtle change that may be present in the hypothalamus of the obese person is at the moment beyond our reach; it may be there, but we lack the tools for detecting it.

METABOLIC ABNORMALITIES: POSSIBILITIES. Let us suppose that there is some metabolic abnormality outside the hypothalamus, and that overeating is not the cause of the abnormality but the result of it. What defects could there be? In general, one would think of:

1. Intrinsic defects of adipose tissue.
    A. Adipose tissue takes up or makes too much fat.
    B. Adipose tissue releases too little fat.

2. Defects in the regulators of fat in adipose tissue.
   A. There is an excessive stimulus on adipose tissue to make and/or store fat.
   B. Fat-mobilizing factors are deficient.

Is there evidence for any of these types of defects? In man, not much; but in humans *and* other species, enough overall so that these possibilities cannot be dismissed. What evidence there is in each category is summarized here:

1A. *Adipose Tissue Defect: Excessive Uptake or Synthesis of Fat.* In some genetically obese rats the adipose tissue takes up more free fatty acid and incorporates more of it into triglyceride than does normal adipose tissue. There seems to be more uptake of triglyceride (via an increased lipoprotein lipase) by adipose tissue in some people with obesity.

Overeating alone may be associated with increased lipogenesis (conversion of glucose to fatty acids); this may, however, be an effect and not a cause. Increased fat might result from an increase in α-glycerophosphate (α-GP) or in the enzyme catalyzing its formation, glycerokinase; in either case, more fatty acids would be converted to triglycerides. Experimentally, some recent work suggests that the mitochondria of an obese person's adipose tissue oxidize less α-GP than normal adipose mitochondria, perhaps leaving more α-GP available for the synthesis of triglycerides.

Other work indicates that the adipose tissue in human obesity does not show increased lipogenesis nor is it any faster in converting glucose to either the glycerol or fatty acid moieties of triglyceride. A key point here may be that the obese person has more fat cells overall, and each is larger than normal and stuffed with triglyceride. The cells may not convert glucose to fat any faster but they may convert *more* of it because of the larger size of the cell. The process of triglyceride synthesis needs more investigation.

Although the size of the adipose cell in an obese person returns to normal after weight loss, there are still more adipose cells than normal. This condition probably explains the ease with which the weight is regained; obese people who have lost weight are notorious for regaining the lost weight, and it may be a matter of many cells filling up with fat sooner and easier than few cells. It is not clear, however, which comes first, the obesity or the increased number of cells.

1B. *Adipose Tissue Defect: Deficient Release of Fatty Acids.* A genetically obese mouse appears to release free fatty acids (FFA) from its adipose tissue more slowly than expected, as is the case with the genetically obese rat in 1A. One might postulate a defective lipase, although when some obese rats were tested, no such defect was found. Another possibility is an abnormal receptor site for lipolytic hormones or a poor synthesis of cAMP, the mediator of catecholamine-induced lipolysis. A genetically obese rat seems to have, in fact, a deficiency in cAMP synthesis, but there is little to support the presence of any of these specific defects in human obesity.

On a more general basis, workers have studied the response of plasma FFA to injections of catecholamines. Most obese people have a normal or high plasma FFA in the resting state. Yet some studies showed that, when given epinephrine, many of these patients show a poor rise in plasma FFA. This seemed particularly to be the case when compared to the number of fat cells in the body, and the same poor rise may be seen with fasting. All of which suggests a deficient adipose tissue response to catecholamines as a cause of obesity. Closer examination of the data showed, however, some differences in methods used with the obese group and with the control group; when the study was repeated, no defect was found. Furthermore, there seems to be no such defect when the obese adipose tissue is studied in vitro. The plasma FFA respond normally to growth hormone as well. One must seriously question the existence of a defective response to lipolytic agents in obesity.

Other work, assessing the ability of the obese person to mobilize fatty acids without giving an exogenous lipolytic agent, shows (1) that release of FFA is normal during exercise, (2) that on the basis of surface area or oxygen consumption there is actually better than normal mobilization of fatty acids, and (3) that overall fatty acid oxidation is normal.

Despite the work in animals, looking for defective release of fatty acids as a cause of human obesity does not seem too fruitful.

2A. *Excess Stimulus on Adipose Tissue to Make or Store Fat.* In a sense, overeating could be included here. It seems in some unknown way to increase lipogenesis (in rats, at least), particularly if the day's food is eaten all at once and not divided into multiple feedings. Work with intact animals also shows that the percentage of body weight that is fat is less with multiple feedings. So the timing of food intake may be an important factor.

As discussed before, obese people have a certain degree of insulin resistance, even when not diabetic, and their plasma insulin is higher than normal particularly after a glucose meal. If adipose tissue were responsive to insulin but muscle were not, one would expect more glucose to be converted to fatty acids and triglycerides. One might then explain the mild insulin resistance, the higher plasma insulin, and the obesity all at once. Unfortunately, the obesity would be explained only if the insulin resistance were present *before* obesity occurred. This has not been shown. Furthermore, when obese people lose weight the insulin resistance disappears, the suggestion being that the obesity causes the insulin resistance and not the other way around. Finally, studies with isolated adipose cells from obese patients show that the cells are *less* responsive to insulin; this may in fact be one cause of the higher plasma insulin: The pancreas secretes more insulin to overcome the deficient response of both muscle and adipose tissue to insulin. It would seem, then, that the basic cause of obesity does not lie here.

The obese person also secretes more hydrocortisone, which would diminish glucose uptake by muscle and further enhance fat deposition because of the secondary rise in insulin. The excess hydrocortisone secretion disappears when the weight is lost, so again it is probably secondary to the obesity.

2B. *Deficient Fat-Mobilizing Factors. Inactivity,* noted above, fits here, since exercise is a known stimulant of FFA mobilization.

*Pituitary fat mobilizers* might be lacking. If growth hormone is the significant fat mobilizer in man, there is some support for this thesis, since obese people do not release growth hormone as well as normal people.

*Poor sympathetic nervous system function* could be a cause, with either not enough stimuli getting to the nerve ending of adipose tissue or not enough catecholamines getting to the fat cells. There is no good evidence one way or the other.

*Deficient thyroxine secretion,* often suggested as a cause of obesity, rarely has anything to do with it. If the patient is hypothyroid, proper thyroid tests should be done and treatment given for the hypothyroidism and not the obesity. Many obese people are treated with thyroid hormone. Few are hypothyroid. Thyroid hormone may be a useful adjunct to treating euthyroid obesity, but it must be used with care and it may simply make the patient irritable and difficult to live with.

Some have suggested that *poor heat loss* by the body may be at fault; this could also be a deficiency in β-adrenergic function since heat loss depends on adequate vasodilation. There is little evidence for the proposal. The same is true for the suggestion that *decreased blood flow* through adipose tissue might account for obesity.

A big problem with human obesity, of course, is that one never knows whether the observed apparent defect is a cause or a result of the obesity. Another problem is that obesity may be many different diseases and there may be no such thing as *the* cause.

If deficient lipolysis or increased fat synthesis, whatever the cause, is the basic difficulty, or if for some reason the hypothalamus is insensitive to the usual appetite-suppressing stimulus, then *eating continues* and *obesity results*. Perhaps in most moderately obese people excessive eating continues only until the adipose tissue as a whole enlarges to the point where overall FFA release is normal, or is enough to shut off the hypothalamic "appestat."

*Treatment of Obesity*

There is little to do but *eat less*. This should not be a cause of lack of enthusiasm; the interest of the physician often determines the success of the diet. Obese children should be treated particularly vigorously (although they are a more difficult problem) since they do not "grow out of it" but rather become obese adults who find it even harder to lose weight.

Some observations have suggested that a high-fat diet causes more weight loss than an isocaloric high-carbohydrate diet. On the face of it, this makes no sense and is thermodynamically impossible. It may in fact be true, however, since calories may be lost in the urine or feces (as ketone bodies or citrate) that could have been used by the body. The point is not settled because of a lack of quantitative information on the caloric loss. Furthermore, a diet high in fat tends to suppress the appetite more than a diet made up largely of carbohydrate; the diet as usually given to the patient may therefore not be truly isocaloric.

In extreme obesity, *total fasting* except for water (the "zero-calorie diet") may be used. Hunger as we know it disappears in about two days. This is an effective method when indicated, though close supervision is required (there are a number of possible complications) and the real success rate is not yet known.

Ideally, the weight loss should be just in adipose tissue, but some loss of protein (and thus muscle) is acceptable since the lean-body mass in gross obesity is increased for the obvious reason that more muscle is needed to carry all that weight. Severely restricted diets, such as the "zero-calorie" one, may, however, cause excessive loss of protein. It is perhaps better, unless there is a pressing need, to give a diet containing some calories. The usual practice is to prescribe a diet containing 400 to 800 calories to grossly obese patients. Not only is net protein loss diminished, but the diet is usually more acceptable to the patient and just as much fat may be lost.

*Multiple meals* containing few calories may blunt the appetite more or less continually and cut down total caloric intake. *Eating slowly* might also cause satiety before too much food is eaten.

*Drugs* have been widely used; amphetamine derivatives are the common ones. None of these derivatives gives more than short-term benefit, and the number available suggests that none is superior. They should be used only as adjuncts and for short or intermittent periods of time, and then only under careful supervision. Other agents being investigated include bile salts to decrease appetite and thyroid hormone to keep basal metabolism up to a normal level. It remains to be seen whether or not a better long-term success rate will result.

Overall results are not impressive. Once a person is obese, he really is not normal even when weight is reduced to its proper level. The number of fat cells remains excessive. The tendency to gain weight is still there, and in fact most patients do become obese again. The cycle is often repeated, first gaining, then losing, only to gain again. Thus, we have what has been called the "rhythm method of girth control." Though the prospects might seem depressing, treating obesity *is* worth the effort since many people feel much better, both physically and mentally, once they have lost weight, and one never knows which patient will gain again and which will not.

## BIBLIOGRAPHY

Ball, M. F., Kyle, L. H., and Canary, J. J.   Comparative effects of caloric restriction and metabolic acceleration on body composition in obesity. *J. Clin. Endocr.* 27:273, 1967.

Friend, D. W.   Weight gains, nitrogen metabolism, and body composition of rats fed one or five meals daily. *Canad. J. Physiol. Pharmacol.* 45:367, 1967.

Issekutz, B., Jr., Bortz, W. M., Miller, H. I., and Wroldsen, A.   Plasma free fatty acid response to exercise in obese humans. *Metabolism* 16:492, 1967.

Krzywicki, H. J., and Chinn, K. S. K.   Human body density and fat of an adult male population as measured by water displacement. *Amer. J. Clin. Nutr.* 20:305, 1967.

Salans, L. B., Knittle, J. L., and Hirsch, J.   The role of adipose cell size and adipose tissue insulin sensitivity in the carbohydrate intolerance of human obesity. *J. Clin. Invest.* 47:153, 1968.

# Appendix I

## GENERAL REFERENCE WORKS

### Basic Physiology

Harris, R. S., Thimann, K. V., and others. *Vitamins and Hormones.* New York: Academic, published annually.

Pincus, G. (Ed.). *Recent Progress in Hormone Research.* New York: Academic, published annually. Beginning 1968, edited by E. B. Astwood.

Pincus, G., Thimann, K. V., and Astwood, E. B. (Eds.). *The Hormones* (5 vols.). New York: Academic, 1948, 1950, 1955, 1964.

Tepperman, J. *Metabolic and Endocrine Physiology* (2d ed.). Chicago: Year Book, 1968.

Turner, C. D. *General Endocrinology* (4th ed.). Philadelphia: Saunders, 1966.

Wolstenholme, G. E. W., and O'Connor, M. (Eds.). *Ciba Foundation Colloquia on Endocrinology,* vols. 1–16. Boston: Little, Brown, 1952–1967.

### Clinical Endocrinology

Astwood, E. B., and Cassidy, C. E. (Eds.). *Clinical Endocrinology. II.* New York: Grune & Stratton, 1968.

Danowski, T. S. *Clinical Endocrinology* (4 vols.). Baltimore: Williams & Wilkins, 1962.

Schwartz, T. B. (Ed.). *Year Book of Endocrinology.* Chicago: Year Book, published annually.

Stanbury, J. B., Wyngaarden, J. B., and Fredrickson, D. S. (Eds.). *The Metabolic Basis of Inherited Disease* (2d ed.). New York: Blakiston Div., McGraw-Hill, 1966.

Williams, R. H. (Ed.). *Textbook of Endocrinology* (4th ed.). Philadelphia: Saunders, 1968.

### Methods

Dorfman, R. I. (Ed.). *Methods in Hormone Research* (5 vols.). New York: Academic, 1962–1966.

Eckstein, P., and Knowles, F. (Eds.). *Techniques in Endocrine Research.* New York: Academic, 1963.

Zarrow, M. X., Yochim, J. M., and McCarthy, J. L. *Experimental Endocrinology: A Sourcebook of Basic Techniques.* New York: Academic, 1964.

## History

Bloomfield, A. L.   *A Bibliography of Internal Medicine. Selected Diseases.*
Chicago: University of Chicago Press, 1960. Includes chapters on the
history of diabetes mellitus, diabetes insipidus, Addison's disease (adrenal
insufficiency), Graves' disease (hyperthyroidism), myxedema (hypothyroidism), tetany, and hyperparathyroidism.
Rolleston, H. D.   *The Endocrine Organs in Health and Disease with an
Historical Review.* London: Oxford University Press, 1936. Over 30 years
old and long out of print.

## Journals

Articles pertinent to endocrinology appear in many journals not specifically devoted to endocrinology. However, there are several journals that
publish large numbers of endocrine articles; if one is to keep up with the
field, these must be read.

*Endocrinology*
*Journal of Clinical Endocrinology and Metabolism*
*Metabolism*
*Acta Endocrinologica*
*Journal of Endocrinology*
*Journal of Clinical Investigation*

# Appendix II

Endocrinology is so shot through with abbreviations and acronyms that it sometimes resembles a table of organization for some bureau of the government. These stunted words, usually capitalized as if to make up in height what they have lost in length, are understood easily enough by those "in the business" but may be mystifying to the newcomer. The following list will then be a source of solace. At the end is a listing of abbreviations of units and weights. Not included are the standard abbreviations of the amino acids.

| | |
|---|---|
| AcCoA | acetyl-coenzyme A |
| acetyl-CoA | acetyl-coenzyme A |
| ACTH | adrenocorticotropic hormone (same as corticotropin) |
| acyl-CoA | fatty acid–coenzyme A |
| ADH | antidiuretic hormone (same as vasopressin) |
| ADP | adenosine diphosphate |
| $\alpha$-GP | $\alpha$-glycerophosphate |
| AMP | adenosine monophosphate |
| ATP | adenosine triphosphate |
| B | compound B or corticosterone |
| B/F | bound-to-free ratio (in immunoassay) |
| BMR | basal metabolic rate |
| BW | body weight |
| cAMP | cyclic 3′,5′-adenosine monophosphate |
| CNS | central nervous system |
| CoA | coenzyme A |
| cortisol | hydrocortisone, compound F |
| $C_p$ | phosphate clearance |
| CRF | corticotropin-releasing factor |
| CSF | cerebrospinal fluid |

| | |
|---|---|
| DHEA | dehydroepiandrosterone |
| DHF | dihydrohydrocortisone |
| DHT | dihydrotestosterone |
| DIHPPA | diiodohydroxyphenylpyruvic acid |
| DIT | diiodotyrosine |
| DNA | deoxyribonucleic acid |
| DOC | deoxycorticosterone |
| DOPA | dihydroxyphenylalanine |
| DPN | diphosphopyridine nucleotide (same as NAD) |
| DPNH | reduced DPN |
| E | compound E, cortisone (sometimes used for epinephrine, though not common) |
| $E_1$ | estrone |
| $E_2$ | 17β-estradiol |
| $E_3$ | estriol |
| ECF | extracellular fluid |
| EPI | epinephrine |
| EPS | exophthalmos-producing substance |
| F | compound F, hydrocortisone, cortisol |
| FFA | free fatty acids |
| FSH | follicle-stimulating hormone |
| FSH-RF | FSH-releasing factor |
| GFR | glomerular filtration rate |
| GH | growth hormone (see HGH) |
| GH-RF | GH-releasing factor |
| GI glucagon | gastrointestinal glucagon |
| α-GP | α-glycerophosphate |
| G-6-P | glucose-6-phosphate |
| G-6-PD | glucose-6-phosphate dehydrogenase |
| GRF | same as GH-RF |
| HCG | human chorionic gonadotropin |
| HGH | human growth hormone |
| HMP shunt | hexose monophosphate shunt |
| HPL | human placental lactogen |
| ICSH | interstitial cell–stimulating hormone (same as luteinizing hormone or LH) |
| ILA | insulin-like activity |
| $K_A$ | association constant, an index of tightness of binding |
| LATS | long-acting thyroid stimulator |

| | |
|---|---|
| LH | luteinizing hormone |
| LH-RF | LH-releasing factor |
| LTH | luteotropic hormone, luteotropin (often used as synonym for prolactin) |
| MIT | monoiodotyrosine |
| mRNA | messenger RNA |
| MSH | melanocyte-stimulating hormone |
| MSH-IF | MSH-inhibiting factor |
| Mt | mitochondria |
| NAD | nicotinamide–adenine dinucleotide (same as DPN) |
| NADH | reduced NAD (same as DPNH) |
| NADP | nicotinamide–adenine dinucleotide phosphate (same as TPN) |
| NADPH | reduced NADP (same as TPNH) |
| NE | norepinephrine |
| OAA | oxaloacetate |
| 17-OHCS | 17-hydroxycorticosteroids |
| OT | oxytocin |
| PBI | protein-bound iodine |
| PEP | phosphoenolpyruvate |
| PFK | phosphofructokinase |
| PGE | prostaglandin E |
| PGF | prostaglandin F |
| PIF | prolactin-inhibiting factor |
| P/O ratio | ratio of high-energy phosphate bonds formed per oxygen atom used |
| PTH | parathyroid hormone |
| PYR | pyruvate |
| RNA | ribonucleic acid |
| S | compound S, 11-deoxycortisol |
| SNS | sympathetic nervous system |
| sRNA | soluble RNA (generally synonymous with tRNA) |
| STH | somatotropic hormone (same as growth hormone or GH) |
| $T_3$ | triiodothyronine |
| $T_4$ | thyroxine |
| TBG | thyroxine-binding globulin |
| TBPA | thyroxine-binding prealbumin |
| TBW | total body water |

| TCA cycle | tricarboxylic acid cycle, Krebs cycle |
|-----------|----------------------------------------|
| TCT | thyrocalcitonin |
| TGB | thyroglobulin |
| THB | tetrahydrocorticosterone, tetrahydro-B |
| THE | tetrahydrocortisone, tetrahydro-E |
| THF | tetrahydrohydrocortisone, tetrahydro-F |
| THS | tetrahydrodeoxycortisol, tetrahydro-S |
| TPN | triphosphopyridine nucleotide (same as NADP) |
| TPNH | reduced TPN (same as NADPH) |
| TRF | thyrotropin-releasing factor (same as TSH-RF) |
| TRIAC | triiodothyroacetic acid |
| tRNA | transfer RNA |
| T/S | thyroid/serum ratio |
| TSH | thyroid-stimulating hormone, thyrotropin |
| TSH-RF | TSH-releasing factor |
| VMA | vanillylmandelic acid |

*Units and Weights*

| mU | milliunit (1/1000 of a unit) |
|-----|------------------------------|
| μU | microunit (1/1000 of a mU, or $10^{-6}$ unit) |
| g | gram |
| mg | milligram (1/1000 of a gram) |
| μg | microgram (1/1000 of a mg, or $10^{-6}$ g) |
| mμg | millimicrogram (1/1000 of a μg, or $10^{-9}$ g) |
| ng | nanogram (modern term for millimicrogram [mμg]) |
| μμg | micromicrogram (1/1000 of a mμg or of a ng, or $10^{-12}$ g) |
| pg | picogram (modern term for micromicrogram [μμg]) |
| mOsm | milliosmol |

# Index

References to pages containing illustrations are in *italics*